P9-CCX-447

INTEGRATING
SPIRITUALITY
INTO TREATMENT

INTEGRATING SPIRITUALITY INTO TREATMENT

RESOURCES FOR PRACTITIONERS

EDITED BY WILLIAM R. MILLER

AMERICAN PSYCHOLOGICAL ASSOCIATION

WASHINGTON DC

Copyright © 1999 by the American Psychological Association. All rights reserved. Except as permitted under the United States Copyright Act of 1976, no part of this publication may be reproduced or distributed in any form or by any means, or stored in a database or retrieval system, without the prior written permission of the publisher.

Fifth printing, January 2010

Published by
American Psychological Association
750 First Street, NE
Washington, DC 20002

Copies may be ordered from
APA Order Department
P.O. Box 92984
Washington, DC 20090-2984

In the U.K., Europe, Africa, and the Middle East, copies may be ordered from
American Psychological Association
3 Henrietta Street
Covent Garden, London
WC2E 8LU England

Typeset in Goudy by EPS Group Inc., Easton, MD

Printer: Maple-Vail Books
Cover Designer: Drymon Design, Washington, DC
Technical/Production Editor: Rachael J. Stryker

Library of Congress Cataloging-in-Publication Data
Integrating spirituality into treatment : resources for practitioners
  / [edited] by William R. Miller.—1st ed.
      p.   cm.
   Includes bibliographical references and index.
   ISBN 1-55798-581-2 (casebound : acid-free paper)
   1. Psychotherapy—Religious aspects.   2. Spirituality.
  I. Miller, William R.
  RC489.R46I58   1999
  616.89'14—dc21   99-12572
                                                          CIP

British Library Cataloguing-in-Publication Data
A CIP record is available from the British Library.

Printed in the United States of America

To George Keen Shortess, PhD,

my first mentor in psychology,
who taught me to love and to integrate its
history, scientific rigor, creativity, and spirituality.

CONTENTS

CONTRIBUTORS

Jennifer Booth, San Diego State University and University of California, San Diego

Brenda S. Cole, Bowling Green State University

Gerard J. Connors, Research Institute on Addictions, Buffalo

Richard L. Gorsuch, Fuller Theological Seminary

Jean L. Kristeller, Indiana State University

Ernest Kurtz, University of Michigan

David B. Larson, National Institute for Healthcare Research

Marsha M. Linehan, University of Washington

G. Alan Marlatt, University of Washington

John E. Martin, University of California, San Diego

Michael E. McCullough, National Institute for Healthcare Research

William R. Miller, University of New Mexico

Kenneth I. Pargament, Bowling Green State University

P. Scott Richards, Brigham Young University

John M. Rector, Brigham Young University

Cynthia Sanderson, Cornell University Medical College

Carl E. Thoresen, Stanford University

Alan C. Tjeltveit, Muhlenberg College

J. Scott Tonigan, University of New Mexico

Radka T. Toscova, Albuquerque Family and Guidance Center

Carolina E. Yahne, University of New Mexico

PREFACE

In the fall of 1965, George Shortess welcomed a wide-eyed and confused freshman into his experimental psychology laboratory at Lycoming College. It was an inner sanctum of equipment workbenches, warehoused apparatuses, and lively animal colonies—not at all what I had in mind by majoring in psychology. I wanted, as a preministerial student, to understand what motivates people and, ultimately, of course, to understand myself. A visionary researcher with an artist's heart, George saw some possibilities in me, patiently mentoring and nurturing me through countless hours of intriguing discussion that spanned the breadth of human experience. Over the next four years he taught me by example, not only the science of psychology but also the humanity of a scientist.

As often happens in college, my young faith began to crumble. In retrospect, I understand it more as the breaking open of a seed pod, but at the time it was a tumultuous shaking of my foundations. I grew disenchanted with the institutional church as I understood it then and found myself strongly drawn in the direction of clinical psychology. As I write this I remember our college chaplain, Paul Neufer, to whom I confessed the troubled agnosticism that was emerging in my senior year, as my simple childhood faith spun its cocoon for adulthood. He offered me not judgment, but compassion and hope. "Being unsure is a difficult but wonderful place to be," he said. "You can grow from there." And so I did.

The Vietnam war interrupted my graduate education, and as a conscientious objector I served as an aide at Mendota State Hospital. It was there in Madison, Wisconsin, that I met my wife, Kathleen Jackson, who for three decades has consistently pulled me out of the ivory tower, helping me to maintain some semblance of contact with earthly reality. A counselor by profession, she exuded a vibrant, practical spirituality, and once again a faith community became my extended family. We enjoyed, and continue to enjoy, what is so easily taken for granted—public worship and practice of religion.

When I resumed graduate study, I found that my faith again needed to go underground, this time for external rather than internal reasons. It did not take long for me to discover that in many psychological circles spirituality was an unwelcome topic in the 1970s. I chose through my graduate training and junior faculty years to stay fairly quiet about spirituality, to keep my spiritual side and religious practice to myself. I lived in two worlds, each occupied by a different group of friends. In the world of psychology I spoke little about spirituality, except with a few colleagues and undergraduate students.

In the world of religion, on the other hand, I found great interest in my scientific and professional discipline. Recognizing the overlap and complementary of my two worlds, I began to look for ways to share within religious circles some of what I was learning about psychology. Kathy and I started giving talks and classes, first for lay audiences and then for clergy. We developed a week-long workshop for pastors, a blend of Rogerian listening skills and practical cognitive–behavioral counseling methods. The latter proved to be particularly popular because clergy are rarely exposed to behavioral psychology in any favorable way during their professional training. The short-term and specifiable nature of behavior therapies seemed especially well suited to the context of pastoral counseling. Over the years, we developed a 5-inch–thick stack of handouts for the workshop.

In the year that I received tenure, I came out of the closet and began writing about psychology and spirituality. First we turned our handouts into a book called *Practical Psychology for Pastors*, which has evolved into a second edition. For laity I wrote a short book (*Living as If*) communicating some insights of cognitive therapy language and terminology that are familiar to people of faith.

A few years later I found myself in the opposite situation, interpreting spirituality to a psychological audience. My colleague John Martin, who that year was chairing the program committee for the annual conference of the Association for Advancement of Behavior Therapy (AABT), persuaded me to co-chair with him a panel on spiritual and religious aspects of therapy. My own paper focused on how one can adapt cognitive therapy in a way that respects and integrates clients' religious beliefs. The first of its kind for AABT, the symposium drew a large audience, resulting in both an edited book titled *Behavior Therapy and Religion* and a special interest group within AABT on spiritual and religious issues in behavior change.

From there on, I have found myself with ever more fascinating opportunities to stand in the doorway between spirituality and psychology, passing things back and forth. I supervised and taught psychology to pastoral counselors and incorporated the spiritual side of human nature into my teaching of psychology. I served on a national panel to develop a denomination's first major policy statement on alcohol since the repeal of Prohibition. I began incorporating some spiritual constructs, measures, and questions into my treatment research and writing more frequently on spirituality and addictions. Then came opportunities to convene two stimulating expert panels to advance the development of scientific research on spirituality within my chosen field of addictive behavior.

All of that led to the doorstep of this book. There are many ways to write and think about spirituality and psychotherapy. For transpersonal and existential psychologists, spiritual issues are old familiar territory. Since Freud's initial essays on the subject, psychodynamic thinkers have sought to incorporate spirituality through writings for public and professional audiences. Almost wholly separated from clinical practice, the psychology of religion continues to flourish through empirical studies of spiritual and religious behavior. The professional field of pastoral psychology in turn remains relatively isolated from behavioral science. What is new is the emergence of interaction between clinical science and spirituality, each informing the other. A taboo on incorporating spirituality in psychotherapy seems to be lifting, and nowhere has this taboo been stronger than in empirically oriented, scientist–practitioner circles.

This book reflects a scientist–practitioner approach to the integration of spirituality and psychotherapy. Its authors appreciate both the value of scientific method as a way of knowing and the spiritual side of human nature that eludes reductionism. It makes for fascinating discourse. The challenge is not unlike that of trying simultaneously to understand subjectively the rich experience of psychotherapy and to comprehend something of its process and outcome through the more objective lens of scientific methodology.

Like the empirical study of psychotherapy, the integration of spirituality and psychotherapy is not wanting for detractors. Hard-nosed empiricists may despair at something as gaseous as spirituality. Others may scoff at attempts to understand spirituality through methods so grounded in materialism and reductionism. My own view is that both frames of reference are fruitful, like the context of discovery and the context of justification.

Yet it is our clients who offer us perhaps the most persuasive reasons for such integration. To the clinician, the client comes first. I try to bring to my clinical work the best that science has to offer, to be informed by what scientific method has revealed about the effectiveness of treatment approaches. I count on my physician to do the same. Clients also bring with them a rich world of meaning, seeking, believing, and wondering. For most, the world of spirit is a reality, and for many it is central to how they understand and live their lives. They expect, or at least hope, to be understood and treated as a whole person. This is one of the things that I appreciate about my own physician, who has cared for me across three decades.

That challenge of integration is what brought me to assemble this book. It is part of my own lifelong search to integrate the spiritual and scientific aspects of my life and to pass insights back and forth through the doorway. It is also part of my quest to be a scientist–practitioner who treats and trains individuals in a manner that deeply respects their own spirituality. We are, I think, only beginning to tap the healing resources that are available to us. I want to search wherever I can—within and without, in the world of spirit and the world of science—to find ways of being compassionate. If that is your search, too, I am glad that you have found this book.

BILL MILLER

ACKNOWLEDGMENTS

A book, like a life, is the product of many influences. I would not be doing the work that I do were it not for the faithful examples of my family and of so many pastors who have been companions on the way. Particularly important in my own journey were Rev. Rob and Sharon Craig, Don Gall, Eduardo Guerra, Paul Hopkins, Sherry Johnston, Norman Marden, Mark Rutledge, Barbara Troxell, and George Wilson. I also recall the many professional colleagues who over the years have engaged me in stimulating discussions about psychology and spirituality. In addition to the contributing authors of this book, to whom I am most grateful, I think now of Drs. John Allen, Melanie Bennett, Allen Bergin, Stephanie Brown, Harold Delaney, Susan Gilmore, Harold Holder, Richard Longabaugh, Margaret Mattson, Ricardo Muñoz, Peter Nathan, Scott Walker, and Allen Zweben. I appreciate my editor at the American Psychological Association (APA), Margaret Schlegel, who met the idea of this book with such contagious enthusiasm and coaxed me along through the process. Thanks also to Theodore Baroody, Linda McCarter, and the production staff at APA who took the project from a pile of manuscripts and disks to the book that you hold in your hand. Finally, no one stretches me quite like my students. In Norwegian and several other languages, "to teach" and "to learn" are the same verb, and that is just how I experience the process of education. I have had the privilege not only of being mentored by but also of mentoring so many extraordinary human beings. Each one has taught me and changed me in some way, and for them all I am grateful.

INTRODUCTION

For as long as people have been able to record their thoughts, they have conceived of reality in a way that is not limited to sensory experience and intellectual knowledge. Most generations and cultures have taken for granted that "this is not all there is," that there is a spiritual dimension of reality and of human nature beyond this material world we know through our senses. To be sure, the degree of emphasis on spirituality varies in pendulum fashion over the years. At the moment, in American culture at least, we seem to be coming out of a period of extreme materialism, experiencing anew the hunger for that which is transcendent in and beyond us.

There are many ways to understand and experience that transcendence. Some call it by the name *spiritual*, and others do not. Some seek it through the historical avenues of religion. Some worship a deity or higher power; others find ultimate meaning in commitment to certain values or in creating gifts that will outlive them.

It is an underlying theme in this book that an understanding of people, individually and collectively, is incomplete without knowing about their spirituality. Like personality, the term *spirituality* is broadly defined in this book, in a way that incorporates all people. The training of psychologists and other mental health professionals is expected to include education about cultural and individual diversity—preparation to work competently with a broad spectrum of people—and such diversity surely includes varieties of spirituality. In a longer historical perspective, the roots of psychology lie in philosophy and are thereby intertwined with theology. William James, recognized as a founder of American psychology, found it natural to study "the varieties of religious experience" and wrote a substantial book on the subject.

Yet, somewhere along the way, spirituality and religion became unwelcome topics for health professionals in general and for mental health professionals in particular. I was trained in the era when psychology had lost both its mind and its soul. There have been influential figures, such as Sigmund Freud and more recently Albert Ellis, who were decidedly hostile toward religion. Yet, I sense that they simply reflected a deeper rift, as though the developing disciplines needed to assert their separateness and independence from parents. Since the trial of Galileo, one can easily find historical examples of direct opposition between science and religion, and there is a clear need for scientists to distance themselves from personal biases, spiritual and otherwise.

Now it seems that psychology's disciplinary development has moved on and that there is a quest to integrate rather than alienate the spiritual side of human nature. This quest is seen in a plethora of new books, in professional organizations, and in a more general resurgence of interest in religion and things spiritual, reflected even in the popular press. About 95% of Americans say that they believe in God. For many, spirituality and religion are important sources of strength and coping resources, and not infrequently people name them as the most important aspect of their lives, central to their meaning and identity. Many special populations cannot be understood at all without appreciating the history and centrality of religion in their community. It is a serious blind spot, then, not to understand or even ask about spirituality in our clients' lives.

Perhaps one source of discomfort is that religious involvement and theistic beliefs are dramatically underrepresented among mental health professionals relative to the general population. Note that sensitivity and responsiveness to spiritual diversity do not require that one personally be a believer or share in clients' perspectives, any more than one must change skin color to respect and communicate across racial differences. This should be obvious from the variety of other ways in which we work with a broad range of clients despite striking personal differences. Yet, I suspect that there is sometimes the sense that if one is not personally a believer, it is best not to raise the subject at all. It would be difficult to find another topic that has been more taboo for therapists. We ask clients about their emotional, physical, mental, sexual, financial, family, vocational, legal, and social lives, but we so often remain silent when it comes to spirituality. It is as though the hallowed American separation of state from church somehow applied to what one may discuss in counseling and psychotherapy.

This book is one of several books published by the American Psychological Association to encourage therapists' responsiveness to clients' spiritual and religious diversity. The focus of this book is practical. Its authors are established scientists who bring important pieces of this puzzle for clinicians. They vary in discipline, context, approach, writing style, and certainly in personal perspective on spirituality and religion. What they all share is an openness, curiosity, and respect for the spiritual side of human nature.

The four parts of this book focus on interrelated aspects important for integrating spirituality in treatment. Part I provides some background and context, exploring the relationship of spirituality to health, tracing the common history of spirituality and psychotherapy, and considering ways in which spiritual dimensions can be assessed. Part II offers a set of practical ways in which spirituality can be addressed and incorporated in the process of treatment. Part III considers particular issues with spiritual overtones, broad themes that often arise in treatment: control, acceptance and forgiveness, hope, and serenity. Finally, Part IV is concerned with ways in which the training of future therapists can be changed to provide better preparation for clients' spiritual and religious diversity.

Thus the book begins with the past and ends with the future. There is a long common history to serve as a basis for integrating spirituality into treatment. Much thought has already gone into operational definitions and a plethora of measures of spirituality, and there is a large body of research on spirituality and health. The distinguished authors of this book describe ways in which spiritual issues are already being incorporated successfully in a range of therapeutic approaches. Yet consideration of spirituality remains the exception rather than the rule in health care. In part, this is because diversity education has largely ignored this topic in professional training. Each new generation of therapists thus enters practice with no models or guidelines for how to incorporate this important side of human nature. It is the professional elephant in the living room: Everyone knows it is there, but no one talks about it above an occasional whisper. If this book accomplishes nothing more than stimulating some open professional discussion about spirituality and treatment, it will have been well worth the journey.

I

SPIRITUALITY AND TREATMENT

1

SPIRITUALITY AND HEALTH

WILLIAM R. MILLER AND CARL E. THORESEN

> Seeking for the Divine . . . has been a major aspiration and force in all cultures and periods of history, yet it has been virtually ignored by traditional psychology. . . . Regular people with ordinary problems who are also on a spiritual path . . . are looking for therapists who will honor their seeking for something sacred and who can respect their whole being—in its psychological and spiritual fullness—rather than belittling or minimizing their spiritual seeking, as much of traditional psychotherapy has historically done.
>
> (Cortright, 1997, pp. 13–14)

Long before there were science-based health care professions, people were served by culturally defined healers. The functions of healing were often blended with those of spiritual leadership within the community, as in the native *shaman*, the Mexican *curandero* and *curandera*, and pilgrimage shrines such as those at Lourdes and at Chimayo, New Mexico. The modern professions of pastoral care, chaplaincy, and pastoral counseling echo the common historical source of spiritual, physical, and mental health care (Miller & Jackson, 1995; Pattison, 1978; Vande Kemp, 1985; cf. chap. 2 in this book).

As scientific methodology increasingly came to guide medical treatment, the health professions became differentiated, first as secular, then as a proliferating array of subspecialties. A medical-technological model emerged as the dominant paradigm in medicine as well as psychology and other health professions that emulated it (Engel, 1977). Implicit assumptions of this view are that (a) differential diagnosis (i.e., the identification of the disease or disorder) is a crucial first step; (b) each disease has a definable specific cause; (c) there is an identifiable best treatment to eradicate the cause; and (d) technological specialization is optimal in the treatment of disease. This model has been effective in treating certain (e.g., infectious) diseases, although even there it may fail by overlooking social, psychological, environmental, and behavioral dimensions of illness. In addressing chronic health problems that account for a majority of medical visits, however, the limitations of a technological model have become obvious (Thoresen & Eagleston, 1985; Thoresen & Hoffman Goldberg, 1998).

The shortcomings of a technological approach are similarly apparent in addressing psychological and behavioral problems, most of which are continuously distributed rather than falling into discrete diseases or disorders. Multiple interrelated causes are common. Furthermore, comparative treatment outcome studies often fail to reveal one superior therapeutic approach (Orlinsky & Howard, 1986). Even attempts to match treatments differentially to client characteristics have met with relatively little success (e.g., Project MATCH Research Group, 1997). Health outcomes are influenced by a broad array of factors beyond the particular treatment delivered (Moos, Finney, & Cronkite, 1990).

WHAT IS HEALTH?

"How are you?" If one reflects on a thorough answer to this question, rather than regarding it as a routine greeting, it opens up the complexity of health and well-being. There are many possible answers. Some of them reflect the absence of aversive states: "OK, not bad." Yet, as wisdom is not merely the absence of ignorance, nor courage the absence of fear, so health is surely more than a lack of disease. A large component of health is subjective, which is what differentiates *disease* (a biomedical concept) from *illness* (subjective feeling states such as weakness, pain, or nausea). People may experience illness in the absence of detectable disease (a common problem in medical care) and can experience wellness despite terminal disease. Even a single continuum, ranging from perfect health to death, fails to capture the richness of experienced wellness.

Health is better conceived of as a *latent construct* like personality, character, or happiness, a complex multidimensional construct underlying a broad array of observable phenomena. The number of component dimensions is a subject of both discussion and study. For illustrative purposes, we propose that health could be conceptualized in three broad domains: suffering, function, and coherence (cf. Antonovsky, 1979). The first of these does typically define health by the absence of an experience, the other two by presence. *Suffering* is one consensual form of unhealth and is a common reason for seeking help. Such suffering may take a variety of forms, including physical pain, anxiety, depression, or distress. Yet, in a larger sense, we have known many healthy people who have lived with chronic pain or who exuded health even as they approached death from disease (e.g, Albom, 1997). The continuum of suffering, from none to severe, is only one domain of health. It is also possible to conceptualize this domain not merely as the absence of suffering but as the presence of certain qualities such as pleasure, happiness and joy, and energy and enthusiasm.

A second meaningful domain of the latent construct of health is *functional ability* versus degree of impairment. Here, too, there are multiple dimensions because there are many kinds of functional ability and many kinds of impairment. In physiological functions, one might attend to dimensions such as immune competence, neuroendrocine function, blood pressure, muscle strength, physical flexibility, and blood cell count, judging an individual's functioning relative to norms or previous performance. Cognitive, emotional, sexual and reproductive, and psychomotor functions are also important parts of health. The impairment or loss of a particular function may be devastating to one person and irrelevant to another depending on the importance placed on it. Cognitive impairment of orientation as to three-dimensional space will be much more disabling to a brain surgeon or an architect than to a writer or a psychotherapist. Flexibility or adaptability to changing conditions is another important element of this functional domain, as is the ability to give and receive love (Antonovsky, 1979; Thoresen & Eagleston, 1985). Again, functional ability is only one aspect of health. One can imagine high-functioning but unhealthy individuals as well as people with great functional impairment who vary widely on other aspects of health.

A subjective sense of *inner peace* or *coherence* in life is a third commonly discussed domain of health. Antonovsky (1979) defined coherence as a global sense of predictability (even with little controllability) of one's internal and external environment and as an optimism that things will work out as best as is reasonable. Others have discussed this as hardiness (Wiebe & McCullum, 1986), resilience (Cicchetti, Rogosch, Lynch, & Hott, 1993; Rutter, 1987), learned optimism (Seligman, 1990), or a sense of meaning and purpose in life (Crumbaugh & Maholick, 1964, 1969; Yalom, 1980). All of these have to do with one's broad subjective perspective on life.

If health is more than the absence of disease, and broader than the single dimension of suffering, then a healer's task is larger than the detection and eradication of a specific disease state. It has to do with quality of life, with the richness that is invoked when we truly ask and answer the question, "How are you?"

WHAT IS SPIRITUALITY?

For at least as long as history has been recorded, humankind has assumed that reality is not limited to the material, sensory world. Belief in a spiritual reality continues to characterize a large majority of Americans, be it belief in a supreme being or order, life after physical death, an ultimate reality, or supernatural beings like angels or demons. Whatever behavioral scientists and health care professionals may themselves believe, the spiritual side of human nature remains important to many or most clients. A substantial minority, at least, describe spirituality as the most important source of strength and direction in their lives. Many prominent voices in the history of psychology have raised up spirituality as a proper subject for scientific study (e.g., Allport, 1961; James, 1902/1985).

Like personality and health, spirituality is complex. It is not adequately defined by any single continuum or by dichotomous classifications; rather, it has many dimensions. Spirituality is better understood as multidimensional space in which every individual can be located (Larson, Swyers, & McCullough, 1997). This avoids the misleading classification of people as "spiritual" versus "not spiritual," or as more versus less spiritual.

Differentiating spirituality from religion can be helpful. However defined, whether broadly as consciousness (Helminiak, 1996) or in relation to transcendence (Miller & Martin, 1988; Thoresen, 1998), spirituality (like personality or character) is an attribute of individuals. Religion, in contrast, is an organized social entity. To be sure, individuals can be characterized for their religiosity, their particular beliefs and practices relative to religion. It is also the case that the exploration of spirituality is one historic purpose of world religions (Smith, 1994). Thoresen (1998), drawing on recent work examining working definitions of spiritual and religious perspectives (Larson et al., 1997), suggested that some characteristics are shared, such as a search for what is sacred or holy in life, coupled with some kind of transcendent (beyond the self) relationship with God or a higher power or universal energy.

Differences clearly exist, however, with *religious* factors focused more on prescribed beliefs, rituals, and practices as well as social institutional features. *Spiritual* factors, on the other hand, are concerned more with individual subjective experiences, sometimes shared with others (cf. Zinnbauer et al. (1997). Maslow (1976) similarly differentiated "the subjective and naturalistic religious experience and attitude" (p. viii; here termed *spiritual*) from institutional organized religions. Religion is characterized in many ways by its boundaries and spirituality by a difficulty in defining its boundaries. Religion involves an organized social institution with, among other things, beliefs about how one relates to that which is sacred or divine. Spirituality does not necessarily involve religion. Some people experience their spirituality as a highly personal and private matter, focusing on intangible elements that provide vitality and meaning in their lives. In what has been described as a "the new spirituality" arising apart from organized religion in recent decades (e.g., Roof, Carroll, & Roozen, 1995), spirituality may be conceptualized in ways that do not assume any reality beyond material existence. In such an individualistic perspective, each person (regardless of religious involvement) defines his or her own spirituality, which might center on material experiences such as mountain biking at dusk, quiet contemplation of nature, reflection on the direction of one's life, and a feeling of intimate connection with loved ones (e.g., "Spirituality in Silicon Valley," 1998). Clearly, spirituality and religion are not the same.

Religion and religiosity can, in fact, interfere with a person's spiritual growth. Some teachings warn that the spiritual purpose of religious practice can be lost in obsessional piety or in political and economic agendas that focus on power and prestige. Spirituality, then, can be defined apart from religion, and the relationships between the two become a matter for empirical study. Before leaving this point, though, it is worthwhile to note that this sharp distinction between spirituality and religion that some currently make has not always been emphasized. When William James (1902/1985) wrote the book, *The Varieties of Religious Experience*, a century ago, he was clearly describing the broader domain that is now called *spirituality*.

So what are the dimensions of this multidimensional space of spirituality? These are a matter of both debate and scientific study. For the present purposes, we propose three broad measurement domains: practice, belief, and experience. In so doing, we acknowledge that others have described a larger number of dimensions. Glock and Stark (1965), for example, described four elements or domains, all of which are associated with the context of religion: the experiential, the ritualistic, the intellectual, and the consequential. Capps, Rambo, and Ransohoff (1976) offered a somewhat different breakdown of six spiritual dimensions within religion: the mythological, ritual, experiential, dispositional, social, and directional. The three domains that we describe here—spiritual practices, beliefs, and experiences—are meant to characterize spirituality more generally, whether inside or outside the context of religion. These broad domains are consistent with a psychosocial perspective that is sensitive to cultural, ethnic, socioeconomic, and religious differences. Each domain, such as practices, can encompass a wide range of constructs and variables. Each is amenable to a variety of qualitative and quantitative assessment approaches (e.g., biographical and autobiographical material, narrative interviews, physiological measures, self-report questionnaires).

The first of these three dimensions is perhaps the easiest to measure because it focuses on overt observable behavior (e.g., Connors, Tonigan, & Miller, 1996). People can be described by the extent to which they engage in spiritual practices such as prayer, fasting, meditation, and contemplation. Also included here would be participation in specifically religious activities such as worship, dance, scriptural study, singing, confession, offerings, and public prayer.

The second domain of spiritual beliefs is large, and its content varies with culture (Smith, 1994). Directly pertinent here are beliefs about transcendence (e.g., soul, afterlife), deity, and the reality of a spiritual dimension beyond sensory and intellectual knowledge. Personal morality and endorsed values are also part of this domain (Rokeach, 1973). Transcending "the *me* factor" (i.e., I, me, my, mine) in personal values has been a common quest in many religions (Bracke & Thoresen, 1996; Easwaren, 1989). The concept of God (where one is present) is an interesting dimension here (e.g., whether the nature, image, and intentions of a supreme being are seen as being fundamentally loving, indifferent, or punitive toward humankind).

The third domain, spiritual experience, offers perhaps the greatest challenges for valid measurement, yet it is fundamental to an understanding of spirituality. Many would regard this experiential dimension as the fundamental and defining nature of spirituality (Helminiak, 1996). Such experiences might be roughly divided into routine, everyday encounters of the transcendent or sacred, versus exceptional spiritual and mystical experiences (although this distinction will break down for some whose daily reality is mystical). At least two perplexing problems of definition emerge. The first is the problem of defining which experiences *are* spiritual. Among individuals who have had sudden, dramatic, and transforming life experiences, for example, some describe them in spiritual language and others do not (Miller & C'deBaca, 1994). Believers and nonbelievers may have essentially parallel experiences, but they differ in the understanding of their meaning and nature. A second challenge is empirical description of the experiences themselves. Whether they are labeled as "spiritual," there appears to be a relatively common topography to certain numinous phenomena including mystical (Bucke, 1923; Oates, 1973), transformational (Loder, 1981; Miller & C'deBaca, 1994), and near-death experiences (Kellehear, 1996).

Before moving on, we acknowledge that this scientific way of thinking and speaking about spirituality will seem strange to many readers. Those who equate spirituality with the experiential dimension may prefer phenomenological metaphors to operational definitions. To speak of "spiritual behavior" appears to reduce spirituality to nothing more than behavior. This is not our intention. Words are unquestionably inadequate to fully describe so complex a phenomenon, and, being defined in distinction from material reality, spirituality is particularly difficult to define. Other complex constructs such as personality can similarly be described as having at least three dimensions—behavioral, cognitive, and experiential—none of which (or their sum) fully characterizes the phenomena to which the word *personality* refers. The upcoming discussion of *spiritual variables* may likewise be jarring both to those who prefer a phenomenological and purely subjective approach to spirituality and to behavioral scientists for whom the term may seem a scientific oxymoron. Yet, we believe that it is important to include clients' spirituality in treatment, and clinical practice is increasingly guided by the fruits of scientific method (e.g., "empirically validated" treatments). We contend that these are compatible and complementary frames of reference, with each offering perspectives that can enhance and enrich the other.

SPIRITUALITY AND CLINICAL PRACTICE

Although these perspectives are compatible, their borders have been characterized as a "no man's land" in which clients can get lost (Wick, 1985). When health problems also have spiritual dimensions, it is often unclear from whom one should seek help. The common border is exemplified by concerns such as value issues, guilt, forgiveness and grace, hope, acceptance, and developmental events that have been described as "spiritual emergencies" (Hendlin, 1985) that, unfortunately, can be mistaken for psychosis. These are currently subsumed under "religious and spiritual problems" in the fourth edition of the *Diagnostic and Statistical Manual of Mental Disorders* (American Psychiatric Association, 1994). Significantly, such problems are no longer assumed to be pathological but extend to the genuine concerns of normal people (Thoresen, 1998). Lacking the needed diversity training, practitioners are often ill-prepared to deal with the spiritual and religious aspects of such concerns (see chap. 13 in this book; Richards & Bergin, 1997). Yet, referral to clergy or other spiritual specialists can also be problematic. Many pastors and spiritual directors lack the psychological expertise to negotiate this border region, which is not the exclusive province of either spiritual or health professionals.

How can this dilemma be resolved? One approach is to help clergy increase their knowledge of contemporary clinical and counseling psychology (Miller & Jackson, 1995). A second approach is the one represented in this book: to provide health professionals with the knowledge, understanding, and skills to competently handle counseling at the border. A third valid possibility is for spiritual and health professionals to collaborate and coordinate their care. Still another possibility is represented by specialized clinics, centers, and practice groups that offer physical and mental health services provided by "bilingual" professionals who are competent in both domains. Such services are sometimes limited to a particular religious perspective, whereas other agencies (such as the Samaritan Centers in the United States) seek to provide professional psychotherapy in a context that is accessible and sensitive to a broad range of faith perspectives.

We believe that it is not necessary (or even feasible) for health professionals to be trained in the specifics of the broad array of spiritual and religious perspectives that may be represented among their clients. What a clinician needs, beyond appropriate initial and continuing professional education, is a set of culturally sensitive proficiencies.

- A nonjudgmental, accepting, and empathic relationship with the client.
- An openness and willingness to take time to understand the client's spirituality as it may relate to health-related issues.
- Some familiarity with culturally related values, beliefs, and practices that are common among the client populations likely to be served.
- Comfort in asking and talking about spiritual issues with clients.
- A willingness to seek information from appropriate professionals and coordinate care concerning clients' spiritual traditions.

It is also wise to be aware of psychotherapy issues that may be especially important or problematic for clients who are committed to a particular religious perspective. Assertiveness training, for example, may raise special issues for some Christian and Islamic clients, for whom assertion can be confused with aggressiveness and appear to conflict with central religious teachings about humility and turning the other cheek. Helpful writings by clinicians with expertise in both psychology and religion are available. Such individuals have thought through issues, such as assertiveness and forgiveness, from the perspective of clinical practice (e.g., Augsberger, 1979; Rayburn, 1985; Sanders & Maloney, 1985; Thoresen, Harris, and Luskin, in press). Part III of this book focuses particularly on such border-crossing issues.

SPIRITUALITY AND HEALTH

Is it a coincidence that spiritual leadership and healing have historically been vested in a common role within so many cultures (Smith, 1994)? One possible reason for this convergence is that people experience their own physical, mental, and spiritual well-being as being interrelated. Indeed, in an era of managed health care and technical specialization, there seems to be a hunger to be understood as a whole person. For many Americans, the first professional sought out in time of crisis is still a member of the clergy, often their own pastor, priest, or rabbi. Medical patients often wish that their doctors would talk with them about spiritual matters, even pray with them, and many draw on spiritual coping resources in times of illness (Daaleman & Neare, 1994; Marwick, 1995; Pargament, 1996, 1997). The desire is to be understood and treated not as a liver, or a depression, or an addiction but as a complete and integrated person. Spirituality, like personality or immune competency, is one facet and one way of thinking about a person, none captures the whole. In this way, it is possible to think of spiritual health as one part of a comprehensive picture. Doing so is part of the historic role played by hospital chaplains and more recently mirrored in the requirement by the U.S. Joint Commission for Accreditation of Healthcare Organizations (JCAHO) that accredited facilities assess spirituality as part of health care.

There are reasons, however, to think of spirituality not only as a dependent variable but also as an independent variable in human health. We had the privilege of participating in a series of expert panels focused on scientific research on spirituality and health, convened in 1996 and 1997 by the National Institute for Healthcare Research (Larson et al., 1997). These panels were composed of prominent scientists from their respective fields, spanning a range of spiritual and religious perspectives. Three of the panels focused, respectively, on the relationship of spirituality to physical health, to mental health, and to alcohol and drug problems. Each panel was asked to address four questions: (a) What is already known from scientific research about spirituality in relation to this area of health? (b) What do we need to know—what are the pressing questions to be asked next? (c) What scientific methods could be used to answer these questions? (d) What barriers impede research in this area?

After reviewing current evidence, all three panels reached the same basic conclusion. When spiritual and religious involvement has been measured (even poorly), it has with surprising consistency been found to be positively related to health and inversely related to disorders. This relationship holds both in correlational studies at the same point in time and in longitudinal or prospective studies in which spiritual and religious involvement is predictive of later health outcomes. These findings hold across physical (Levin, 1994), mental (Bergin, 1983; Larson, Pattison, Blazer, Omran, & Kaplan, 1986; Larson et al., 1992), and substance use disorders (Gorsuch, 1995). The panels also concurred that the reasons for this protective relationship are poorly understood at present and represent a high priority for future study.

SPIRITUALITY AND TREATMENT

Much more limited has been research on the effectiveness of spiritual interventions for health problems, although studies are accumulating here as well. For example, in a comprehensive review of spiritual and religious factors related to psychological outcomes, only 6% of more than 150 studies involved treatments (Worthington, Kurusu, McCullough, & Sanders, 1996). The chapters in this book reflect some frontiers of such work. The evidence to date does not suggest that current scientifically based health care methods should be replaced by spiritual approaches. Indeed, to do so would reflect a narrow vision of the nature of health. Rather, the evidence emphasizes the importance of incorporating spirituality into modern health care. This includes considering clients' spirituality as a component of health (as dependent variables) as well as drawing on spiritual resources in the process of healing (as independent variables). The possible impact of treatment in altering spiritual factors, for example, deserves careful attention, especially the issue of whether changes in specific spiritual behaviors, beliefs and experiences promote improved health and reduce the risk of disease (Thoresen, 1998; Thoresen, Luskin, & Harris, 1998; Thoresen et al., 1997).

This raises an immediate concern for the health care professional: What if I do not share the client's spiritual perspective or religious belief system? Indeed, psychologists, physicians, and scientists are not representative of the populations they serve when it comes to spiritual beliefs and religious involvement (Bergin & Jensen, 1990; Maugans & Wedland, 1991; Shafranske, 1996). A specialist's approach would be to call in qualified clergy to deal with spiritual aspects of a client's care, and there are distinct advantages to interprofessional collaboration. Yet, as already noted, clients generally do not want to be understood just in parts but as a whole person, and we believe (with JCAHO) that all health care providers should know something of their clients' spirituality to develop a comprehensive understanding of their problems and design an appropriate treatment plan.

There is good news. Just as one does not need to be a recovering alcoholic or drug addict to treat substance use disorders effectively (McLellan, Woody, Luborsky, & Goehl, 1988), one need not be a believer to help clients discuss spiritual features of their condition and their care. Profound respect for spiritual, religious, and cultural diversity is called for here. A clinician who regards all religious belief to be pathogenic is not only disregarding the weight of empirical evidence but also is likely to manifest this prejudice in practice (Bergin, 1980; Richards & Bergin, 1997). Clinicians need to understand something about their clients' spiritual beliefs, practices, and experiences, particularly when these factors are related to what brings them into therapy or what may be helpful in the process of treatment. Within a professional atmosphere of mutual respect and acceptance, there is room for fruitful collaborations that include the client's spirituality (Miller & Martin, 1988).

Propst (1980, 1988; Propst, Ostrom, Watkins, Dean, & Mashburn, 1992), for example, found in randomized trials with religiously oriented clients that the effectiveness of cognitive–behavioral therapy for depression was substantially increased when their spiritual perspectives were incorporated into the treatment. This was true whether the clinicians were themselves religiously oriented. Spiritual content can be incorporated into scientifically based treatment approaches without dramatically reshaping them, thereby rendering them more accessible (and effective) to clients for whom spirituality is of central importance (Johnson & Ridley, 1992; Worthington, 1988).

A number of major health intervention studies have already incorporated what is essentially spiritual material (e.g., Friedman et al., 1986; Nowinski, Baker, & Carroll, 1992; Ornish et al., 1990; Spiegel, Kaplan, Kraemer, & Gottheil, 1989). Spirituality related themes raised in these contexts have included the sense of direction, meaning, and purpose in life; feelings of connectedness with oneself, with others, and with God or a higher power; clarifying what is trivial and what is truly vital in life; reducing self-critical and hostile cognitions; and fostering love, compassion, and forgiveness (Thoresen, 1998; Thoresen, Luskin, & Harris, 1998). Such concerns may not have been labeled as spiritual—they are often referred to as personal values or philosophy of life issues—but their spiritual relevance seems clear. To illustrate, in the Recurrent Coronary Prevention Program (Friedman et al., 1986), coronary patients in the psychosocial treatment were asked to practice listening with their heart to others, to verbally express their love and compassion for others, and to spend time alone in experiencing nature. Each week they were also asked to reflect on spiritually related quotations, such as "It is only with the heart that one can see rightly. What is essential is invisible to the eye" (St. Exupery, 1943, p. 9). Rarely have such themes been central, however, and they often have been given little or no emphasis. Equally rare has been a careful assessment of client spiritual and religious factors to study their impact on health outcomes within the context of intervention research.

What if a client should ask, "What are *your* religious beliefs?" It is a fair question, and an open summary of your pertinent beliefs and values can be an appropriate response (see chap. 7 in this book). Often, however, the underlying concern is more general and is similar to that of the client who asks a younger-looking clinician, "Just how old are you?" What may be most needed is your reassurance that even if there are areas where your values and beliefs may differ, you will respect the client's beliefs, and such differences ordinarily do not impede working together effectively (Malony, 1985). You can also indicate that should either of you find that this becomes a problem, you would make an appropriate referral.

SUMMARY

Spiritual well-being is an important and too often overlooked dimension of health. Much is already known. Spiritual and religious involvement is not only common but is often important in clients' lives and has been generally linked to positive health outcomes. A client's spiritual perspectives may be relevant in understanding his or her problems and useful in the process of treatment. Although seldom taught in the training of health professionals, there is a large literature on the assessment of spirituality and religiousness. Incorporating spiritual perspectives in secular treatment has been found to improve outcomes for religiously oriented clients. Spiritually rooted interventions and collaboration with spiritual professionals may also enhance successful treatment.

Yet, a great deal remains to be done. With regard to assessment, the dimensions and measures that are most pertinent for treatment are yet to be defined. Although there appears to be a general protective effect of spiritual and religious involvement, little is known about why this occurs or how it interacts with the processes and outcomes of specific treatments. The scientific evaluation of interventions with a spiritual focus has barely begun. Clients themselves, as well as a broad body of research, tell us that spirituality is a significant dimension in health and may hold important keys in understanding healing. As that understanding expands, it will become clearer how best to address spiritual and religious factors in treatment. This book is one step in that direction.

REFERENCES

Albom, M. (1997). *Tuesdays with Morrie*. New York: Doubleday.

Allport, G. (1961). *The individual and his religion*. New York: Macmillan.

American Psychiatric Association. (1994). *Diagnostic and statistical manual of mental disorders* (4th ed.). Washington, DC: Author.

Antonovsky, A. (1979). *Health, stress, and coping*. San Francisco: Jossey-Bass.

Augsberger, D. W. (1979). *Anger and assertiveness in pastoral care*. Philadelphia: Fortress Press.

Bergin, A. E. (1980). Psychotherapy and religious values. *Journal of Consulting and Clinical Psychology, 48*, 95–105.

Bergin, A. E. (1983). Religiosity and mental health: A critical reevaluation and meta-analysis. *Professional Psychology: Research and Practice, 14*, 170–184.

Bergin, A. E., & Jensen, J. P. (1990). Religiosity of psychotherapists: A national survey. *Psychotherapy, 27*, 3–7.

Bracke, P. E., & Thoresen, C. E. (1996). Reducing type A behavior patterns: A structured-group approach. In R. Allen & S. Scheidt (Eds.), *Heart and mind* (pp. 255–290). Washington, DC: American Psychological Association.

Bucke, R. M. (1923). *Cosmic consciousness*. New York: E. P. Dutton.

Capps, D., Rambo, L., & Ransohoff, P. (1976). *Psychology of religion*. Detroit, MI: Gale Research.

Cicchetti, D., Rogosch, F. A., Lynch, M., & Hott, K. D. (1993). Resilience in maltreated children: Processes leading to adaptive outcome. *Development and Psychopathology, 5*, 629–647.

Connors, G. J., Tonigan, J. S., & Miller, W. R. (1996). A measure of religious background and behavior for use in behavior change research. *Psychology of Addictive Behavior, 10,* 90–96.

Crumbaugh, J. C., & Maholick, L. T. (1964). An experimental study in existentialism: The psychometric approach to Frankl's concept of noogenic neurosis. *Journal of Clinical Psychology, 22,* 200–207.

Crumbaugh, J. C., & Maholick, L. T. (1969). *The Purpose in Life Test.* Chicago: Psychometric Affiliates.

Daaleman, T. P., & Neare, D. E., Jr. (1994). Patient attitudes regarding physician inquiry into spiritual and religious issues. *Journal of Family Practice, 39,* 564–568.

Easwaran, E. A. (1989). *Meditation.* Tomales, CA: Nilgiri Press.

Engel, G. (1977). The need for a new medical model: A challenge for biomedicine. *Science, 196,* 129–136.

Friedman, M., Thoresen, C. E., Gill, J. J., Ulmer, D., Powell, L. H., Price, V. A., Brown, B., Thompson, L., Rabin, D. D., Breall, W. S., Bourg, E., Levy, R., & Dixon, T. (1986). Alteration of Type A behavior and its effect on cardiac recurrences in postmyocardial infarction patients: Summary results of the Recurrent Coronary Prevention Project. *American Health Journal, 112,* 653–665.

Glock, C. Y., & Stark, R. (1965). *Religion and society in tension.* Chicago: Rand McNally.

Gorsuch, R. L. (1995). Religious aspects of substance abuse and recovery. *Journal of Social Issues, 5*(12), 65–83.

Helminiak, D. A. (1996). A scientific spirituality: The interface of psychology and theology. *International Journal for the Psychology of Religion, 6,* 1–19.

Hendlin, S. J. (1985). The spiritual emergency patient: Concept and example. *The Psychotherapy Patient, 1*(3), 79–88.

James, W. (1985). *The varieties of religious experience: A study in human nature.* Cambridge, MA: Harvard University Press. (Original work published 1902)

Johnson, W. B., & Ridley, C. R. (1992). Source of gain in Christian counseling and psychotherapy. *The Counseling Psychologist, 20,* 159–175.

Kellehear, A. (1996). *Experiences near death.* New York: Oxford University Press.

Larson, D. B., Pattison, E. M., Blazer, D. G., Omran, A. R., & Kaplan, B. H. (1986). Systematic analysis of research on religious variables in four major psychiatric journals, 1978–1982. *American Journal of Psychiatry, 143,* 329–334.

Larson, D. B., Sherrill, K. A., Lyons, J. S., Craigie, F. C., Jr., Thielman, S. B., Greenwold, M. A., & Larson, S. S. (1992). Associations between dimensions of religious commitment and mental health reported in the *American Journal of Psychiatry* and *Archives of General Psychiatry:* 1978–1989. *American Journal of Psychiatry, 149,* 557–559.

Larson D. B., Swyers J. P., & McCullough M. E. (Eds.). (1997). *Scientific research on spirituality and health: A consensus report.* Rockville, MD: National Institute for Healthcare Research.

Levin, J. S. (1994). Religion and health: Is there an association, is it valid, and is it causal? *Social Science and Medicine, 38,* 1175–1182.

Loder, J. E. (1981). *The transforming moment: Understanding convictional experiences.* New York: Harper & Row.

Malony, H. N. (1985). Assessing religious maturity. *The Psychotherapy Patient, 1*(3), 25–33.

Marwick, C. (1995). Should physicians prescribe prayer for health? Spiritual aspects of well being considered. *Journal of the American Medical Association, 273,* 1561–1562.

Maslow, A. H. (1976). *Religions, values, and peak-experiences.* New York: Penguin Books.

Maugans, T. A., & Wedland, W. C. (1991). Religion and family medicine: A survey of physicians and patients. *Journal of Family Practice, 32,* 210–213.

McLellan, A. T., Woody, G. E., Luborsky, L., & Goehl, L. (1988). Is the counselor an "active ingredient" in substance abuse rehabilitation? An examination of treatment success among four counselors. *Journal of Nervous and Mental Disease, 176,* 423–430.

Miller, W. R., & C'deBaca, J. (1994). Quantum change: Toward a psychology of transformation. In T. Heatherton & J. Weinberger (Eds.), *Can personality change?* (pp. 253–280). Washington, DC: American Psychological Association.

Miller, W. R., & Jackson, K. A. (1995). *Practical psychology for pastors: Toward more effective counseling* (2nd ed.) Englewood Cliffs, NJ: Prentice Hall.

Miller, W. R., & Martin, J. E. (Eds.). (1988). *Behavior therapy and religion: Integrating spiritual and behavioral approaches to change.* Newbury Park, CA: Sage.

Moos, R. H., Finney, J. W., & Cronkite, R. C. (1990). *Alcoholism treatment: Context, process, and outcome.* New York: Oxford University Press.

Nowinski, J., Baker, S., & Carroll, K. (1992). *Twelve step facilitation therapy manual: A clinical research guide for therapists treating individuals with alcohol abuse and dependence* (Vol. 1, Project MATCH Monograph Series). Rockville, MD: National Institute on Alcohol Abuse and Alcoholism.

Oates, W. E. (1973). *The psychology of religion.* Waco, TX: Word Books.

Orlinsky, D. E., & Howard, K. I. (1986). Process and outcome in psychotherapy. In S. L. Garfield & A. E. Bergin (Eds.), *Handbook of psychotherapy and behavior change* (3rd ed., pp. 311–381). New York: Wiley.

Ornish, D., Brown, S. E., Scherwitz, L. W., Billings, J. H., Armstrong, W. T., & Ports, T. A. (1990). Can coronary artery disease be reversed? *Lancet, 336,* 129–133.

Pargament, K. I. (1996). Religious methods of coping: Resources for the conservation and transformation of meaning. In E. P. Shafranske (Ed.), *Religion and the clinical practice of psychology* (pp. 215–239). Washington, DC: American Psychological Association.

Pargament, K. I. (1997). *The psychology of religion and coping.* New York: Guilford Press.

Pattison, E. M. (1978). Psychiatry and religion circa 1978: Analysis of a decade, Part 1. *Pastoral Psychology, 27*, 8–25.

Project MATCH Research Group. (1997). Matching alcoholism treatments to client heterogeneity: Project MATCH posttreatment drinking outcomes. *Journal of Studies on Alcohol, 58*, 7–29.

Propst, L. R. (1980). The comparative efficacy of religious and nonreligious imagery for the treatment of mild depression in religious individuals. *Cognitive Therapy and Research, 4*, 167–178.

Propst, L. R. (1988). *Psychotherapy within a religious framework: Spirituality in the emotional healing process*. New York: Human Sciences Press.

Propst, L. R., Ostrom, R., Watkins, P., Dean, T., & Mashburn, D. (1992). Comparative efficacy of religious and nonreligious cognitive-behavioral therapy for the treatment of clinical depression in religious individuals. *Journal of Consulting and Clinical Psychology, 60*, 94–103.

Rayburn, C. A. (1985). The religious patient's initial encounter with psychotherapy. *The Psychotherapy Patient, 1*(3), 35–45.

Richards, P. S., & Bergin, A. E. (1997). *A spiritual strategy for counseling and psychotherapy*. Washington, DC: American Psychological Association.

Rokeach, M. (1973). *The nature of human values*. New York: Free Press.

Roof, W. C., Carroll, J. W., & Roozen, D. A. (Eds.). (1995). *The post-war generation and establishment religion*. Boulder, CO: Westview Press.

Rutter, M. (1987). Psychosocial resilience and protective mechanisms. *American Journal of Orthopsychiatry, 57*, 316–331.

Sanders, R. K., & Maloney, K. N. (1985). *Speak up! Christian assertiveness*. Philadelphia: Westminster John Knox.

Seligman, M. E. P. (1990). *Learned optimism: How to change your mind and your life*. New York: Pocket Books.

Shafranske, E. P. (1996). Religious beliefs, affiliations, and practices of clinical psychologists. In E. P. Shafranske (Ed.), *Religion and the clinical practice of psychology* (pp. 149–162). Washington, DC: American Psychological Association.

Smith, H. (1994). *The world's religions: A guide to our wisdom traditions*. San Francisco: HarperCollins.

Spiegel, D., Kaplan, G. A., Kraemer, H. C., & Gottheil, E. (1989). Effects of psychosocial treatment on survival of patients with metastatic breast cancer. *Lancet, 14*, 888–891.

Spirituality in Silicon Valley. (1998, May 14). *San Jose Mercury News*, p. A1.

St. Exupery, A. (1943). *The little prince*. New York: Harcourt, Brace & World.

Thoresen, C. E. (1998). Spirituality, health and science: The coming revival? In S. Roth-Roemer, S. Kurpius Robinson, & C. Carmin (Eds.), *The emerging role of counseling psychology in health care* (pp. 409–431). New York: Norton.

Thoresen, C. E., & Eagleston, J. R. (1985). Counseling for health. *The Counseling Psychologist, 13*, 15–87.

Thoresen, C. E., & Hoffman Goldberg, J. (1998). Coronary heart disease: A psychosocial perspective. In S. Roth-Roemer, S. Kurpius Robinson, & C. Carmin (Eds.), *The emerging role of counseling psychology in health care* (pp. 94–136). New York: Norton.

Thoresen, C., Harris, A. A. H., & Luskin, F. (in press). Forgiveness, health and disease: Is there a relationship? In M. McCullough, K. Pargament & C. Thoresen (Eds.), *The frontiers of forgiveness*. New York: Guilford Press.

Thoresen, C. E., Luskin, F., & Harris, A. O. (1998). Science and forgiveness interventions: Reflections and recommendations. In E. Worthington (Ed.), *Dimensions of forgiveness* (pp. 163–192). Philadelphia: Templeton Foundation Press.

Thoresen, C., Worthington, E., Swyers, J., Larson, D., McCullough, M., & Miller, W. R. (1997). Religious/spiritual interventions. In D. Larson, J. Swyers, & M. McCullough (Eds.), *Scientific research on spirituality and health: A consensus report* (pp. 104–128). Rockville, MD: National Institute on Healthcare Research.

Vande Kemp, H. (1985). Psychotherapy as a religious process: A historical heritage. *The Psychotherapy Patient, 1*(3), 135–146.

Wick, E. (1985). Lost in the no man's land between psyche and soul. *The Psychotherapy Patient, 1*(3), 13–24.

Wiebe, D. J., & McCullum D. M. (1986). Health practices and hardiness as mediators in the stress-illness relationship. *Health Psychology, 5*, 425–438.

Worthington, E. L. (1988). Understanding the values of religious clients: A model and its application to counseling. *Journal of Counseling Psychology, 35*, 166–174.

Worthington, E. L., Kurusu, T. A., McCullough, M. E., & Sanders, S. J. (1996). Empirical research on religion and psychotherapeutic processes and outcomes: A 10-year review and research prospectus. *Psychological Bulletin, 119*, 448–487.

Yalom, I. D. (1980). *Existential psychotherapy*. New York: Basic Books.

Zinnbauer, B. J., Pargament, K. I., Cole, B., Rye, M., Butter, E. M., Belavich, T. G., Hipp, K. M., Scott, A. S., & Kadar, J. L. (1997). Religion and spirituality: Unfuzzying the Fuzzy. *Journal for the Scientific Study of Religion, 36*(4), 549–564.

2

THE HISTORICAL CONTEXT

ERNEST KURTZ

Some 90 years ago, at the time of the birth of modern psychotherapy in the United States as marked by Sigmund Freud's visit to Clark University, the philosopher Josiah Royce warned against "confusing theology with therapy." Royce observed that much of the American debate over psychotherapy seemed to establish the health of the individual as the criterion of philosophical (and, by implication, theological) truth. Replying to that claim, Royce pointed out that "whoever, in his own mind, makes the whole great world center about the fact that he, just this private individual, once was ill and now is well, is still a patient" (Royce, cited in Holifield, 1983, p. 209).

Patient, however, is a therapeutic term. Might Royce with equal justice have observed that "whoever, in her own mind, makes the whole world center about the fact that she, just this private individual, once sinned but is now saved, is still far from the kingdom of heaven"? With what other variations of vocabulary might we conjure in this context?

Whatever the vocabulary used, discussion of the relationship between psychotherapy and spirituality occurs within the larger context of the re-

Ernest Kurtz is a retired historian (PhD in History of American Civilization from Harvard University, 1978) who currently holds visiting scholar privileges at the University of Michigan in Ann Arbor. He may be reached by electronic mail at kurtzern@post.harvard.edu.

lationship between science and religion. That relationship has often been less than happy. Ian Barbour's (1966) *Issues In Science and Religion* and Philip Rieff's (1966) *The Triumph of the Therapeutic* remain useful summaries. Yet, even this generalization will draw disagreement, for *spirituality* and *psychotherapy* are two terms shrouded in diverse denotations and confusing connotations.

According to usage within the American Psychological Association, the term *psychotherapy* refers to a young science, which claims to have some qualities of an art, that originated with Sigmund Freud and "the discovery of the unconscious" (Freedheim, 1992; Shafranske, 1996). The history of psychotherapy, then, is not the story of "the insane" or their treatment. That is a different history. In a pre–*Diagnostic and Statistical Manual of Mental Disorders* (4th ed.; *DSM–IV*) vocabulary, my concern here is the story of neurotic rather than psychotic individuals. As understood in what follows, the goal of psychotherapy is the alleviation of mental and emotional distress that may have biological referents but the sources of which are thought to be in some way in a person's relationships, past or present, with other persons. The method of psychotherapy is a relationship with some other person or persons, which relationship in some way changes the style if not the nature of other relationships. In an age of biological psychiatry and chemical comforting, this description may seem naive. However, the present age's discoveries and enthusiasms will also be integrated into some larger understanding, and psychotherapy as portrayed above will remain.

The term *spirituality* has its own fascinating history, but it is generally currently used to denote "certain positive inward qualities and perceptions" while avoiding implications of "narrow, dogmatic beliefs and obligatory religious observances" (Wulff, 1996, p. 47). Historians of the spiritual such as Edward Kinerk (1981), Philip Sheldrake (1991), and Bernard McGinn (1991), as well as theological commentators such as Don Browning (1980) and Donald Capps (1993), would agree. The goal of spirituality is the alleviation of mental, emotional, and spiritual distress thought to be at least in part caused by the lack of an appropriate relationship with ultimate reality, most often signaled by and reflected in inappropriate relationships with other people and things. Spirituality is less a method than an *attitude*, a posture of one's very being that allows seeing not different things but everything differently (Edwards, 1755/1960; Holifield, 1983, p. 88).

Just as every psychotherapy applies some psychology, some understanding of how the human mind and emotions work, any spirituality is a lived theology, a posture that positions one within total reality. Neither psychologies nor theologies need be formalized, but everyone has them, however implicitly. And just as a genuine psychology can never be the possession of any "school," theology may be mediated by, but is never the captive of, any religion.

As the terms *psychotherapy* and *spirituality* are most often currently used, comparisons or contrasts of them involve a category error. Spirituality is best glimpsed in synonyms such as *sanity, sanctity, serenity, health, wholeness, holiness*: It is, simply, that for which all persons strive. Medicine and religion, therapies and ritual, each aim to ease access to that reality. Jerome Frank (1974) has defined the components of psychotherapy as including a socially sanctioned healer, a sufferer who seeks relief, and a circumscribed series of contacts that are designed to afford the sufferer relief, certainly characteristics better fitting religion and medicine than spirituality.

However, all these terms—even *spirituality* and *therapy*—today come freighted with such baggage that we best begin by leaving aside such specifications and opening the story with the observation that every human society has had its healers, those who alleviated distress by in some way "making whole" sufferers who sought them out. And in every society, there has been the realization that this making whole takes place both within the individual sufferer and in that person's relationships with the larger world. Early societies usually found both facets in one healer. More recent cultures are pulled by opposing tendencies to integrate and to separate them, but both modern spiritualities and modern psychotherapies opt for integration, seeing the fullness of human be-ing as comprising the *physical,* the *mental,* the *emotional,* and the *spiritual,* although one or another of those facets may be ignored for a time, and there seems to be an enduring tendency to fold one or another of those four into one of the others.

Hoping to avoid argumentative caricatures, what follows will take both psychotherapy and spirituality in their ordinary expression. All practices have aberrations. Focusing on them results in little beyond polemic pain. Remaining with the *real,* then, I concentrate on the ideal for which it always strives rather than on the deviations into which it sometimes lapses. Within this understanding, I propose that the difference between psychotherapy and spirituality relevant to this chapter is that which is more commonly construed as a reflection of the different approaches of science and religion. The former, the "scientific approach," relies on the human and especially the self, agreeing with Protagoras that "man is the measure of all things." It studies that which is verifiably perceivable by the five human senses. The latter approach, that of the religious or spiritual insight, insists on the reality and significance of some power outside of the self and in some way greater than the human individual and transcendent of ordinary sense experience.

What follows is less a complete narrative of the relationship between these two realities than a series of glimpses at significant moments in that history. To attempt to tell of all the interactions would require too superficial a treatment of each. Instead, then, I choose to examine in some depth a series of historical moments—less "events" than broader happenings that are significant to how scholars view the relationship between psychotherapy and spirituality on the threshold of the third millennium of the common era. The earliest of these moments occurred before the birth of psychotherapy and so tell directly of events in the history of spirituality that bear on later understandings of the promise and perils of the human condition. In the latter part of this chapter, I cover roughly the past 150 years and directly discuss interactions between representatives of the two traditions, spirituality and psychotherapy.

ANCIENT GREECE

The earliest forms of what may be viewed as psychotherapy came in the garb of philosophy rather than that of medicine, although holistic assumptions blurred even that distinction (Boethius, 524/1927; Nicholson, 1995). Within the history that most shaped the culture within which we live, the distinction that interests us first emerged with some explicitness in classical Greece, wherein was recognized a differentiation between mythological and rationalist explanations. Although this division was not precisely parallel to the later distinction between psychotherapy and spirituality, it was founded in a similar vision that there was a basic difference between seeking help from beyond, outside the self, and insistence that the only reliance is on the human and especially the self. Dodds (1951), who commented on this dawn of rationalism and the reaction against it after 432 B.C.E., adduced as evidence for his interpretation "the increased demand for magical healing which within a generation or two transformed Asclepias from a minor hero into a major god" (p. 193).

Rather than explore diverse understandings of *mythology* and *rationalism* or the mental state of the Delphic Pythia, one gains a better sense of the concerns specific to psychotherapy and spirituality by looking to the answers offered in later Greek, Hellenistic, and Roman culture to the questions "What is 'the good life'? How is it attained and how destroyed?" Alhough answers varied, those who contemplated such queries offered at least implicit and often explicit listings of what came to be termed by both philosophers and theologians the *virtues* and *vices*: the habits of thinking and acting that make us who and what we are, some constructively, others destructively.

Zeno's philosophy of Stoicism, which is among the earliest, set the pattern. Stoicism began as a radical criticism of conventional moral attitudes, insisting that the good for humans is not to be found in the identification of happiness with worldly success. Strictly speaking, Zeno argued, only virtue and vice are good and bad: Virtue (a wholesome state of mind) is always beneficial, and vice (an unwholesome state of mind) is always harmful. Everything else is indifferent for happiness because wealth or health (for instance) can be used well or badly. Zeno and virtually all the other ancients included civic responsibility, a sense of obligation for the good order of one's society, among the most desirable good habits and practices. Beyond this quality but related to it, what were later termed *the cardinal virtues* of courage, justice, prudence, and moderation were commonly encouraged, although more consistently by the philosophers than by the devotees of the religions of the place and era (Colish, 1985; Inwood, 1985).

How were these qualities and this information conveyed? By the presentation of models who were to be (or not to be) imitated, as the writings of Plutarch, both his *Lives and Moralia* reflect (Plutarch, c. 101/1949, c. 100/1971). Moderns term this *mentoring*, a word borrowed from the name of Mentor, the trusted tutor of Telemachus, Odysseus's son, in Greek mythology. The connection with the story is even clearer if we recall how the goddess Athena took on the appearance of Mentor to offer Telemachus not only guidance but "good words of comfort and courage" (Hamilton, 1969, p. 206). Distant as this mythic episode may seem from later understandings of "the indwelling of the Spirit," the story does foreshadow what would become one interpretration, in the Christian context, of the practice of "spiritual direction," which becomes one root of what would still later be termed *psychotherapy*.

EARLY CHRISTIAN MONASTICISM

The advent of Christianity, however momentous in other ways, brought little change but considerable specification in these practices. Mentoring shifted from the political to the spiritual life, which became in the Christian vocabulary a facet of *cura animarum*—"the care of souls." Religion was enlisted in explicit support of the classic virtues, and a list of capital vices was set forth. Because distances of time and place tend to make the early Christian ascetics seem weird to modern understanding, the fountainhead role of these individuals in what will become both spirituality and psychotherapy justifies pausing to make them intelligible.

The "desert fathers" (there were also "desert mothers"; cf. Ward, 1987) took to the desert less as a form of escape from a world they deemed corrupt and corrupting than in search of a setting that would allow them to explore the nature of the human be-ing that their faith told them had been "redeemed." The desert became their laboratory for studying what it means to be human, thus merging therapeutic philosophy into a therapeutic theology. The wastelands of Egypt and the hillsides of Palestine may seem distant from our times and concerns, but these ancient teachers shaped themes that would be analyzed and reformulated through the centuries and into our own time (Brown, 1988; McGinn, 1991; Tugwell, 1986).

Three practices, each in its own way significant to later psychotherapeutic thought, characterized this early Christian pursuit of spirituality: the *imitatio* that sought personal change and growth in a process of identification with outstanding exemplars of the qualities one sought to develop, the *asceticism* that reminded of the reality of divided human nature, and the practice of *spiritual direction* that is docility before a chosen mentor.

Understanding these practices and their relationship to modern psychotherapy requires a grasp of the monastic age's understanding of the virtues and vices, the wholesome and unwholesome states of mind, the qualities deemed desirable or dangerous for living a truly human life. The philosophers had their lists and examples, as reflected in the complementary biographies presented by Plutarch, whose *Lives* affords a useful bridge to understanding the early Christian emphasis on *imitatio*: less "imitation" than an actual *putting on* of the habits, postures, and attitudes of those, preeminently Jesus of Nazareth himself, who were recognized as holy, sane, and healthy in the fullest sense that others wanted to "be like" them. Sanctity, sanity, spirituality, or serenity is that which we want when we see it—we want to "be like that" (Brown, 1987).

The Christian tradition from its beginning urged such modeling: "Learn of me, for I am meek and humble of heart" [Mt. 11:29]. The foundation of that facet of the Christian spiritual tradition that most closely resembles the later invention of psychotherapy, "spiritual direction," was laid by Anthanasius's "Life of Anthony" (List, 1930). Because spirituality is an experience, it is best studied in the lives of those who do experience it. This does not mean that "the saints" are perfect. Classic sanctity and sanity are instead rooted in awareness and conviction of one's own *imper*fection. This is, after all, the reason for spiritual direction: Because of the many weaknesses of human nature, the ease with which it can deceive itself, even someone convinced of his or her own direct contact with God must submit that claim to the scrutiny of some other (Tugwell, 1985).

All spiritualities offer both centering practices and mirroring practices. Among the former are not only prayer and meditation and chanting but also the asceticisms of self-denial, and it was on these practices that the "desert monks" concentrated. The mirroring practices of reading and telling and hearing the stories of the saints, begun by Athanasius (List, 1930), were also developed in the practice of spiritual direction, of telling some other who had the qualities one wanted of one's efforts to attain them. In such "holy conversations," we find evidence of both the didactic instruction of practical suggestions and the offering of illustrations from one's own experience, usually in service to discerning between "good spirits" and "bad spirits" in categories not too unlike many differently named modern diagnoses (McGinn, 1991; Sellner, 1983, 1990).

The idea of a personal guide or "director" meant simply someone who was already experienced in what one wished to attain, as the terms *venerable* or *elder* or *old one* convey. "Abba," in Greek *geron*, also implies a need for insight and discernment in the practice of "disclosure of thoughts" (Louf, 1982; Ware, 1986). The point here is twofold: (a) the long-standing suspicion of self-instruction in the area of spirituality (or, later, psychotherapy, Freud's self-analysis being the only accepted exception) and (b) an awareness that one can learn from another's experience as well as one's own. Basic to all civilization is the realization that each one need not learn everything for himself or herself: Each generation builds on what those who went before discovered.

Equally misunderstood by moderns is the practice of asceticism. Not only in Christianity but in all spiritualities of which there are records, asceticism is not world rejecting but is seen within the metaphor of the discipline of training for participation in competitive sport and as a practice exercise of the kind of "detachment" better captured by the German *Gelassenheit*, which carries the connotation of letting go *and* letting be.

Over time, these practices produced more. As finally codified by Evagrius Ponticus near the end of the 4th century, the early Christian anchorites developed a catalog of *logismos*. Although often confused with "the capital sins" and indeed the basis for that later listing, the term *logismos* is better translated as "bad attitudes." These were the ways of thinking, the patterns of organizing experience, the postures of being, that experience taught these men and women were the key impediments to attaining the sanctity, the wholeness, that they sought (Tugwell, 1985).

Any spirituality has, likely more explicitly than any psychotherapy, a catalog not so much of "do's and don't's" as of the *ways of thinking* that get one in trouble. A later popular vocabulary would label them *toxic*. Rational–emotive therapists name them *irrational beliefs*, and cognitive therapists term them *cognitive distortions*. But however designated within the disciplines that would help us find wholeness, all these endeavors suggest that there are virtues and vices, habits helpful to and practices harmful to one's deepest well-being. Among the "vices" listed by Evagrius were the later-named "capital sins," but it is important to note their meaning here, in the setting of their original monastic tradition. Reading Evagrius empathetically, the reader senses the presence of a wise, experienced, compassionate cognitive–behavioral therapist who also happens to be familiar with the depth psychologies.

The problem, Evagrius took care to point out, lay not in "bad thoughts" but in a process of *bad thinking* that is really *wrong vision*—seeing things from the perspective of one's fears and fantasies (*un*realities) rather than seeing things truly. *Logismos* involve *choosing* to see the bad—*bad* in the sense of "unreal," not fitting reality. *Logismos* are the archenemies of the soul, the demons from within that destroy proper perspectives on the world and thus prevent people from concentrating on the actual reality of their lives, leading them farther and farther from their actual condition, making them try to solve problems that have not yet arisen and need never arise.

Of the eight *logismos* charted by Evagrius (in Tugwell, 1985), four merit brief attention in this context. *Avarice* did not signify "materialism" as moderns think of it, "but futile planning for an unreal future" (p. 26). He defined *avarice* not as pure material greed but as the principle of thinking about what does not yet exist, a preoccupation with hopes and fears, with imaginary or future things in more modern terms, with abstract numbers rather than with empirical knowledge.

Envy stands at an opposite extreme from avarice: It involves obsession not with the future but with the past, a haunting remembrance of "the old days" as those "happy days" now gone and never to return. Evagrius expanded the Greek term *lype*, which signified distress over deprivation, to include a kind of *depression*, a cultivated sorrow. Much of the pain of spiritual suffering, he suggested, comes from wallowing in fantasies of things being other than how they are.

Anger came next, and by *anger*—not *ira* but *iracundia*—Evagrius meant not the emotion but a *clinging to* its fervor, the resentment that refuses forgiveness. As an example, he offered the experience of *obsession* with someone who has wronged us, the situation of being "unable to think of anything else" (p. 27). Such fixations can ruin our health, even—Evagrius warned—give us nightmares. As always, the trouble comes from failing to see the real issue. Anger, which is inevitable, is not to be squandered by focusing attention on the wrongs of others; rather, it should be directed at our own faults, especially at how we have wronged others, thus moving us to make amends, to right the scales of justice and so bring peace to our relationships.

After anger came the classic trap, the "noonday demon" (p. 27) *acedia*—a kind of listlessness or boredom in which nothing engages interest or appeals. The translation of *acedia* truest to Evagrius's thought is *self-pity*, a far more accurate term than *laziness* or *sloth*, for it conveys both the utter melancholy of this condition and the self-centeredness on which it is founded.

Spirituality's understanding of "sin," then, began far from that reality's modern caricatures. In fact, it much more resembles the kinds of thinking traps that many clients bring to the psychotherapist's office. And the ancient spiritual guide, like the modern psychotherapist, although not ignoring actions, saw them as being far less significant than *orientation*—the dispositions and postures, the *patterns of thinking* that bring harm.

FROM THE FALL OF ROME TO THE DAWN OF THE ENLIGHTENMENT

Much of medieval life remains veiled by ignorance and stereotypes (Cantor, 1991). High points such as the rediscovery of Greek medicine from Islamic sources and the spread of accurate anatomical knowledge in the universities, the Renaissance and the Reformation, the voyages to the Americas and trade with Asia and Africa, are less important to our story of the relationship between psychotherapy and spirituality than are echoes of the themes already seen, echoes that bridge these insights into the modern age.

From the early medieval period well into the 19th century, diverse kinds of individuals acted as local healers. The practices of medicine, spirituality, and psychology were intertwined by the naive holism of people who enjoyed firsthand familiarity with wild and domestic animals, with crops and seasons and all the vagaries of a nature they were certain was ordered despite all the chaos that confronted them. Images for the spiritual life, for human life, became standardized: the journey, warfare, a ladder (Miles, 1988). Some trends that took shape in earlier Christianity were reinforced by Islamic importations: The 14th-century "letters of spiritual guidance" by Ibn 'Abbad were popular, and the Sufi *maqam* offered a modernizing catalog of virtues on the way to becoming "stages" (Ibn 'Abbad, 1332/1986; Renard, 1996).

The late 11th and early 12th centuries saw the appearance in Spain of Jewish contributors to the ongoing story of the healing of the mind and spirit. Bahya ben Joseph ibn Pakuda (c. 1080/1996) produced one of the most popular books of Jewish spiritual literature, *Guidance to the Duties of the Heart*, which combines a traditional theology with a moderate mysticism inspired by the teachings of the Muslim Sufi mystics. This work compares the commandments of the heart—those relating to thoughts and sentiments—with the commandments of the limbs, the Mosaic commandments enjoining or prohibiting certain actions, more evidence of the perdurance in variations of the holistic understanding of human being.

For well over a thousand years, then, *cura animarum*—the care of souls—embraced the emotional, the mental, and the spiritual life of people, for rather than being differentiated, these were seen as aspects of one unified human life. However, the practitioners of the *cura animarum* were not only, and in some locations were not mainly, authorities constituted by the church. "Local healers," people who were recognized as able to heal, to make whole, flourished. Some were mountebanks and some were quacks, but far more were sincere individuals who in one way or another had learned how to tap the natural healing powers of herbs and suggestions, various forms of exercise, and persuasion (Frank, 1974). Most often, in the culture of the time, these people operated from a worldview shaped by religious imagery, sometimes but not always guided by church, synagogue, or mosque authority.

In time, both the Reformation and the witchcraft craze, and even more the economic changes connected with both, undercut such practices, and the Renaissance gave way to the Age of Enlightenment. It is worth noting, however, before leaving this 1,200-year era, that near its end Robert Burton's (1621/1989) *Anatomy of Melancholy* reproduced and reinforced Galen's distinction between "true afflictions of conscience and a melancholy that occurred when gross elements in the blood" (in Holifield, 1983, p. 61) malfunctioned, with recommendations for the treatment of both, separate, conditions.

THE ENLIGHTENMENT

Studies of art and anatomy as well as of the Islamic preservation of and additions to Aristotle's science led to the Renaissance rediscovery of the differentiation among the unity of the physical, mental, emotional, and spiritual. This and the rediscovery of classical alternatives to the Christian vision eventually led to the Reformation in religion and to the modern mode of thinking that arose in the Enlightenment era, which, for my purposes, I will date at roughly equivalent to the 18th century, more specifically from Bayle's (1697/1952) *Dictionary* to Kant's (1797/1969) *Foundations* or, in the American context, from the denouement of the Salem witch trials in 1692 to the dawning of the Second Great Awakening at Cane Ridge, Kentucky, in 1801 (H. F. May, 1976).

Enlightenment thinkers expected an Age of Reason to replace the Age of Faith, but that process proved slow and difficult, and many—from mid-19th century Romantics to late 20th-century postmodernists—questioned the expectation's validity (Berman, 1981). In an ironic twist, although its science displaced planet Earth from the center of the physical universe, Enlightenment psychology revived the Protagorean vision that placed human beings at the center of the moral universe. If this freed from faith, it did not liberate from gullibility. The twin development of science and secularization instead saw the emergence of "a company of scientific magicians who purveyed to the credulity of the eighteenth-century public" (Bromberg, 1975, p. 162). Anton Mesmer, who was, in all innocence, one of those "scientific magicians," was also a grandparent of modern psychotherapy.

The Age of the Enlightenment was also the age of magnetism and electricity, and the concept of "force" began what becomes a regular appearance in discussions of psychotherapy, witness to a tacit assumption that some kind of superior force is required to overcome mental symptoms. Mesmer's "animal magnetism" fit well into the aspirations of the era (Fuller, 1982). Solving a spiritual problem through science was "quintessentially Victorian," and mesmerism, especially as imported to the United States after his death, became "simply the first in a long line of attempts to heal the psychological problems, spiritual hunger, and moral confusion of the American unchurched" (Cushman, 1992, p. 31).

The Romantic reaction against Enlightenment assumptions offered few real alternatives in the area of mental healing. In the United States, Emersonian transcendentalism, the Fox sisters' spiritualism, the Oneida and other perfectionists, each demonstrated anew the quick path from mysticism to obscurantism, from a dollop of scientific insight to a flood of quack exploitation. Within professional medicine, George Miller Beard's neurasthenia and S. Weir Mitchell's rest cure reflected the gender assumptions of a population recently riven by a civil war that had slain or maimed so many of its young men just as a modern economy unfolded under the pressures of immigration, industrialization, and urbanization. Psychotherapy, as we know it, came to being in a world of confusing tumult—a world convinced, with more validity than are some other ages, that it was undergoing change at an unprecedented rate (Douglas, 1977; Meyer, 1965/1980).

THE UNITED STATES IN THE 19TH CENTURY

Mesmerism was brought to the United States by Charles Poyen in 1836. Its major underlying tenet, the same as that of all the embryonic psychotherapies of the time, "was a belief in the accessibility and availability of the realm of the spirit in a nontraditional and experiential setting" (Cushman, 1992, p. 31). Although left undefined, "spirit" tended to feature "a secular universalism and a valorization of self-expression that was rooted in the larger Romantic and Counter-Enlightenment movements in Europe" (ibid.; Fuller, 1982).

There were differences in the American context, however, as subsequent history makes clear. Although pristine Puritanism soon deceased, the evangelical impulse of the two Great Awakenings of the 1740s and the 1800s pulsed through American society throughout the 19th century and beyond (McLoughlin, 1978). In the United States more than in the northern Europe, from which newly professionalizing Americans drew their modern identity, "the care and cure of souls" was a pastoral function, in colleges as well as in churches and congregations. Yet, already, before the advent of psychotherapy, a process of change was under way (Bledstein, 1976).

As summarized by Holifield (1983), what unfolded was a

> story of changing attitudes toward the "self" [that] proceeds from an ideal of self-denial to one of self-love, from self-love to self-culture, for self-culture to self-mastery, for self-mastery to self-realization within a trustworthy culture, and finally to a later form of self-realization counterposed against cultural mores and social institutions. (p. 12)

The story emerged in stages, and any understanding of the healing of "self" that is personality change and how this process came to be understood in American culture must begin here in the early 19th century, with Charles Grandison Finney and Horace Bushnell. Although carried on in theological terms, their differing visions encapsulate much later dialogue between psychotherapy and spirituality.

"The outstanding revivalist in America for almost half a century," Finney propounded "New Measures" in his classic *Revivals of Religion*, especially his lecture, "How to Promote a Revival" (Finney, 1835/1962; McLoughlin, 1968). Underlying Finney's vision was the Jacksonian Age's go-getting answer to the classic theological quandary over the relationship between divine sovereignty and human free will. The Great Awakening of the 1740s had shown that revivals, although the work of God, could be "called down." Those revivals, however, although sparked into flame by a traveling evangelist such as George Whitfield, were likely to catch fire only in tinder long prepared by the regular exertions of a believing parish minister and his flock (Heimert, 1966).

Finney's conversions were "called down" differently. The gathering of strangers into groups far larger than any parish, the preparatory admonitions, the recital of vivid testimonies, the anxious bench for those wavering, the reaction to those first "struck down" by the Spirit: Assuming that people wanted to change, no more effective means of convincing them that they have been changed has yet been devised. Finney's ideas did not arise out of vacuum. Early 19th-century theology, which was, for all purposes, a practical psychology, followed the science of the time in abounding in "schemes of classification" and particularly in efforts to "classify the stages in the order of salvation" (Holifield, 1983, p. 127; Rosenberg, 1976).

There are different kinds of "stages," however. Horace Bushnell, pastor of the well-to-do North Congregational Church of Hartford, Connecticut, from 1833 to 1876, believed "Growth, not Conquest, the True Method of Christian Progress," as he titled an 1844 essay. Two years later he began his "Discourse on Christian Nurture," in which he suggested that rather than expecting some dramatic conversion experience, a child of Christian parents should grow up not knowing himself or herself as other than Christian. Education, not conversion, according to Bushnell, was the normal way of attaining change and wholeness (Bushnell, 1861/1916; McLoughlin, 1968; Smith, 1965).

We are still some way from today's "psychotherapy" and "spirituality." Yet, if what has been characterized as the mid-19th-century "spiritual emptiness, moral confusion, and a yearning for intense experience" issued in "a new type of religious or spiritual practice," then that "institution of popular, unchurched religious psychology" remains with us (Cushman, 1990; Fuller, 1989). Some may think its expressions confined to TV preachers or the "self-help" sections of bookstores, but elements of this approach may also be found in many therapeutic and more traditional religious settings. Unsurprisingly, those who ignore this possibility seem to become the most inextricably entangled in it (MacIntyre, 1981; Mercadante, 1996; Meyer, 1965/1980).

This presents a difficulty for any effort to be judicious. The story of the relationship between psychotherapy and spirituality may easily be viewed as either tragedy or comedy, and it cannot be told without seeming the one or the other. For rarely in American history have psychotherapy and spirituality, in their interaction, been represented by the best in either's tradition or expression. No doubt due in part to the democratic style of American society, a kind of cultural Gresham's law dictates that debased popularizations override careful analyses, with the result that both psychotherapy and spirituality know each other mainly by caricature. Although we are interested in neither tent-revival jerkings nor phrenology's racism, neither the panentheism of imported gurus nor the victimology of pop-media psychology, it is within the echoes of these excesses that we find the real story of psychotherapy and spirituality in the United States, and so I ask readers of both camps to be patient with the elements of caricature that necessarily intrude into what follows.

For "the institution of popular, unchurched religious psychology" did not stop with spiritualism and mesmerism. The line of faith healers and mind cures that runs from hypnotism and spiritualistic seances through New Thought, the theosophy of Madame Blavatsky, and the Unity School of Lee's Summit, Missouri, reached a temporary culmination in Mary Baker Eddy and Christian Science (Braden, 1963). The mind-cure approach at that point diverged into two streams: those who clung to spirituality as their chief therapeutic tool (New Thought, etc.) and those who sought to bond with the newly emerging medical science that was studying personality dissociation as a phenomenon indicative of the subconscious mind (Emmanuel movement). Those engaged in these endeavors contested whether faith cures and moral therapeutics of neurotics were the same or to be distinguished, but meanwhile, "both disciplines taught methods for attaining serenity and peace of mind; both charged themselves with the task of resolving basic concepts of psychotherapy with correlative ones from Christian and Jewish doctrine" (Bromberg, 1975, p. 176; Meyer, 1965/1980).

But the story is even more complex, for the Emmanuel movement, one grandparent of the self-help mutual-aid movement pioneered by Alcoholics Anonymous, had solid ties with the medical establishments of Boston and Harvard. Emmanuel has been styled "the first serious effort to transform the cure of souls in light of the new psychology," the core expression of "theology becomes therapy," but its form was uniquely shaped by the medical context of the turn-of-the-century northeastern United States (Holifield, 1983, p. 201).

In late 19th-century Europe, Kraft-Ebbing, Nordau, and Lombroso were setting forth ominous visions of human nature—of a dangerous self, sexual and aggressive. Although Americans still relied on George Miller

Beard and S. Weir Mitchell, whose moral exhortation became the backbone of the first generation of explicitly medical and psychological rather than religious advice manuals, Sigmund Freud began by the end of the century to dominate the European scene (Cushman, 1992; Hale, 1971a). From the perspective of the history of understandings of the meaning of "human," Freud did not so much offer a new departure as he reflected a classical reaction against Romantic, 19th-century optimism. Despite his animus against all forms of religious belief, Freud's recognition and embrace of "human doubleness" fit well with classic spiritual insight. Similarly, "the discovery of the unconscious," if stripped of the hermeneutics of suspicion, cohered well albeit in different imagery with the *logismos* of the 4th-century desert monks as well as with traditional understandings of "demons" and even "original sin" (Balint, 1968; Dodds, 1951; Rieff, 1966). Carl Jung, enamored of a still more different imagery involving archetypes, would achieve that stripping, but his apparent identification of the unconscious with the divine presented a different pile of problems that, ironically, opened the door of the modern imagination to even greater romanticisms (Greenwood, 1990; Noll, 1995; Rieff, 1966; Satinover, 1994).

THE UNITED STATES IN THE 20TH CENTURY

In the United States, however, and especially in the neighborhood of Boston, the advent and popularity of Christian Science challenged and even frightened the medical profession, which found itself—in this era before Abraham Flexner—losing patients to a methodology that some found as effective while less painful and costly. This context lay behind the extension of the work with groups begun by Joseph Hershey Pratt for patients with TB in 1905 to other homebound chronic sufferers, a project furthered by Richard Cabot and others of almost-as-awesome name at Massachusetts General Hospital. In the same year, two ministers at Boston's Emmanuel Church, Samuel McComb and Ellwood Worcester, who had been trained in the Leipzig laboratories of Gustav Fechner, began a clinic in which they sought to blend pastoral counseling with the latest medical and psychological knowledge and techniques. Soon, not only Pratt and Cabot but also psychiatrists Isador H. Coriat and James Jackson Putnam were cooperating with the Emmanuel Mission (Hale, 1971a; Holifield, 1983; McCarthy, 1984).

That cooperation began to sour in 1908 and was terminated in 1909, the year Sigmund Freud visited the United States to speak at Clark University. Freud's ideas were embraced with enthusiasm by a psychiatric profession uncertain of its identity at the dawn of its own professionalization. The acceptance of Freud, as the writings of Putnam make clear, was aided in no small degree by the threat posed by Christian Science and the frustration of the Bostonians' experience with the Emmanuel Mission (Hale, 1971a, 1971b).

There was yet another ingredient in this early 20th-century mix out of which psychotherapy as we know it developed. The mental hygiene movement—"the watershed of mental healing"—took life from Clifford Beers's 1908 autobiography, *The Mind That Found Itself*, a book that led noted psychiatrist Adolf Meyer to comment that "it looks at last as if we have what we need . . . a man for a cause" (Bromberg, 1975, p. 211; Beers, 1908; Dain, 1980).

Preparing the way for all this and at times assisting it along was the psychology of William James, a Harvard professor who deeply respected the experience of "ordinary people," as his classic *Talks to Teachers* (James, 1899/1958a) brilliantly attests. Philosopher as well as psychologist, James blended laboratory findings with common sense. His reliance on introspection and his respect for diverse and at times questionable manifestations of "the spiritual" rendered William James for many decades an unlikely avatar of "psychologist." James's clear identification with "the sick soul" and lightly veiled autobiographical references may indeed make him seem a forerunner of late 20th-century popular psychologies, as Donald Meyer accused, or even the protoprogenitor of what has been termed *recovery porn* (Kurtz, 1996; Meyer, 1965/1980). There was, however, more to the William James whose courage Freud admired and confessed to envying. James was a philosopher of the spirit attempting to revivify the classic virtues, not a panderer of therapies attempting to lure the masses into buying his books (Barzun, 1983; Browning, 1980; Zaleski, 1993–1994).

The rediscovery by Pratt and Worcester and others of the power of groups as settings wherein individuals may in some way be "made whole" fit well with the insights of the Progressive era of the first 19 years of the American 20th century. However, it also reflected the religiospiritual focus on "gathered community" that has found so many expressions throughout history, from "chosen people," to *ecclesia*, to the development of cenobitic monasteries out of the desert anchorite experience, to the construction of the "city on a hill" that John Winthrop understood the Puritan adventure of colonizing New England to be, to the utopian communities and later communes that continually pop up on the American scene, although not in the decade of the 1920s. For both spirituality and psychotherapy followed the larger culture in losing sight of that communitarian vision in the decade that followed the blunting of Progressive insight in the aftermath of World War I.

THE 1920s TO THE 1950s

In the 1920s, according to the familiar stereotype, the inhabitants of the United States passed through a prolonged adolescence, testing newly found freedoms in a context of mood swings that ranged from carefree exuberance to disillusioned cynicism, but virtually always styled with self-conscious posturing (Leuchtenburg, 1958). Although a victorious power that had made the world "safe for democracy," America became isolationist, as signaled by the halt of immigration by the Johnson acts of 1921 and 1924. A buoyant consumer economy was maintained, for a time, by the continuing move from farms to cities and the new availability of consumer credit with which to purchase new "consumer durables" such as automobiles, refrigerators, radios, and more that poured off factory assembly lines untroubled by a labor movement effectively squelched in the postwar "Red scare" (Bernstein, 1966).

As false for most Americans as were the stereotypes of Jazz Age flappers and wide stock ownership, that broader population also changed during this decade, largely as a result of the relentless drumbeat of new advertising techniques pioneered by Edward Bernays, who rarely let clients forget that he was a nephew of Sigmund Freud. If the elite embraced Freudian psychoanalysis or their understanding of it, which emphasized the evil of repression and the power of sex, the greater part of the population became laboratory specimens for the behaviorist manipulations of followers of John Broadus Watson (Baritz, 1960; Lears, 1994; Susman, 1984). To critics such as T. S. Eliot, what united both apparently contradictory psychologies—psychoanalysis and behaviorism—was their demeaning of human freedom and thus of human beings (Eliot, 1943). In a decade when eugenic thought was chic as well as prevalent and the concept of "lesser races" undergirded immigration "reform," few noticed that demeaning, except for the Blacks and Catholics and Jews thrust into that category, all of whom also just happened to adhere to religious visions that rejected such ideologies (Broderick, 1963; Cone, 1984; Frazier, 1964; Rosenberg, 1976).

The self-conscious adulthood of 1920s adolescence also embraced disillusionment, often without much analysis of whether what was rejected was really illusion. Under the impact of the birth of Fundamentalist religion with the publication of *The Fundamentals* between 1905 and 1910, the Protestant churches, the usual vehicles of spirituality in the United States up to that time, became mired in the politics of "the Fundamentalist controversy" and increasingly irrelevant for a significant part of the American people (Furniss, 1954). The works of psychologist James Henry Leuba and others, meanwhile, more and more seemed less to explain religion than to explain religion away (Wulff, 1991, pp. 47ff).

More significantly for the relationship between psychotherapy and spirituality, the 1920s gave a twist to the Progressive Age's faith in experts, who seemed to many to progressively become more dictators than helpers (Bledstein, 1976; Lubove, 1965). As cultural historian Christopher Lasch has detailed, the extension of psychology's focus from child guidance to child rearing devalued immigrant religious traditions and shifted the prestige of expert authority from the extended family to professionals, a doctrine assiduously spread through the public school system (Lasch, 1977). The mental hygiene movement, in summary, "applied the bourgeois values of quantification, objectification, and cleanliness to the realm of emotional and psychological complaints" (Cushman, 1995, p. 152).

The popular psychologies of the decade were hardly better. Followers of Dubois and Coué pursued their goals, convinced of the power of implanted ideas over the will (Coué, 1922). A decade supposedly ruled over by the contradictory insights of Watson's behaviorism and Freud's psychoanalysis actually found most citizens completing a change begun in the 1890s: From a valuing of *character*, the focus shifted to *personality* and eventually to the enthronement of celebrity personalities whose ability to sell products made them more and more a dominant force in American society (Lears, 1994; Susman, 1984).

And what of spirituality? In the seminaries, the influence of John Dewey (1916), especially his *Democracy and Education*, shaped the nascent pastoral care movement. In the same period, clergyman Anton Boisen, supported by the enduring *noblesse oblige* of the Harvard hospitals' Richard Cabot, began training seminary students at Worcester State Hospital, a program that would evolve into clinical-pastoral training (Boisen, 1936/1971; Holifield, 1983, pp. 222–229).

This impetus to the merging of psychotherapy and spirituality was blunted if not broken by the Great Depression that followed the Great Crash of October 1929, bringing to America the vision of human finitude that had dawned on Europe in August 1914 (Barrett, 1958). The Depression of the 1930s dampened the ardor of most clergy and "applied psychologists," but the more extreme religiophilosophical movement rolled on. Divine Science, Universal Science, Life Science, Jewish Science, and later Scientology, served thousands (Braden, 1963; Bromberg, 1975, p. 179).

But more was going on. In 1932, the same year his brother Reinhold published *Moral Man and Immoral Society*, Yale's Helmut Richard Niebuhr translated Paul Tillich's *The Religious Situation*, which argued that genuine religion was antithetical to the illusion that cultural values, even those of human health and well-being, were the values of God (Niebuhr, 1932; Tillich, 1932/1956). Some psychotherapists took to heart the insights of these "crisis theologians." Rollo May's 1939 *The Art of Counseling*, for example, presented human beings as "finite, imperfect, and limited," their consequent insecurity driving them to prideful self-will. May expressed wariness of optimism about "growth" and its attendant assumptions that more enlightenment, education, and ethics could transform the personality. Reflecting the formulations of neo-orthodox thinkers, he suggested that human life was marked by an unending conflict between freedom and determination (R. May, 1939).

However, the twin victories over the Depression and the Axis powers soon restored confidence in experts and heightened reliance on professionals. Still, there were doubters, and psychological and theological thinkers alike wrestled with the realities of the roles taken by Europe's most "civilized" peoples in the extermination camps of the Holocaust (Litton, 1986).

THE POST–WORLD WAR II SCENE

Chastened by the Holocaust and the realities of nuclear power in an era of cold war, a variant of existentialist insight emerged in the psychotherapeutic thought of the postwar period, a variant that blended psychotherapeutic and spiritual insight in ways not seen before. Set forth most explicitly by concentration camp survivors such as Viktor Frankl, this understanding of the human condition and its emotional disturbances cohered well with the neo-orthodox theology that had emerged in the 1930s, and it gained slow adherence in the 1950s when it was overtaken by the "peace of mind, heart, and soul" of popularizers Norman Vincent Peale, Fulton J. Sheen, and Joshua Loth Liebman, in what became the customary Herbergian *Protestant, Catholic, Jew* formulation (Frankl, 1955, 1959; Herberg, 1955; Liebman, 1946; Peale, 1948, 1952; Sheen, 1949). In some ways the Eisenhower decade of the 1950s marked both the high and low points of American religious spirituality, as evidenced less in the addition of "under God" to the Pledge of Allegiance or of "In God We Trust" (with large unconscious irony) to American coinage, than by President Dwight David Eisenhower's heartfelt affirmation that "Our government makes no sense unless it is founded in a deeply felt religious faith *and I don't care what it is*" (quoted, and emphasis added by, Herberg, 1955, p. 84, citing the *New York Times* of December 23, 1952).

At various times in this era, a "third psychiatric revolution" was proclaimed. The term signified for some the revolt of psychologists against the medical model, the new emphasis on "a full life" issuing in new schools of psychotherapy that had a somewhat sociological flavor (Bromberg, 1975, p. 276). Others used the phrase to denote a restoration of religious insight to psychotherapy (Stern, 1954) or the growth of a spiritually based group therapy (Mowrer, 1964a, 1964b). Perhaps most significant in the late 1950s, however, was theologian Wayne Oates's critique of the positive thinkers for treating personality as a reflex mechanism subject to prudential ethics and wishful voluntarism. Such an approach, Oates (1955, 1957) observed, ignored the self's internal contradictions, overlooked the necessity for people to accept their limitations, and presented religion merely as a crutch to be used for narrowly personal benefits.

The decade of the 1960s, with its assassinations, flower children, and anti-Vietnam war agitation, marked the beginning of a kind of confluence between psychotherapy and spirituality. In the wake of such as Peale and Blanton and the "peace movement" of Liebman and Sheen, an American psychotherapy derived from Karen Horney and Harry Stack Sullivan and an "ego psychology" largely imported from Britain seemed to open new possibilities (Guntrip, 1973; Horney, 1950; Sullivan, 1947/1953). Finding both classic spirituality and classic Freudian insight "too dark and gloomy," sufferers and therapists and spiritual guides united in rediscovering the "goodness" of the self. Classic thought, whether Freudian, Christian, or Jewish, had a deep awareness of the human potential for evil, a reality increasingly ignored by 1960s and later psychotherapeutic thought, both popular and academic. Both Freud and the classic psychologies as well as the classic spiritualities, that is to say, remained profoundly aware of human duality, a vision lost or obscured by emergent expressions of psychotherapy and spirituality less rooted in history than in the day's tie-dyed T-shirt, inspirational poster, and smiley-button markets. (Wulff, 1996, pp. 55ff, offered a useful summary from the viewpoint of psychology.)

Meanwhile, from the National Training Laboratory for Group Development emerged the "encounter" and "growth" movements, "T-groups," "sensitivity training," and a humanistic psychology that, although in some ways "spiritual," soon became virtually indistinguishable from the utopianisms that had flourished with similar brevity in earlier ages. The "human potential movement" offered a therapeutic ethic that insisted on the distinction between the conventional public self and the true inner self. Such a distinction found expression in a persistent tendency to exalt the values of "honest" self-expression and a communal intimacy that furthered the ongoing repeal of reticence. The decade saw a by-now familiar litany of honorific words became part of the popular vocabulary of what might still be loosely called *virtue*: openness, honesty, tolerance, sensitivity, and self-realization (Bromberg, 1975; Gurstein, 1996; Holifield, 1983, p. 310).

The psychoanalysis of Carl Jung, meanwhile, emphasized the "process of individuation" and recognized that religious ideas had a place in psychotherapy. Many spiritually inclined individuals found help in Jungian insight; many others found Jungian quasi-theism less mystical than obscurantist. Similar difficulties confronted those who turned to Asian spiritualities. In contrast to the rational psychotherapy of the Western world, which seeks causes and attempts adjustment to the social environment, and in contrast to the traditional spiritualities of the Western world, which glory in the goodness of creation, Eastern philosophies are therapeutic in that insight into the essential emptiness of the universe leads to freedom from desire, misery, and anxiety (Bromberg, 1975, pp. 334ff). Such approaches have always appealed to some; they rarely are embraced by many.

For those concerned about spirituality, the emphasis on *self-realization* and its synonyms soon lay bare the problems of the flirtation of the spirituality of the pastoral theology movement with psychotherapy. Following the lead of the neo-Freudians, many theologians adopted an ethic of self-realization that defined "growth" as the primary ethical good, a vision directly contrary to much spiritual insight. Then the oil-price shocks of the later 1970s and increasing concern about ecology began to call into question such assumptions (Page, 1996; Schumacher, 1973).

The following memorable scene described by Holifield (1983, p. 332) captures the divide that existed between spirituality and psychotherapy in this era. Theologian Paul Tillich's final public appearance was a dialogue with psychologist Carl Rogers. The two disagreed about the ambiguity of human nature. Rogers believed that "estrangement" was imposed by cultural institutions. Tillich held that it was a tragic and inevitable component in any process of maturation. Rogers argued that for the modern world, God was dead, and he wondered why Tillich continued to use a religious vocabulary. Tillich insisted that scientific language is always limited in scope and that only the language of religious symbol and myth could point beyond itself to the unconditioned ground of all existence (Holifield, 1983; Tillich, 1952).

More was going on even at the time, however. The late 1950s saw the beginnings of a psychotherapeutic revolt against the medical model (Bromberg, 1975, p. 276). O. Hobart Mowrer denounced "acceptance" as "cheap grace," and the later 1960s saw a movement by the explicitly spiritually rooted away from what came increasingly to be regarded as a psychological approach criticized by Holifield (1983) as "a sterile and introverted Narcissism of I for Me by Myself" (p. 320). Without abandoning the ideal of acceptance, some pastoral writers began to talk about the importance of "confronting" people with the need to face and change their destructive patterns of living. Two decades later, this approach encountered its own limits when the overextension of the Twelve Step program pioneered by Alcoholics Anonymous became ensnared with an ever-broadening concept of "addiction" (Bregman, 1996; Kurtz, 1996; G. G. May, 1988; Mercadante, 1996).

THE CURRENT SCENE ON THE EVE OF THE MILLENNIUM

Other essays in this book detail the current scene. I hope to tie together the broad story limned above by concluding with a few observations suggested by study of the history of the relationship between psychotherapy and spirituality. From Hans Selye on stress in the 1950s, through 1960s' transcendental meditation and "the relaxation response" as presented by Herbert Benson in the 1970s and after, through the efforts to harness ecstasy by Richard Bucke, Edgar Cayce, Carlos Casteneda, Alan Watts, and Timothy Leary; to the popularizations of Larry Dossey, Depak Chopra, Joan Boryshenko, and Caroline Myss, as well as renewed interest in American

Indian spiritual healing practices, the continuing assumption of an inter-face connecting physical medicine as well as psychotherapy with spirituality leads some to see dawning a new and promising rapprochement among them (Siegmund, 1965). This vision was furthered financially by Sir John Templeton, whose munificence in awarding prizes and sponsoring publications and conferences on the topic helps the willingness of students to immerse themselves in this still academically unpromising area.

The federal Office of Alternative Medicine meanwhile scandalizes some even as it brings hope to others. Modern scientific medicine—and psychotherapy claims to be scientific even if not strictly medical—was born out of the rejection of what Ahlstrom (1975) termed *harmonial religion*, a view of the world "in which spiritual composure, physical health, and even economic well-being are understood to flow from a person's rapport with the cosmos" (p. 528). Is such harmonialism a necessary sequella of holistic vision? Someday, perhaps, efforts to prove the existence of God will have a *DSM* diagnostic category—which will likely suit the age's saints just fine: Mystical and spiritual experience exists in a different category than "proof." Still, some will always be intrigued by attempts to demonstrate the material effects of some spiritual cause. Given that most individuals intuit in them-selves some unity of the physical, mental, emotional, and spiritual, there is always hope that people can know more about those aspects and their relationship, especially in themselves.

Others will no doubt continue to resist such trends, seeing them as just another in the long parade of the spiritually deprived attempting to fashion in their own image a "God of the gaps." More impressed by the mystical tradition than by rational psychologies, these rejoice in an ecu-menism that makes it possible for those rooted in varying religious traditions to draw on the spirituality of each other. In part inspired by Jungian insight and its Campbellian popularization, others incorporate in-sights from East Asian religions into current mental healing techniques (Bromberg, 1975, pp. 334ff.; Campbell, 1988). At least since the 1960s also, "new religions" have converged on the idea of altering human con-sciousness. "Altering human consciousness" can, of course, be attempted with or without chemical assistance (Bromberg, 1975, p. 336; Clark, 1969; James, 1902/1958b). However, as Martin Marty observed, "Wheresoever two or three yoga or Zen students gathered, conversation almost never had to do with intellectual constructs but with liberation from them" (Marty, 1989, p. 142).

For those who primarily observe, thus falling under harsh strictures from many representatives of both psychotherapy and spirituality, the main question today is "*Which* psychology, *which* spirituality?" Large differences remain unresolved in understandings of the relationships between asceti-cism and repression, a problem hardly solved by the careless calling of medieval saints "anorexic" or the lazy labeling of monasticisms as vehicles for escape (Wulff, 1991).

Another area of divergence between at least some forms of psychotherapy and spirituality involves discretion, reticence, and privacy. The psychotherapeutic mind-set, rejecting "repression," tends to favor the free expression of thoughts and feelings (Bromberg, 1975, pp. 270ff). At first, this applied only or mainly in the therapeutic setting, but popularization of these ideas has extended the practice variously named "letting it all hang out" and "honest sharing" to all areas of life and experience. Spirituality, because its concern is a different kind of human vulnerability, in general retains a mistrust of sheer spontaneity not because it is "evil" or to be "repressed" but out of a hesitancy to intrude on others, a concern lest the destruction of privacy and the devaluing of the sense of shame issue in the progressive loss of those traits and characteristics that are precisely the most human as well as the most humane (Gurstein, 1996).

Related to this divergence is a different emphasis on the relationship of "rights" to "responsibilities" and the ways of thinking about the wrongs done to one. Influenced by contemporary legalism, psychotherapy tends to present its insights in terms of "rights" and "empowerment." Spirituality has always been more aware of *responsibilities*. Not unrelatedly, the psychotherapeutic approach, especially in its more popular manifestations, attends to how one has been wronged. Although the term *victim* may be eschewed, discovering experiences of victimization seems to be what much contemporary psychotherapy is all about. The classic tradition of spirituality, although it does not advise ignoring injuries received, suggests that these be viewed in the context of the injuries one has inflicted on others. "Self-esteem" seems to be the highest goal of many psychotherapies; spiritualities usually present "self-centeredness" as the bane of spiritual existence. Those two visions are compatible, but often those promoting one or the other seem to ignore that reality (Adelson, 1996; Glendon, 1991).

And so I conclude with more questions than answers. Can the classic virtues and vices retain any meaning in a culture that worships "the market" as God, a system that defines greed and envy as economic necessities? Spirituality in all its forms has always begun by urging renunciation. Can psychotherapy, which is essentially the tool of any culture it serves, share that vision (Cushman, 1992, 1995)? Both psychotherapy and spirituality have to do with the acceptance of realistic limits. But what of the unbridled valuing of human control, a linchpin of psychotherapy, as opposed to spirituality's concern to preserve the sense of awe in the presence of mystery and an awareness of the strengths tapped by an admission of powerlessness? The first prayer, like the first call to a therapist, is a cry for help. But what comes next, if these two view helplessness differently (Tiebout, 1949)?

The critiques of psychotherapy offered by such as Rieff (1959, 1966), Laing (1965, 1971; Collier, 1977), Szasz (1973, 1976), and Cushman

(1990, 1992, 1995) stand irritatingly unanswered. The critiques of spirituality offered by serious thinkers who have the misfortune to wander into the "self-help and psychology" section of any large bookstore grow increasingly strident. Where do we go from here? I have not the foggiest idea: Historians are not prophets. However, I offer this chapter in the hope that the frame it provides may assist the other chapters in this book to further meaningful movement in something approximating a direction that will contribute to the sanity of humankind.

REFERENCES

Adelson, J. (1996). Down with self-esteem. *Commentary, 101,* 34–38.

Ahlstrom, S. E. (1975). *A religious history of the American people* (Vol. 2). Garden City, NY: Doubleday.

Bahya ben Joseph ibn Pakuda. (1996). *The duties of the heart.* Northvale, NJ: Jason Aronson. (Original work published circa 1080)

Balint, M. (1968). *The basic fault: Therapeutic aspects of regression.* New York: Brunner/Mazel.

Barbour, I. G. (1966). *Issues in science and religion.* Englewood Cliffs, NJ: Prentice Hall.

Baritz, L. (1960). *The servants of power.* Middletown, CT: Wesleyan University Press.

Barrett, W. (1958). *Irrational man: A study in existential philosophy.* New York: Doubleday.

Barzun, J. (1983). *A stroll with William James.* New York: Harper & Row.

Bayle, P. (1952). *Selections for Bayle's Dictionary.* Princeton, NJ: Princeton University Press. (Original work published 1697)

Beers, C. W. (1908). *A mind that found itself.* New York: Longmans, Green.

Berman, M. (1981). *The re-enchantment of the world.* Ithaca, NY: Cornell University Press.

Bernstein, I. (1966). *The lean years.* Baltimore: Penguin Books.

Bledstein, B. J. (1976). *The culture of professionalism.* New York: Norton.

Boethius. (1927). *De consolatione philosophiae.* London: Oxford University Press. (Original work published 524)

Boisen, A. T. (1971). *The exploration of the inner world: A study of mental disorder and religious experience.* Philadelphia: University of Pennsylvania Press. (Original work published 1936)

Braden, C. S. (1963). *Spirits in rebellion.* Dallas, TX: Southern Methodist University Press.

Bregman, L. (1996). Psychotherapies. In P. H. Van Ness (Ed.), *Spirituality and the secular quest* (Vol. 22, pp. 251–276). New York: Crossroad Herder.

Broderick, F. L. (1963). *Right reverend new dealer, John A. Ryan*. New York: Macmillan.

Bromberg, W. (1975). *From shaman to psychotherapist*. Chicago: Regnery.

Brown, P. (1987). The saint as exemplar in late antiquity. In J. S. Hawley (Ed.), *Saints and virtues* (pp. 3–14). Berkeley: University of California Press.

Brown, P. (1988). *The body and society*. New York: Columbia University Press.

Browning, D. S. (1980). *Pluralism and personality: William James and some contemporary cultures of psychology*. Lewisburg, PA: Bucknell University Press.

Burton, R. (1989). *The anatomy of melancholy* . New York: Oxford University Press. (Original work published 1621)

Bushnell, H. (1916). *Christian nurture*. New Haven, CT: Yale University Press. (Original work published 1861)

Campbell, J. (1988). *The power of myth*. New York: Doubleday.

Cantor, N. F. (1991). *Inventing the Middle Ages*. New York: Morrow.

Capps, D. (1993). *The depleted self: Sin in a narcissistic age*. Minneapolis, MN: Fortress Press.

Clark, W. H. (1969). *Chemical ecstasy*. New York: Sheed & Ward.

Colish, M. L. (1985). *The Stoic tradition from antiquity to the early Middle Ages*. Leiden, The Netherlands: Brill.

Collier, A. (1977). *R. D. Laing: The philosophy and politics of psychotherapy*. New York: Pantheon Books.

Cone, J. H. (1984). *For my people: Black theology and the Black church*. Maryknoll, NY: Orbis Books.

Coué, E. (1922). *Self mastery through conscious autosuggestion*. New York: American Library Service.

Cushman, P. (1990). Why the self is empty: Toward a historically situated psychology. *American Psychologist, 45,* 599–611.

Cushman, P. (1992). Psychotherapy to 1992: A historically situated interpretation. In D. K. Freedheim (Ed.), *History of psychotherapy: A century of change* (pp. 21–64). Washington, DC: American Psychological Association.

Cushman, P. (1995). *Constructing the self, constructing America: A cultural history of psychotherapy*. Reading, MA: Addison-Wesley.

Dain, N. (1980). *Clifford W. Beers: Advocate for the insane*. Pittsburgh, PA: University of Pittsburgh.

Dewey, J. (1916). *Democracy and education*. New York: Macmillan.

Dodds, E. R. (1951). *The Greeks and the irrational*. Berkeley: University of California Press.

Douglas, A. (1977). *The feminization of American culture*. New York: Knopf.

Edwards, J. (1960). *The nature of true virtue*. Ann Arbor: University of Michigan Press. (Original work published 1755)

Eliot, T. S. (1943). *Four quartets*. New York: Harcourt, Brace.

Finney, C. G. (1962). *Revivals of religion*. Chicago: Moody Press. (Original work published 1835)

Frank, J. D. (1974). *Persuasion and healing*. New York: Schocken Books.

Frankl, V. E. (1955). *The doctor and the soul: An introduction to logotherapy*. New York: Knopf.

Frankl, V. E. (1959). *From death camp to existentialism*. Boston: Beacon Press.

Frazier, E. F. (1964). *The Negro church in America*. New York: Schocken Books.

Freedheim, D. K. (1992). Preface. In D. K. Freedheim (Ed.), *History of psychotherapy: A century of change* (pp. xxvii–xxi). Washington, DC: American Psychological Association.

Fuller, R. C. (1982). *Mesmerism and the American cure of souls*. Philadelphia: University of Pennsylvania Press.

Fuller, R. C. (1989). *Alternative medicine and American religious life*. New York: Oxford University Press.

Furniss, N. F. (1954). *The fundamentalist controversy, 1918–1931*. New Haven, CT: Yale University Press.

Glendon, M. A. (1991). *Rights talk*. New York: Free Press.

Greenwood, S. F. (1990). Emile Durkheim and C. G. Jung: Structuring a transpersonal sociology of religion. *Journal for the Scientific Study of Religion, 29*, 482–495.

Guntrip, H. (1973). *Psychoanalytic theory, therapy, and the self*. New York: Basic Books.

Gurstein, R. (1996). *The repeal of reticence*. New York: Hill & Wang.

Hale, N. G., Jr. (1971a). *Freud and the Americans*. New York: Oxford University Press.

Hale, N. G., Jr. (1971b). *James Jackson Putnam and psychoanalysis*. Cambridge, MA: Harvard University Press.

Hamilton, E. (1969). *Mythology*. New York: New American Library.

Heimert, A. (1966). *Religion and the American mind*. Cambridge, MA: Harvard University Press.

Herberg, W. (1955). *Protestant, Catholic, Jew*. Garden City, NY: Doubleday.

Holifield, E. B. (1983). *A history of pastoral care in America*. Nashville, TN: Abingdon Press.

Horney, K. (1950). *Neurosis and human growth*. New York: Norton.

Ibn 'Abbad Muhammad ibn Ibrahim. (1986). *Letters on the Sufi path*. New York: Paulist Press. (Original work published 1332)

Inwood, B. (1985). *Ethics and human action in early Stoicism*. New York: Oxford University Press.

James, W. (1958a). *Talks to teachers*. New York: Norton. (Original work published 1899)

James, W. (1958b). *The varieties of religious experience*. New York: Norton. (Original work published 1902)

Kant, I. (1969). *Foundations of the metaphysics of morals*. Indianapolis, IN: Bobbs–Merill. (Original work published 1797)

Kinerk, E. (1981). Toward a method for the study of spirituality. *Review for Religious, 40*, 3–19.

Kurtz, E. (1996). Twelve-Step programs. In Peter H. VanNess (Ed.), *Spirituality and the secular quest* (pp. 277–302). New York: Crossroad Herder.

Laing, R. D. (1965). *The divided self*. Baltimore: Pelican.

Laing, R. D. (1971). *Self and others*. Baltimore: Pelican.

Lasch, C. (1977). *Haven in a heartless world*. New York: Basic Books.

Lasch, C. (1978). *The culture of narcissism*. New York: Norton.

Lears, T. J. J. (1994). *Fables of abundance*. New York: Basic Books.

Leuchtenburg, W. E. (1958). *The perils of prosperity: 1914–1932*. Chicago: University of Chicago Press.

Liebman, J. L. (1946). *Peace of mind*. New York: Simon & Schuster.

Lifton, R. J. (1986). *The Nazi doctors*. New York: Basic Books.

List, J. (1930). *Das Antoniusleben des hl. Athanasius d. Gr: eine literarhistorische studie zu den anfangen der byzantinischen hagiographie*. Athens, Greece: P. D. Sakellarios.

Louf, A. (1982). Spiritual fatherhood in the literature of the desert. In John R. Sommerfeldt (Ed.), *Abba: Guides to wholeness and holiness East and West* (pp. 37–63). Kalamazoo, MI: Cistercian.

Lubove, R. (1965). *The professional altruist*. Cambridge, MA: Harvard University Press.

MacIntyre, A. (1981). *After virtue*. Notre Dame, IN: University of Notre Dame Press.

Marty, M. E. (1989). Religion in America 1935–1985. In D. W. Lotz (Ed.), *Altered landscapes: Christianity in America 1935–1985* (pp. 1–16). Grand Rapids, MI: Eerdmans.

May, H. F. (1976). *The enlightenment in America*. New York: Oxford University Press.

May, G. G. (1988). *Addiction and grace*. San Francisco: Harper & Row.

May, R. (1939). *The art of counseling: How to gain and give mental health*. Nashville, TN: Cokesbury.

McCarthy, K. (1984). Psychotherapy and religion: The Emmanuel Movement. *Journal of Religion and Health, 23*(2), 92–105.

McGinn, B. (1991). *The foundations of mysticism*. New York: Crossroad Herder.

McLoughlin, W. G. (1968). *The American evangelicals, 1800–1900*. New York: Harper & Row.

McLoughlin, W. G. (1978). *Revivals, awakening, and reform*. Chicago: University of Chicago Press.

Mercadante, L. A. (1996). *Victims and sinners*. Louisville, KY: Westminster John Knox Press.

Meyer, D. (1980). *The positive thinkers*. New York: Doubleday. (Original work published 1965)

Miles, M. R. (1988). *Practicing Christianity*. New York: Crossroad Herder.

Mowrer, O. H. (1964a). Alcoholics Anonymous and the "third" reformation. *Religion in Life, 34*, 383–397.

Mowrer, O. H. (1964b). *The new group therapy*. New York: Van Nostrand.

Nicholson, S. (1995). The expression of emotional distress in Old English prose and verse. *Culture, Medicine and Psychiatry, 19*, 327–339.

Niebuhr, R. (1932). *Moral man and immoral society*. New York: Scribner.

Noll, R. C. (1995). *The Jung cult*. Princeton, NJ: Princeton University Press.

Oates, W. E. (1955). *Religious factors in mental illness*. New York: Association Press.

Oates, W. E. (1957). *The religious dimensions of personality*. New York: Association Press.

Page, R. (1996). Theology and the ecological crisis. *Theology, 99*, 106–114

Peale, N. V. (1948). *A guide to confident living*. New York: Prentice Hall.

Peale, N. V. (1952). *The power of positive thinking*. New York: Prentice Hall.

Plutarch. (1949). *Plutarch's moralia*. Cambridge, MA: Harvard University Press. (Original work published circa 101)

Plutarch. (1971). *Plutarch's lives*. Cambridge, MA: Harvard University Press. (Original work published circa 100)

Renard, J. (1996). *Seven doors to Islam*. Berkeley: University of California Press.

Rieff, P. (1959). *The mind of the moralist*. New York: Doubleday-Anchor.

Rieff, P. (1966). *The triumph of the therapeutic: Uses of faith after Freud*. New York: Harper & Row.

Rosenberg, C. E. (1976). *No other gods*. Baltimore: Johns Hopkins University Press.

Satinover, J. B. (1994). Jungians and gnostics. *First Things, 46*, 41–48.

Schumacher, E. F. (1973). *Small is beautiful*. New York: Harper & Row.

Sellner, E. C. (1983). Soul friend: Guidance on our sacred journeys. *Spiritual Life, 29*, 73–83.

Sellner, E. C. (1990). *Mentoring: The ministry of spiritual kinship*. Notre Dame, IN: Ave Maria.

Shafranske, E. P. (1996). Introduction. In E. P. Shafranske (Ed.), *Religion and the clinical practice of psychology* (pp. 1–17). Washington, DC: American Psychological Association.

Sheen, F. J. (1949). *Peace of soul*. New York: Whittlesey House.

Sheldrake, P. (1991). *Spirituality and history*. New York: Crossroad Herder.

Siegmund, G. (1965). *Belief in God and mental health*. New York: Desclee.

Smith, H. S. (1965). Introduction. In H. S. Smith (Ed.), *Horace Bushnell* (pp. 3–39). New York: Oxford University Press.

Stern, K. (1954). *The third revolution*. New York: Harcourt, Brace.

Sullivan, H. S. (1953). *The interpersonal theory of psychiatry*. New York: Norton. (Original work published 1947)

Susman, W. (1984). *Culture as history: The transformation of American society in the twentieth century*. New York: Pantheon Books.

Szasz, T. (1973). *The second sin*. New York: Doubleday-Anchor.

Szasz, T. (1976). *Karl Kraus and the soul doctors*. Baton Rouge: Louisiana State University Press.

Tiebout, H. M. (1949). The act of surrender in the therapeutic process. *Quarterly Journal of Studies on Alcohol, 10*, 48–58.

Tillich, P. (1952). *The courage to be*. New Haven, CT: Yale University Press.

Tillich, P. (1956). *The religious situation*. New York: Meridian Books. (Original work published 1932)

Tugwell, S. (1985). *Ways of imperfection*. Springfield, IL: Templegate.

Tugwell, S. (1986). The Eastern fathers: Evagrius and Macarius. In C. Jones, G. Wainwright, and E. Yarnold (Eds.), *The story of spirituality* (pp. 168–175). New York: Oxford University Press.

Ward, B. (1987). *Harlots of the desert*. Kalamazoo, MI: Cistercian.

Ware, K. (1986). The Eastern fathers: Introduction. In C. Jones, G. Wainwright, and E. Yarnold (Eds.), *The story of spirituality* (pp. 159–160). New York: Oxford University Press.

Wulff, D. M. (1991). *Psychology of religion: Classic and contemporary views*. New York: Wiley.

Wulff, D. M. (1996). The psychology of religion: An overview. In E. P. Shafranske (Ed.), *Religion and the clinical practice of psychology* (pp. 43–70). Washington, DC: American Psychological Association.

Zaleski, C. (1993–1994). Speaking of William James to the cultured among his despisers. *Journal of Psychology and Religion, 2–3*, 127–170.

3

ASSESSING SPIRITUALITY

RICHARD L. GORSUCH AND WILLIAM R. MILLER

For some, assessing (let alone measuring) *spirituality* sounds like an oxymoron. As noted in chapter 1, spirituality by its very nature defies material limits and thus might be thought to elude operational definition and measurement. Yet, spirituality, if the term has interpersonal meaning and therefore communicates, poses no greater (or lesser) challenges than those inherent in measuring other latent constructs such as personality, health, intelligence, or love. No single approach is likely to be adequate to the task or meet the different nuances important to various theories or investigators. Instead, assessment proceeds by defining relevant domains within the broader construct and identifying reliable ways to assess them.

Although the psychology of religion is not often covered in the training of health professionals, research in this discipline has wrestled for decades with the complexities of measuring spiritual constructs, and there is already a large psychometric literature on which to draw. Indeed, given the multitude of instruments already developed, there is less need for creating new scales than for using and understanding existing measures, at least with regard to religious constructs (see reviews by Gorsuch, 1984, 1990; Hall, Tisdale, & Brokaw, 1994; Hill, Butman, & Hood, 1999; McDonald, LeClair, Holland, Alter, & Friedman, 1995; Richards & Bergin, 1997). Less developed are scientifically sound ways of assessing spirituality that do not rely on religious contexts and constructs.

This practically focused chapter begins with a brief consideration of why clinicians should assess clients' spirituality. The main body of the chapter is devoted to recommendations on how to assess spirituality in ways that are relevant to treatment. We start with broader approaches and proceed to more specific measures organized around the three broad assessment domains—cognitive, behavioral, and experiential—outlined in chapter 1. Finally, we offer a few general cautionary notes about this area of assessment.

WHY ASSESS CLIENTS' SPIRITUALITY?

The importance of understanding clients' spirituality as part of treatment is discussed throughout this book. For purposes of this chapter, we consider the role of spiritual processes as prognostic, contextual, outcome, and intervention variables in treatment. Consistent with other chapters, we use the term *spirituality* here as the larger construct, within which religious involvement is only one aspect, albeit the one most easily and most often studied. Although spirituality may and often does involve an institutional religion, it is also meaningfully distinct from religion (Shafranske & Gorsuch, 1984).

Prognosis

One simple reason for attending to spirituality is that variables in this domain have been widely shown to be predictive of health outcomes. As discussed in chapter 1, the general finding is that religious involvement in particular is often inversely related to physical, mental, and substance use disorders. In this regard, clinicians ought to be interested in at least a basic understanding of clients' spirituality, much as one assesses other risk and protective factors such as family history, social support, and stress.

The fact that religious involvement is generally a protective factor raises an interesting consideration in clinical intake interviewing. For clients who have had active religious involvement, why did it not protect in their case? There is insufficient research to address this problem in the needed detail, but at least three theoretical possibilities can be entertained:

1. *Their religion was protective but other influences overwhelmed it.* Although religious involvement is an often-confirmed and occasionally the strongest inverse predictor of, for example, substance abuse (Gorsuch, 1994b), many other factors

are also involved (e.g., Gorsuch & Butler, 1976; Miller & Hester, 1995). Such other risk factors may simply be stronger than any protective effect of the client's spirituality. If this is the case, the client's spirituality might be an asset in treatment as other factors are countered.

2. *Their religion had a detrimental effect.* Some evidence suggests that a restrictive religious focus with a condemning deity can exert an adverse influence. In such a case, aspects of the client's current religiosity could represent an obstacle rather than a resource in treatment.

3. *Currently observed religious beliefs or behaviors are a by-product of the client's disorder (e.g., negative self-evaluation in clinical depression).* Other or prior aspects of the client's spirituality may have been benevolent, but these were distorted in part because of the problems that have arisen. In the midst of mental distress such clients may believe, for example, that they have betrayed God or that God is angry at them and is condemning or punishing them. In this case, direct treatment of the disorder may restore a healthier spirituality. Furthermore, a reconnection with and grounding in the original spiritual tradition may promote health. It may contain potentially therapeutic beliefs and rituals for grounding, cleansing, restoration, forgiveness, and reconciliation. Reconnection with these authentic traditions could then reestablish the original benevolent spirituality.

As with any prognostic information, the person's religious history and present sense of spirituality must be considered in sufficient detail and in relation to other available data.

Context

A second reason for understanding clients' spirituality is that, regardless of its relationship to presenting problems, for many people it is an important or even central element of their larger worldviews and life context within which presenting concerns will be addressed. Understanding clients' spirituality can promote clearer communication, offering contextual information that is important to the process of treatment. Clients may bring a broad range of spiritual beliefs and coping resources, ranging from private personal practices (such as prayer or meditation) to involvement in supportive religious communities. The nature of these resources will vary across varieties of religion and spirituality. Understanding the ethics deemed normative within the client's worldview can be important as well, particularly regarding topics on which religious groups differ widely and often passionately (e.g., alcohol and drug use, homosexuality, divorce, and abortion). When such values differ from the therapist's own, disclosure and possible referral become ethical issues (see chap. 7 in this book). An appreciation of the client's spiritual and religious context (i.e., frame of reference) can also illuminate the ways in which he or she uses language. For some, a phrase like "waiting for God's call" refers to everyday decision making, whereas for others it may reflect awaiting clarity on an important choice or even feeling immobilized by uncertainty. For yet others it may reflect psychotic ideation. The client's context spells this out. Of course, no therapist can know all of the varieties of religious context in detail, but it is helpful to be sufficiently knowledgeable to ask the right questions of the right people. Consultation with a clergy representative of the client's tradition may be useful. A problem that occurs with some clients is that they fail to understand their own religious tradition, and this misunderstanding in turn complicates their situation.

For clients who have been involved in a faith community, it can be important to understand how the presenting concerns relate to that community. Clients may see their problems as a barrier to involvement and have curtailed or stopped participating. In this case, a measure of successful treatment might be the extent to which the client has regained his or her former level of engagement in the community (through forgiveness, accepting responsibility, restoring relationships, etc.). A spiritual community also can be an important resource for the client and therapist. People already known to the client may provide useful information, social support, and physical resources to aid in recovery. Clergy may already be acquainted with a client's situation and offer a useful professional resource. Clinical pastoral education has long been part of the training of many clergy, and interprofessional collaboration can be beneficial (Gorsuch & Maylink, 1988; Miller & Jackson, 1995). When a client's problem has important spiritual aspects, clergy may be particularly helpful. It is surprising how many laity simply misjudge the position of their own religion and underestimate the extent of willing support available within their own faith community. Working with clergy can clarify for the therapist a client's particular spiritual tradition and resources. As in any coprofessional involvements, some prior knowledge of the other professional is useful in understanding the degree to which he or she may be helpful in a particular case.

Outcome

Spiritual functioning is not static, but changes over time. Thus, it can be useful to track clients' spirituality through and after treatment rather than assessing it only at intake. Treatment can affect spiritual functioning.

An interesting example for clinical intervention is that of spiritual coping. It is almost a truism that a person needs treatment because of difficulties in coping. Pargament (1996; Pargament & Brant, 1998) has demonstrated links between particular spiritual coping styles and indicators of mental health. Treatment often focuses on changing coping styles toward more adaptive patterns (Folkman et al., 1991; Pargament, 1996). This can and should be done in a manner that is sensitive to and consistent with the client's spirituality (for a case example, see Miller, 1988).

Spiritual variables may also be important mediators or moderators of change (Gorsuch, 1994b). Information from a spiritual history can be useful in deciding what is to be expected of the client's spirituality and what could be monitored for change. As noted earlier, although spiritual and religious involvement is usually found to be associated with a lower risk of substance use disorders, certain spiritual aspects may increase risk or exacerbate problems. A conception of God as loving and forgiving appears to be associated with less risk of substance abuse, whereas a concept of God as wrathful and punitive may be linked to increased risk (Gorsuch, 1994b). (Remember, of course, that such beliefs can also be altered by psychopathology.) Shifts in this domain may thus be pertinent in the course of recovery.

Intervention

The above discussion suggests that spiritual variables can also be pertinent as aspects of intervention. Propst (1980; Propst, Ostrom, Watkins, Dean, & Mashburn, 1992) has described how incorporating clients' own specific spiritual perspectives in cognitive therapy can enhance outcomes in the treatment of depression. This requires some understanding of the client's spirituality and specific strategies for incorporating this information into intervention (Propst, 1988; Richards & Bergin, 1997). For example, if building on the client's spirituality is appropriate, enhancing meditation (see chap. 4 in this book), acceptance or forgiveness (see chap. 10), hope (see chap. 11), or prayer (see chap. 5) could be included as a goal of intervention, and the extent to which it is being practiced could be tracked as part of treatment (see chap. 8). Indeed, a spiritual change is sometimes the most important aspect of an intervention (e.g., Barlow, Abel, & Blanchard, 1977; Gorsuch, 1994b). Involving the client in the positive elements of his or her spirituality may enhance hope, forgiveness, restoration of community, and a renewed sense of self-worth.

SPIRITUAL ASSESSMENT

As with personality, a comprehensive assessment of spirituality can occupy many hours and calls on special expertise (Pruyser, 1976; Richards & Bergin, 1997). Although seldom taught in clinical training, there is already a large literature describing interviewing methods and psychometric instruments for assessing religious and spiritual variables (Hood, Spilka, Hunsberger, & Gorsuch, 1996; Richards & Bergin, 1997).

It is worthwhile here to differentiate between assessment and measurement. Assessing a client's spirituality can be accomplished in a variety of ways, only some of which involve discrete measures or scales. The broad goal of assessment is understanding. A clinical interview, structured or unstructured, is one form of assessment. We start with some broad content that can be incorporated in clinical interviewing and proceed toward more specific measures.

Clinical Interviewing

As a starting point, think of clients' spirituality as one of several broad areas about which you will want to learn in initial clinical interviews. One simple question is, "How important is spirituality or religion in your daily life?" The degree of importance placed on religion or spirituality has been tied to health outcomes, and this question opens the door for exploration of spiritual issues. Follow such a broad question with reflective listening rather than with a barrage of further questions. A simple elaboration is to ask, "Tell me *in what ways* spirituality (or religion) has been important to you."

Also of clinical interest is whether the client currently participates in any religious or spiritually oriented organizations (including the ubiquitous Twelve Step fellowships) and, if not, whether he or she has ever done so. A history of past but not current involvement may be important information as a context for a client's present situation. A few general questions for clinical interviewing include (Woods & Ironson, in press) the following: (a) Do you practice a religion currently? [In what ways?] (b) Do you believe in God or a higher power? [How do you experience (God) in your daily life?] (c) Are there spiritual practices that you follow regularly? [Tell me about them] Some such information can also be collected with a brief questionnaire (e.g., Connors, Tonigan, & Miller, 1996).

A person's overall sense of meaning or purpose in life has also been linked to other health domains. Clinicians often explore the level and nature of subjective meaning in a client's life: (a) What things are most important to you? (b) What gives your life purpose or meaning? Again, brief psychometrically validated instruments are available to assess constructs such as a sense of purpose in life (e.g., Crumbaugh & Maholick, 1969), coherence (e.g., Antonovsky, 1979), and spiritual well-being (e.g., Ellison, 1983).

Meaning in life is often linked to what a person sees as important life goals or values. Clients are sometimes asked to write a personal "mission statement." A related but more specific inquiry focuses on the guiding values in a client's life. Rokeach (1973, 1983) developed a ranking method to assess values, and a card-sorting procedure can also be used to explore current or past values (Miller & C'deBaca, 1994). To what extent are the client's beliefs and behaviors consistent with (working in the service of) these stated core values? It can also be illuminating to compare the conformity or nonconformity of the client's own beliefs and behaviors with those prescribed and proscribed by a particular religious tradition with which the client is or has been affiliated.

For clients who believe in a deity, it can be informative to know how they understand the nature of and their relationship to their God or higher power. Religious involvement is not invariably beneficial and can be harmful (cf. Gorsuch, 1994b).

Spiritual Measures

Measures are usually more specific, related to particular constructs and definitions. They can be as simple as a single item and as complex as qualitative ratings or a factorial instrument. All clients can be characterized on spiritual measures, if only by a lack of specific beliefs, behavior, and experience.

Spiritual Screening Items

For the therapist, assessing spirituality involves a balance of breadth and depth. For two reasons we begin this section with the shallowest approach: a set of single-item measures. The first reason is that they give an overview of the variety of ways in which current scientists operationalize aspects of spirituality. The second reason is that, for initial screening and obtaining a broad overview, it may be desirable to start with a set of simple items. To be sure, there are disadvantages to using single items instead of scales; for example, they are more idiosyncratic and underestimate the size of relationships (Gorsuch & McFarland, 1977). Yet, brief items can provide at least an introduction to your client's worldview on spiritual issues, and having an estimate is better than having no information at all.

Single items parallel the open questions discussed above, which might be used to evoke spiritual material in a clinical interview. The difference is that questionnaire items also have carefully worded answers from which to choose. For some items, there are also published norms with which clients' responses can be compared. When comparison with other samples is desirable, precise wording for these single items is important because the phrasing of both the questions and the answers have been standardized in survey research and affect responses. In any event, a set of paper-and-pencil items on spirituality can be included within broader screening questionnaires.

One of the most commonly used items for religion (Gorsuch & McFarland, 1977) is the following: "How important is your religion to you?" (1 = not at all; have no religion, 9 = extremely important; my religious faith is the center of my entire life). The item can be asked with regard to spirituality more generally: "How important is your spirituality to you?" A simple measure of religious involvement asks how often the person participates in religious worship (Gorsuch & McFarland, 1977). Another common single item inquires about the individual's belief in God, a supreme being, or universal spirit (Gallup, 1990).

It would be helpful to clinicians to have a concise set of such screening items. At the time of this writing, the National Institute on Aging and the Fetzer Institute (1998) were completing work on the development of a core instrument to measure domains of religiousness and spirituality that are most likely to affect health outcomes.[1] In its current form, it is composed of 40 items designed to screen multiple domains including religious preference or affiliation, spiritual experiences, organizational religiousness, private spiritual practices, religious social support, religious coping, beliefs and values, commitment, forgiveness, meaning, and overall self-rankings. This instrument offers promise for some standadization of basic measurement in this area. An initial screen of such items can be followed up with more specific items or scales. For clients who believe in God, for example, it may be useful to understand something of the person's concept of God. For those who are involved in a religion, further information can be useful on the nature of the religious community and on their motivations for involvement. (The National Institute on Aging and the Fetzer core screening instrument will be accompanied by a companion set of scales to assess some of these constructs in greater detail.) In the following sections we suggest some short scales that may be used for follow-up in the clinical assessment of clients' spirituality in the three domains outlined in chapter 1: belief, behavior, and experience.

Spiritual Beliefs and Motivation

From a strict measurement perspective, beliefs consist of a person's convictions about the truth or falseness of the content of a statement. Theoretically, they arise from direct experience and other methods of learning (e.g., modeling, vicarious learning) and are then used to guide decisions and to interpret new experiences (rule-governed behavior). Beliefs provide the *content* for one's reality and so lie at the opposite end of the spectrum from functional definitions of spirituality. This definition of belief is admittedly narrow, but it can be useful to distinguish between specific conceptions of reality and broader attitudes or motivations.

---

[1]For information, contact the Fetzer Institute, 9292 West KL Avenue, Kalamazoo, Michigan 49009-9398.

Psychologists have at times paid too little attention to beliefs, and that is true of the psychology of spirituality as well. This occurs in part because much empirical research on spirituality has been conducted within the context of American Christianity, where, rightly or wrongly, some homogeneity of beliefs is assumed. Two dissertations illustrate the potential importance of specific beliefs. Fulton (1990) found that a literal interpretation of the Bible was predictive of a negative value judgment about homosexual behavior. In examining acceptance of a female pastor, however, Hao (1993) found that beliefs about the Bible were unimportant; it was beliefs about the reactions of possible new church members that were crucial to acceptance.

Another example of the usefulness of more specified belief can be found in research that uses a functional question such as "How important is your relationship with God?" If one stops there, those who conceive of God as loving and forgiving would be grouped with those who conceive of God as vengeful and wrathful. Such lumping could mask important differences, and results could vary depending on a sample's particular mix of believers with the two different concepts of God. A common and simple method for measuring the God image is an adjective checklist with 5- or 7-point Likert scales ranging from *strongly agree* to *strongly disagree* (Gorsuch, 1968; Schaefer & Gorsuch, 1992). A short set of three positive and three negative adjectives (e.g., forgiving, merciful, and loving; cruel, stern, and wrathful) can provide a quick estimate, or the full checklist can be used for more reliable measurement.

Measures of spiritual beliefs tend to be specific to a particular religion or a form of spiritual thought. With largely Christian samples, for example, the Gallup (1990) poll has used single items to assess beliefs about God and the Bible and to ask whether respondents self-identify as a born-again or evangelical Christian. Scales designed to measure beliefs within one religion are unlikely to generalize well across religions. Scales querying monotheistic beliefs, for example, simply do not work with Buddhists or Hindus. Mathew, Mathew, Wilson, and Georgi (1995) developed a cross-cultural scale to assess more generic dimensions of spirituality, including mystical experiences, belief in life after death, valuing of altruism and unselfishness, and belief in paranormal phenomena.

With regard to broader personal perspectives, Gordon Allport (1950) laid the foundation for what is now a classic distinction between intrinsic and extrinsic motivation for engagement in religion, one of the most widely used concepts in this field. Allport really addressed orientation rather than motivation, and his scales mixed belief, motivation, and behavior, and others (Gorsuch, 1994a; Gorsuch & McPherson, 1989) have sought to separate out the motivational component. Extrinsic motivations involve tangible social (e.g., to meet people, to see people I know, for status) or personal (e.g., for personal protection, for healing of an illness, for comfort in times of trouble and sorrow) benefits of participation. Intrinsic motivation, on the other hand, involves spirituality or religion as valued for itself and is integrated and central in the person's life. It is the latter type of intrinsically motivated involvement that is most closely linked to positive health outcomes (Hood et al., 1996). (Indeed, some would argue that motivation is "spiritual" only when it is intrinsic.) Gorsuch and McPherson (1989) have developed and normed a 14-item scale to assess Allport's intrinsic–extrinsic distinction from a motivational perspective.

Spirituality may also give meaning to life and answer needs for a perspective on death and other existential issues. The quest for such answers, in fact, is one possible broad definition of spirituality. For individuals involved in religion, a widely used scale measures this concept of spiritual questing (Batson & Schoenrade, 1991a, 1991b). The Quest Scale includes three motivational subdimensions represented by the following items:

Existential	"I was not very interested in religion till I began to ask questions about the meaning and purpose of my life."
Positive Doubts	"It might be said that I value my religious doubts and uncertainties."
Openness to Change	"I am constantly questioning my religious belief."

The general sense of meaning or purpose in life, useful in both secular and religious contexts, represents another motivational aspect of spirituality that can be pertinent to psychotherapy and related to outcome. Here the most widely used scale is one not explicitly linked to religion: the Purpose in Life Scale (Crumbaugh & Maholick, 1964, 1969). A similar scale with an explicitly theistic content is the Spiritual Well-Being Scale of Paloutzian and Ellison (1991).

Spiritual Behavior

Spiritual practices represent a second major assessment domain. Spiritual behaviors are those that involve a distinct spiritual and transcendent component. Such components can be individually or institutionally oriented. Examples of the former include meditation, fasting, prayer, and spiritually based compassion (whether directly person to person or indirectly as in charitable donations). Examples of institutionally oriented spiritual behavior include public worship and prayer, evangelism, and compassionate service (e.g., feeding and clothing) coordinated by religious groups. It is noteworthy that religious activities are not necessarily spiritual. Participation in organizational committees, for example, may be appropriate for measuring religious institutional commitment, but these may have little or no spiritual component.

As with belief scales, measures of spiritual behavior have often been specific to particular religious contexts. Measures developed within one religious perspective may not apply well outside that context. The proper measurement of worship behavior is influenced by the religious tradition. Buddhist worship is not characterized by formal events as are found in Judeo-Christian circles. The number of times per week a Christian attends worship is a function not only of personal attributes but also of the denomination with which the person is affiliated. Cultural context is also the reason why the most commonly used single-item measure of worship attendance has multiple-choice answers that stop at "once a week or more." Other measures have been developed to assess adherence to spiritual practices prescribed within specific secular groups, such as the Twelve Step programs (see chap. 6 in this book). Connors and his colleagues (1996) developed a brief scale intended to survey the frequency of involvement in somewhat more generic spiritual and religious practices such as prayer and meditation, study of sacred writings, and worship attendance.

An important caution here is that frequency counts, though simple, are usually insufficient to understand much about spiritual and religious behavior. The frequency of prayer, for example, is less related to healthy outcomes than is the *type* of prayer practiced (see chap. 5 in this book). Similarly, as described above, the frequency of religious attendance is often a less sensitive predictor of health than measures that reflect motivations for participation (e.g., intrinsic vs. extrinsic).

Another active line of clinically relevant assessment research has focused on coping behaviors that have spiritual and religious roots. The best known researchers in this area, Pargament and Brant (1998), have identified four major styles of religious coping, represented by these example items:

Collaborative	Work together with God as partners.
Religious Support	Sought support from clergy or church members.
Anger at God	Felt angry that God did not hear my prayers.
Punitive Religious Appraisal	Decided that God was punishing me for my sins.

The first two styles are generally related to positive health outcomes and the latter two to poorer outcomes. A "surrender" coping style (see chap. 9 in this book) has also been described by Paragament (1996) and by Wong-

McDonald and Gorsuch (1997). Scales with adequate reliability and validity are available from the above sources, and state measures are also available (e.g., Scheafer & Gorsuch, 1993). In the context of Alcoholics Anonymous, scales of involvement are available that specifically include the practice of the Twelve Steps, which can be thought of as spiritually based coping behaviors (Montgomery, Miller, & Tonigan, 1995; Tonigan, Connors, & Miller, 1996).

A simple but important point to remember in measuring spirituality behavior (i.e., the practice of spirituality) is that instructions should specify a particular time frame. This is particularly important when measuring changes associated with time, such as the effects of an intervention. Items that are phrased as "Have you ever . . ." are likely to show little change because they reflect lifetime accumulations. Questions specifying a time frame, such as "During the last month, have you . . .," are more sensitive to change. For example, state measures of religious coping can be used to assess change (Scheafer & Gorsuch, 1993). Some scales measure both lifetime and current levels of spiritual and religious behavior (Connors et al., 1996). Most scales can be readily adapted to measure any desired time frame.

Spiritual Experiences

Mystical experience is at the heart of what many would call "spirituality." Its characteristics have been widely documented: The experience is felt as profound, as difficult to communicate, and as having a transcendent dimension. A dramatic conversion experience is one example of mystical experience (Loder, 1981; Rambo, 1993), but such profound experiences also occur outside the context of religion (Miller & C'deBaca, 1994). Hood's (1985; Hood, Morris, & Watson, 1993) scales of mysticism have become standard measures for this domain.

Mystical experiences are necessarily measured by self-report, but more recent attention has been devoted to physiological changes that may occur during specific controllable spiritual experiences. There are, for example, well-documented physiological changes that occur during meditation. The differentiation of types of prayer (see chap. 5 in this book) suggests the question of whether the various types may be associated with different physiological changes. The relationship is also reciprocal, in that certain physiological changes (e.g., drug states or fasting) have been used to facilitate spiritual experiences (Miller, 1998). Questions such as these appear to be important not only in themselves but also for possible mediators of the relationship between spirituality and health.

Finally, note that the phenomena represented by these sections (belief, behavior, and experience) can and do interact with one another. Coping, for example, involves behaviors, beliefs, and motivations (Pargament,

1996). Spiritual coping with stress, for example, might include prayer (see chap. 5 in this book), acceptance and forgiveness (see chap. 10), and "turning it over" to a higher power (see chap. 9). Here, behavioral, cognitive–motivational, and experiential dimensions blend, and a thorough understanding of spirituality will transcend the neat categories differentiated here.

SOME REFLECTIONS ON ASSESSING SPIRITUALITY

In closing, we offer a few general points of observation and advice with regard to assessing spirituality based on experience and past reviews (Gorsuch, 1984, 1990). First, we repeat our plea to avoid creating more homemade scales when there are already psychometrically sound options. New scales are useful if and only if they add incrementally to the currently available measures. Consider devoting psychometric effort to improving already-developed scales to make them more applicable to clinical populations.

Second, we emphasize that the impact of a person's religion or spirituality may be either negative or positive when evaluated by an extrinsic criterion. Historically, spiritual experience and belief encompass both the divine and the demonic. Be mindful of the potential for both types of effects on the person. Whether a particular form of spirituality is beneficial or harmful is an empirical question once definitions of "benefit" and "harm" have been established. The concepts of benefit and harm, of course, can sometimes be as difficult to define as spirituality itself.

Third, when using measurement scales, be conscious of their demographic range of applicability. Many scales were developed in college samples and are of unknown utility with other age groups (e.g., adolescents and many adults) or when educational levels are lower. Generalizability may be threatened by reading difficulty or from question content that is not applicable to the respondent. There are also profound cultural differences in the expression of spirituality, and scales normed in one cultural context may not work well in others. The assessment of spirituality has too often relied on approaches developed in and limited to one religious context. These are prime areas for psychometric development. How can spirituality be measured in ways that are not limited by a particular religious perspective? Will a scale developed for one age, educational, or cultural group apply to other populations, and how do the scale's psychometric properties change? What adaptations are needed to make an assessment approach applicable for a broad range of individuals and groups?

Fourth, the difference between content and function is of import in measuring spirituality. There is specific content in spiritual measures, as in doctrinal beliefs about the nature of God or scripture, or the beyondist

(Cattell, 1972) belief about a current lack of knowledge and the role of the social sciences in providing that knowledge. Function is involved in questions such as the motivation giving rise to a search for meaning. For example, in studying prejudice, fundamentalism has been defined by the content of beliefs (e.g., Fulton, 1990) or functionally in a manner independent of doctrinal content (Hunsberger, 1997). The findings of such studies are likely to vary depending on whether content or function is emphasized in operational definitions.

Fifth, the appropriate scale to use with a particular person or situation may be either culture specific or more general. More generic instruments usually measure function rather than content. For example, a spiritual person may be seen as one who has a clearly defined ultimate concern. The strength of this approach is that it readily applies to a wide range of spirituality because content is not specified. Current work in revising the intrinsic–extrinsic scales takes this into account, encompassing a greater variety of reasons to be religious than Allport (1950) proposed (Gorsuch, Mylvaganam, Gorsuch, & Johnson, 1997) and cross-validating items with a Buddhist sample in Thailand and the United States. Multicultural measures are preferable whenever possible to enhance generalizability and are more likely to be tapping spirituality than a more limited religious perspective.

Finally, with this said, spirituality measures also need to be designed at the appropriate level of aggregation. If an outcome measure is specific to one religious setting, then spirituality ought to be measured in a manner appropriate to that setting. There is little point in assessing the use of the Twelve Steps within groups that do not know about or practice them. Questions in a study of health effects of religious involvement may better focus on the respondent's particular religious community rather than on an amorphous "religion" in general. According to the purpose of its use, a scale about prayer might tell the person to "fill this out only for those times when you pray about your problem." This means that specific instructions for scales may need to be tailored. The reliability and validity of a scale can shift (e.g., from correlations ranging from the .20s to the .60s) depending on the match of aggregation between independent and dependent measures (Fishbein & Ajzen, 1974; Rushton, Brainerd, & Pressley, 1983).

CONCLUSIONS

Like many other latent constructs used in health care and research, spirituality can be carefully and fruitfully measured. It is odd indeed that this aspect of humanity, so often experienced by clients as being central to their well-being, is so rarely measured or even asked about in clinical work. It is not for a lack of reliable measures, although there is certainly room for improvement. What is needed is to bring together psychology and spirituality, two traditions that have for decades worked in relative isolation despite some common roots. It is a larger hope underlying this entire book that such integration will serve to improve the quality of our clients' care and health.

REFERENCES

Allport, G. W. (1950). *The individual and his religion: A psychological interpretation.* New York: Macmillan.

Antonovsky, A. (1979). *Health, stress, and coping.* San Francisco: Jossey-Bass.

Barlow, D. H., Abel, G. G., & Blanchard, E. G. (1977). Gender identity change in a transsexual: An exorcism. *Archives of Sexual Behavior, 6,* 387–395.

Batson, C. D., & Schoenrade, P. A. (1991a). Measuring religion as quest: 1. Validity concerns. *Journal for the Scientific Study of Religion, 30,* 416–429.

Batson, C. D., & Schoenrade, P. A. (1991b). Measuring religion as quest: 2. Reliability concerns. *Journal for the Scientific Study of Religion, 30,* 430–447.

Cattell, R. B. (1972). *A new morality from science: Beyondism.* Elmsford, NY: Pergamon Press.

Connors, G. J., Tonigan, J. S., & Miller, W. R. (1996). A measure of religious background and behavior for use in behavior change research. *Psychology of Addictive Behavior, 10,* 90–96.

Crumbaugh, J. C., & Maholick, L. T. (1964). An experimental study in existentialism: The psychometric approach to Frankl's concept of noogenic neurosis. *Journal of Clinical Psychology, 22,* 200–207.

Crumbaugh, J. C., & Maholick, L. T. (1969). *The Purpose in Life Test.* Chicago: Psychometric Affiliates.

Ellison, C. W. (1983). Spiritual well-being: Conceptualization and measurement. *Journal of Psychology and Theology, 11,* 330–340.

Fishbein, M., & Ajzen, I. (1974). Attitudes towards objects as predictors of single and multiple behavioral criteria. *Psychological Review, 81,* 59–74.

Folkman, S., Chesney, M., McKusick, G., Ironson, G. H., Johnson, D., & Coates, T. (1991). Translating coping theory into an intervention. In J. Eckenrode (Ed.), *The social context of coping* (pp. 239–260). New York: Plenum.

Fulton, A. (1990). *Religious orientation, anti-homosexual sentiment, identity status, and fundamentalism: In search of mature religion.* Unpublished doctoral dissertation, Fuller Theological Seminary, Pasadena, CA.

Gallup, G. (1990). *Religion in America.* Princeton, NJ: Gallup Report.

Gorsuch, R. L. (1968). The conceptualization of God as seen in adjective ratings. *Journal for the Scientific Study of Religion, 7,* 56–64.

Gorsuch, R. L. (1984). Measurement: The boon and bane of investigating religion. *American Psychologist, 39,* 228–236.

Gorsuch, R. L. (1990). Measurement in psychology of religion revisited. *Journal of Psychology and Christianity, 9*(2), 82–92.

Gorsuch, R. L. (1994a). Toward motivational theories of intrinsic religious commitment. *Journal for the Scientific Study of Religion, 33,* 315–325.

Gorsuch, R. (1994b). Religious aspects of substance abuse and recovery. *Journal of Social Issues, 51,* 65–83.

Gorsuch, R., & Butler, M. (1976). Initial drug abuse: A review of predisposing social psychological factors. *Psychological Bulletin, 83,* 120–137.

Gorsuch, R. L., & Maylink, W. D. (1988) Toward a co-professional model of clergy-psychologist referral. *Journal of Psychology and Christianity, 7*(3), 22–31.

Gorsuch, R. L., & McFarland, S. (1977). Single vs. multiple-item scales for measuring religious values. *Journal for the Scientific Study of Religion, 11*(1), 53–64.

Gorsuch, R. L., & McPherson, S. (1989). Intrinsic/extrinsic measurement: I/E-revised and single-item scales. *Journal for the Scientific Study of Religion, 28,* 348–354.

Gorsuch, R. L., Mylvaganam, G., Gorsuch, K., & Johnson, R. (1997). Perceived religious motivation. *International Journal for the Psychology of Religion, 7*(4), 253–261.

Hall, T. W., Tisdale, T. C., & Brokaw, B. F. (1994). Assessment of religious dimensions in Christian clients: A review of selected instruments for research and clinical use. *Journal of Psychology and Theology, 22,* 395–421.

Hao, J. (1993). *Religious beliefs, affects, and values towards supporting women's pastoral leadership: Applying reasoned action and aggregation theories.* Unpublished doctoral disseration, Fuller Theological Seminary, Pasadena, CA.

Hill, P., Butman, R., & Hood, R. (1999). *Measures of religiousness.* Birmingham, AL: Religious Education Press.

Hood, R. W., Jr. (1985). Mysticism. In P. Hammond (Ed.), *The sacred in a secular era* (pp. 285–297). Berkeley: University of California Press.

Hood, R. W., Jr., Morris, R. J., & Watson, P. J. (1993). Further factor analysis of Hood's Mysticism Scale. *Psychological Reports, 3,* 1176–1178.

Hood, R., Spilka, B., Hunsberger, B., & Gorsuch, R. (1996). *The psychology of religion: An empirical approach.* New York: Guilford Press.

Hunsberger, B. (1997). Religious fundamentalism, right-wing authoritarianism, and hostility toward homosexuals in non-Christian religious groups. *International Journal for the Psychology of Religion, 6,* 39–49.

Loder, J. E. (1981). *The transforming moment: Understanding convictional experiences.* New York: Harper & Row.

Mathew, R. J., Mathew, V. G., Wilson, W. H., & Georgi, J. M. (1995). Measurement of materialism and spiritualism in substance abuse research. *Journal of Studies on Alcohol, 56,* 470–475.

McDonald, D. A., LeClair, L., Holland, C. J., Alter, A., & Friedman, H. L. (1995).

A survey of measures of transpersonal constructs. *Journal of Transpersonal Psychology*, 27, 171–235.

Miller, W. R. (1988). Including clients' spiritual perspectives in cognitive behavior therapy. In W. R. Miller & J. E. Martin (Eds.), *Behavior therapy and religion: Integrating spiritual and behavioral approaches to change* (pp. 43–55). Newbury Park, CA: Sage.

Miller, W. R. (1998). Researching the spiritual dimensions of alcohol and other drug problems. *Addiction*, 93, 979–990.

Miller, W. R., & C'deBaca, J. (1994). Quantum change: Toward a psychology of transformation. In T. Heatherton & J. Weinberger (Eds.), *Can personality change?* (pp. 253–280). Washington, DC: American Psychological Association.

Miller, W. R., & Hester, R. K. (1995). Treatment for alcohol problems: Toward an informed eclecticism. In R. K. Hester & W. R. Miller (Eds.), *Handbook of alcoholism treatment approaches: Effective alternatives* (2nd ed., pp. 1–11). Boston: Allyn & Bacon.

Miller, W. R., & Jackson, K. A. (1995). *Practical psychology for pastors: Toward more effective counseling* (2nd ed.) Englewood Cliffs, NJ: Prentice Hall.

Montgomery, H. A., Miller, W. R., & Tonigan, J. S. (1995). Does Alcoholics Anonymous involvement predict treatment outcome? *Journal of Substance Abuse Treatment*, 12, 241–246.

National Institute on Aging and the Fetzer Working Group. (1998). *Measurement scale on religion, spirituality, health and aging.* Unpublished manuscript, Fetzer Institute, Kalamazoo, MI.

Paloutzian, R. F., & Ellison, C. W. (1991). *Manual for the Spiritual Well-Being Scale.* Nyack, NY: Life Advances.

Pargament, K. (1996). *The psychology of religion and coping: Theory, research, and practice.* New York: Guilford Press.

Pargament, K. I., & Brant, C. R. (1998). Religion and coping. In H. G. Koenig (Ed.), *Handbook of religion and mental health* (pp. 112–128). San Diego, CA: Academic Press.

Propst, L. R. (1980). The comparative efficacy of religious and nonreligious imagery for the treatment of mild depression in religious individuals. *Cognitive Therapy and Research*, 4, 167–178.

Propst, L. R. (1988). *Psychotherapy within a religious framework: Spirituality in the emotional healing process.* New York: Human Sciences Press.

Propst, L. R., Ostrom, R., Watkins, P., Dean, T., & Mashburn, D. (1992). Comparative efficacy of religious and nonreligious cognitive–behavioral therapy for the treatment of clinical depression in religious individuals. *Journal of Consulting and Clinical Psychology*, 60, 94–103.

Pruyser, P. (1976). The minister as diagnostician. Philadelphia: Westminster Press.

Rambo, L. R. (1993). *Understanding religious conversion.* New Haven, CT: Yale University Press.

Richards, P. S., & Bergin, A. E. (1997). *A spiritual strategy for counseling and psychotherapy.* Washington, DC: American Psychological Association.

Rokeach, M. (1973). *The nature of human values.* New York: Free Press.

Rokeach, M. (1983). *Rokeach Value Survey.* Palo Alto, CA: Consulting Psychologists Press.

Rushton, J. P., Brainerd, C. J., & Presley, M. (1983). Behavioral development and construct validity: The principle of aggregation. *Psychological Bulletin, 94,* 18–38.

Schaefer, C. A., & Gorsuch, R. L. (1992). Dimensionality of religion: Belief and motivation as predictors of behavior. *Journal of Psychology and Christianity, 11,* 244–254.

Scheafer, C. A., & Gorsuch, R. L. (1993). Situational and personal variations in religious coping. *Journal for the Scientific Study of Religion, 34,* 136–147.

Shafranske, E. P., & Gorsuch, R. L. (1984). Factors associated with the perception of spirituality in psychotherapy. *Journal of Transpersonal Psychology, 16,* 231–241.

Tonigan, J. S., Connors, G. J., & Miller, W. R. (1996). The Alcoholics Anonymous Involvement (AAI) Scale: Reliability and norms. *Psychology of Addictive Behaviors, 10,* 75–80.

Wong–McDonald, A., & Gorsuch, R. (1997, November). *Surrender to God: An additional coping style?* Paper presented at the meeting of the Society for Scientific Study of Religion, San Diego, CA.

Woods, T. E., & Ironson, G. H. (in press). Religion and spirituality in the face of illness: How cancer, cardiac, and HIV patients describe their spirituality/religiousity. *Journal of Health Psychology.*

II

ADDRESSING SPIRITUALITY
IN TREATMENT

4

MINDFULNESS AND MEDITATION

G. ALAN MARLATT AND JEAN L. KRISTELLER

The purpose of this chapter is to illuminate the role of meditation and mindfulness in clinical therapy. Although meditation has also been shown to be helpful in the treatment of physical disease (e.g., cancer and AIDS), the primary application here is in the treatment of psychological and behavioral problems. In this chapter, we draw on our experiences in meditation practice as well as on our research and clinical work and that of others. Our clinical practices have included addictive behaviors, particularly alcoholism and eating disorders, general behavioral medicine, and anxiety and depressive disorders. The clinical approaches described here have also been used with a wide variety of clinical problems including the treatment of personality and conduct disorders as well as relationship problems.

The material in this chapter is organized as follows. The first section is devoted to a discussion of definitions and types of meditation practice, followed by a brief review of theories about how meditation may work (mechanisms of action). In the second section, various applications and examples of meditation practice are reviewed, along with specific instructions on how to implement them in clinical practice. In the third and final section, research designed to evaluate the clinical effectiveness of meditation is reviewed, along with a discussion of future trends. Throughout, there is consideration of how these meditative techniques may relate to issues of spirituality.

MEDITATION AND MINDFULNESS: DEFINITIONS AND THEORIES

Meditation practice is often identified as a relaxation technique (Benson & Proctor, 1984). Although this is certainly a legitimate aspect of meditation, and one that has made these techniques more easily understood, our primary focus is on meditation as an approach to developing mindfulness, whether at a physical, psychological, or spiritual level. The meditation techniques that have gained the most attention within clinical practice in the United States in the past several decades have come from Eastern traditions, in which the physical, psychological, and spiritual aspects of the self are not seen as distinct as they are in Western traditions. Hence, there is sometimes confusion or concern that meditation practices are in some way antithetical to Western or Christian religious or spiritual practice and belief. In fact, virtually all spiritual traditions have created meditative practices.

Although we primarily address clinical and research evidence based on Eastern traditions, we believe that recognizing and acknowledging the universality of this experience are critical. The full value of meditative practices is best understood as tapping into the universal potential for the human mind to transcend its preoccupation with negative experiences—with fears, anxiety, anger, and obsessions—and to become more comfortable with the experiences of compassion, acceptance, and forgiveness (Huxley, 1944).

What is mindfulness? To be fully mindful in the present moment is to be aware of the full range of experiences that exist in the here and now. It is bringing one's complete attention to the present experience on a moment to moment basis. As defined by two leading meditation teachers,

> mindfulness means seeing how things are, directly and immediately seeing for oneself that which is present and true. It has a quality of fullness and impeccability to it, a bringing of our whole heart and mind, our full attention, to each moment. (Goldstein & Kornfield, 1987, p. 62)

Mindful awareness is based on an attitude of acceptance. Rather than judging one's experiences as good or bad, healthy or sick, worthy or unworthy, mindfulness accepts all personal experiences (e.g., thoughts, emotions, events) as just "what is" in the present moment. Mindful acceptance of difficult thoughts or emotional states often transcends their negativity.

> The practice of mindfulness defuses our negativity, aggression, and turbulent emotions. . . . Rather than suppressing emotions or indulging in them, here it is important to view them, and your thoughts, and whatever arises with an acceptance and generosity that are as open and spacious as possible. (Sogyal, 1992, p. 123)

Perhaps the most significant clinical application of mindfulness is the capacity to adopt an "observing self" (Deikman, 1982) that pays careful attention to one's thoughts and feelings as they occur in the present moment. This observing self is also what connects meditation as part of psychotherapy to behavioral techniques such as self-monitoring and to cognitive techniques in which characteristic distorted or dysfunctional thoughts are systematically identified. Although these approaches have documented value, they still leave the individual accepting the conditioning or thought patterns as "themselves." Rather than "overidentifying" with one's thoughts or feelings, mindfulness allows people to see their thoughts as "just thinking," not as personal directives that they must identify with, follow, or give into:

> The practice of mindfulness is not reserved for the meditation cushion. . . . If we are able to wake up, if only occasionally and for a few moments at first, stand back from the ongoing drama of our lives and take an objective look at the habit patterns in which we are caught, then their compulsive hold over us begins to loosen. We dis-identify from them; that is, we begin to see that those thoughts and feelings are not us. They come along accidentally. They are neither an organic part of us nor are we obliged to follow them. (Snelling, 1991, p. 55)

John Teasdale, a professor of psychology in the United Kingdom, conducted a study on mindfulness meditation as a relapse prevention treatment for depression (Teasdale, Segal, & Williams, 1995). In a discussion of his preliminary results, Teasdale (1997) illustrated the difference between the meditation treatment condition included in his study and a more standardized cognitive therapy approach. He first presented the following negative thought as expressed by one of his depressed clients: "My life is a failure; I am miserable and see no reason to go on living." A cognitive therapist would try to help this client change the content of his thoughts, perhaps by suggesting counterexamples to minimize overgeneralization or other cognitive distortions (Beck, Wright, Newman, & Liese, 1993).

In contrast, the aim of meditation therapy is not to change the content of the thought itself but to alter the client's attitude or relationship to the thought, Teasdale stated. Thinking that "my life is a failure" is accepted as just a thought that occurred in the mind. In this sense, the thinking mind is regarded as being similar to one of the five senses that registers (but does not cause) visual, auditory, and other incoming stimuli. Negative thoughts are similarly registered and noticed as "thought stimuli" that are occurring in the mind. As such, negative thoughts are not over-personalized and do not serve as dictators of subsequent feelings and activities (e.g., suicide attempts). As indicated by the title of a recent book on meditation and psychotherapy, *Thoughts Without a Thinker* (Epstein, 1996), thoughts are accepted as the natural behavior of the mind, but not as inherently defining the self.

The meditation literature describes many different meditative practices (Goleman, 1977; Shapiro & Walsh, 1984). Most reviewers of this literature have referred to two basic types of meditation practice: concentrative meditation and mindfulness meditation (Smith, 1975). Mindfulness meditation is also referred to as "opening up," insight, or Vipassana meditation. Concentrative practices focus on a specific object of attention, such as awareness of the breath (paying close attention to the physical sensations of breathing in and out). Other objects of concentration may include a visual target such as a candle flame or mandala, or the sound of a repeated word or mantra. In transcendental meditation (TM), practitioners repeat a Sanskrit term as the focus of their meditation (O'Connell & Alexander, 1994); secularized versions of this method have substituted the word "one" (Benson & Proctor, 1984), or encourage the practitioner to select a word or sound of their choice (Carrington, 1998). An example of a concentrative meditation practice is given below in the section on clinical applications.

In insight or mindfulness practices, the meditator is instructed to develop an awareness of any mental content, including thoughts, imagery, physical sensations, or feelings, as they consciously occur on a moment-to-moment basis. As with concentrative meditation, the overall focus is on paying close attention to one's immediate experience in an attitude of acceptance and "loving kindness." The two types of practice are often combined, as in the teaching of insight or Vipassana meditation (Goldstein & Kornfield, 1987; Kabat-Zinn, 1990). In 10-day Vipassana meditation retreats, the first 3 days are devoted to practicing concentrative meditation (a focus on the breath) before beginning a week of insight meditation (a focus on physical sensations and thoughts as they occur in the moment). Vipassana is the Buddhist tradition from which most mindfulness techniques derive.

Both concentrative and insight meditation techniques are associated with two main processes: (a) the direct experience of "impermanence" or the constantly changing nature of perceived reality, and (b) the ability to self-monitor subjective events from the perspective of an objective or detached observer. Both have important clinical implications.

As an illustration of the first outcome, one of us (G.A.M.) once attended a meditation retreat in which he experienced considerable pain in his knees while seated cross-legged for long hours in meditation. As he later wrote in his journal,

> At one point, the pain became almost unbearable, and I felt compelled to stretch out my legs to release the pressure. The meditation teacher instructed me to resist this strong urge to move my legs, and instead to continue sitting in the same posture while carefully observing the painful sensations I felt in my knees.
>
> At first the pain seemed solid and unyielding in its aversiveness. After "watching" the pain for several minutes, however, I began to notice small changes. Instead of feeling one solid, unchanging block of pain stimuli, I began to notice that the pain signal changed subtly over time. Instead of one solid block of pain, careful attention showed me that the pain signal pulsed in waves of intensity that went up and down. I began to notice periods of "less pain" between pulses of more intense pain in an "in and out" kind of pattern. Once my awareness focused on the spaces of "less pain" that occurred between the more painful pulses, my basic attitude changed as I began to "open up" to the pain experience. Although the pain was still present, it felt less intense, as though my awareness could "see through" the pain to the other side. The spaces between the pain stimuli widened, and I felt my urge to do anything to escape or avoid the pain diminish. The painful sensations rose and fell like waves on the sea, and I was able to find a balance point between the crests of intense sensations. Of course, I was still very thankful when the meditation period was finally over and I could stretch my legs with great relief.

The second process that develops in meditation is the ability to step aside from one's own mental and subjective functioning and to observe the stream of consciousness from the perspective of a vigilant but detached observer. It is in this way that meditation is similar to the behavioral technique of self-monitoring, in which clients are asked to observe or to keep a record of their ongoing thoughts or behavior. Langer (1989) also described a cognitive theory of mindfulness and its relation to health promotion and disease prevention. In all these areas of application, the individual is trained to adopt an objective perspective of self-observation based on an attitude of acceptance and nonevaluation.

The meditative practice of self-monitoring thoughts and other mental events often leads the individual to become less identified with his or her own thought processes ("thoughts without a thinker"), no matter how upsetting or infatuating they may otherwise be. The meditator can learn to develop a sense of equanimity or balance without being absorbed into his or her own mental processes. This process of "mental disidentification" is nicely illustrated in the following passage taken from a book on meditation practice:

> An image about practicing meditation that may be helpful is that of standing at a railroad crossing, watching a freight train passing by. In

each transparent boxcar, there is a thought. We try to look straight ahead into the present, but our attachments draw our attention into the contents of the passing boxcars: we identify with the various thoughts. . . . So, we're looking straight ahead, not distracted by any of the contents, when all of a sudden one of the boxcars explodes as it goes by. We're drawn into that one, we jump into the action in that boxcar. Then we come back with a wry smile full of recognition that it was just an image of an explosion, just a boxcar thought. Then, we notice as we look straight ahead that we're starting to be able to see between the cars. And we begin to see what's on the other side of the train, what is beyond thought. We experience that the process is occurring against a background of undifferentiated openness, that, moment to moment, mind is arising and passing away in vast space. As we experience the frame of reference in which all this melodrama is occurring, it begins freeing us from being so carried away—even by fear. We start seeing. (Levine, 1979, pp. 29–31)

MODELS OF MEDITATION EFFECTS

There are several theoretical models that have been advanced by both researchers and therapists to explain the beneficial effects of meditation (Shapiro & Walsh, 1984). Although space does not permit a full discussion of all approaches, consider the following models in terms of their clinical implications: (a) as a physiological relaxation technique; (b) as a way of changing neurological function; (c) as a type of positive addiction; (d) as a metacognitive intervention; and (e) as promoting spiritual and existential growth.

Relaxation

The first model considers meditation effective to the extent that it elicits a state of deep physical relaxation. Research on the physiological effects of meditation shows that individuals engaged in meditative practice exhibit what has been called a "wakeful hypometabolic state" (Wallace, Benson, & Wilson, 1984), demonstrated by changes such as reduced oxygen consumption, decreased sympathetic activity in the autonomic nervous system, and muscle relaxation (Orme-Johnson, 1984). Changes in brain wave activity, consistent with more relaxation, have also been demonstrated. Because many types of meditation and relaxation procedures produce a similar response, Benson and Proctor (1984) referred to this reaction as the "basic relaxation response." This model is most frequently used when including meditation as a basic behavioral relaxation technique, either as a way to reduce chronic states of tension through daily practice or as a component of treatment in which anxiety-producing mental content may become desensitized through extinction or counterconditioning (Goleman, 1971; Goleman & Schwartz, 1984).

Neurological Processing

Other researchers have developed a model based on studies of electroencephalographic changes that occur during meditation (Glueck & Stroebel, 1984; Kasamatsu & Hirai, 1966) that underlie a sense of altered consciousness. Studies have shown, for example, that meditation is capable of producing changes in hemispheric laterality (Bennett & Trinder, 1984). Pagano and Frumkin (1984) found that meditation selectively influences right-hemisphere functioning. These findings have led some theorists to postulate that meditation may be effective by changing symmetry in hemispheric brain activity (Ley & Smylie, 1989; Ornstein, 1972).

Positive Addiction

Glasser (1976) defined meditation as one of several potential "positive addictions." As with exercise and other lifestyle habits, the regular practice of meditation can become intrinsically rewarding. A "positive" addiction has six characterics: The activity is noncompetitive, it is easily accomplished, it can be done alone, it has positive value, improvement needs to be judged only by the person, and it can be done without self-criticism. Meditation practice has all these characteristics.

Metacognitive Intervention

Many meditation practices have in common the use of a repetitive object of awareness, such as focusing on the breath in mindfulness meditation. A gradual change in one's attitude toward thinking, particularly in terms of how cognitions may give rise to negative or disturbing emotions, appears central to many reports of therapeutic benefit. From this perspective, meditation is primarily a metacognitive practice. Meditation does not involve normal analytical thinking processes (Goleman, 1971), yet a critical aspect of most practices is a sense of heightened but detached awareness of sensory and thought experience. Understanding the therapeutic value of this process may represent a particularly important integration of Eastern and Western psychologies (Walsh, 1996).

Spiritual and Existential Practice

The Eastern meditation practices currently in use in the United States have derived primarily from traditional sources in Hinduism and Buddhism. Disengaging meditation from its Eastern roots as recommended by some authors (Benson & Proctor, 1984; Kabat-Zinn, 1990) may make this practice more appealing and acceptable within Western psychotherapy practice (Carrington, 1998; Shapiro & Walsh, 1984). However, leaving out the spiritual aspect of meditation practice may limit a full understanding of the potential of this practice (Benson & Proctor, 1984; Goldstein & Kornfeld, 1987). To the extent that spiritual experience is a universal human capacity, meditation has been proposed, and experienced by many, as a way to cultivate a sense of inner calm, harmony, and transcendence often associated with spiritual growth (O'Murchu, 1994). Meditation may accomplish this by providing a technique that "turns off" or "bypasses" cognitive processing of usual daily preoccupations and concerns, allowing access to these other aspects of being.

Each of the above models appears to have some merit, based on both research and clinical practice experience. Future research is needed to further clarify the mechanism and effective "active ingredients" of meditation.

MEDITATION TECHNIQUES IN CLINICAL PRACTICE

This section is devoted to the clinical application of meditation. As a global method of stress management, relaxation, and personal centering, we recommend meditation as a method to attain a balanced lifestyle. The topic of lifestyle balance (Marlatt, 1985) can be introduced early in the clinical process. Describe lifestyle balance as a global intervention designed to produce a sense of balance or harmony in one's daily habits and introduce a menu of activities with several options including meditation and exercise. Encourage clients to practice engaging in one or more of these activities throughout each week of therapy until they find the right balance between physical activities (exercise) and mental relaxation (meditation). Both exercise and meditation are described as potential "positive addictions" that can be practiced on a regular basis as a means of achieving greater harmony or balance in daily activities.

For clients who are new to meditation practice, we recommend beginning with instruction in a basic practice of concentrative meditation. After introducing the topic of meditation, the client engages in the technique for a 10-min supervised practice session (described below).

First, explore the client's prior conceptions and associations as well as any experiences with meditation. For those who have already learned a meditation practice, we discuss issues of implementation or possible barriers to regular practice. Newcomers to meditation may hold preconceptions of meditation that range from a romanticized view of it as a "magic" formula to a hostile defensive perception that it represents a foreign religious practice. It may also be seen as simply a relaxation method that has limited value for them. After exploring these beliefs and feelings, it may be useful to reframe meditative techniques as having their source in a wide range of cultural traditions. A common benefit is that meditation elicits both physical and psychological relaxation and fosters a "release" from the types of issues that brought the person to therapy. Using a metaphor that illustrates the idea of letting go or nonattachment can often be useful. For example, describe meditation as being similar to sitting on the bank of a swift-flowing river, observing the flow of the water as it passes by, without getting caught in either the past ("upstream" thoughts) or the future ("downstream" thoughts). Phrases such as finding "inner wisdom" or "inner peace" are relatively nonthreatening but capture a sense of the larger purpose involved.

After discussion and questions about meditation are completed, give the client instructions for a practice session in the office. Then ask the client to practice the technique on a daily basis at home between clinical sessions. Meditating with the client during the first practice session both provides a model and creates less self-consciousness for him or her. Have the client assume a comfortable sitting position, holding the back in a straight, upward position (either sitting in a straight chair with feet on the floor or on a cushion with legs folded). The rationale for this posture is to promote relaxed wakefulness rather than a relaxed state that easily descends into sleep. Eyes are closed or can be left in a half-open position with one's gaze facing ahead and slightly downward. Use variations of the following instructions while sitting in meditation along with the client:

First, take a few deep breaths and notice the flow of air as you inhale, then gently exhale, again noticing the physical sensations of your out-breath. . . . Throughout this time, your job is to pay close attention to your breathing, breath by breath. It is best to breathe in and out through your nose, unless it's more comfortable to breathe through your mouth. Allow your breathing to relax and gradually assume a natural pace and rhythm as you first inhale, then exhale, slowly and deeply. Pay close and deep attention to the physical sensations that accompany each inbreath and outbreath. Notice that your breath is cool as it flows in at the tip of your nose and warm as it flows out. Notice the precise and subtle sensations of your breath as it passes in and out of your nostrils. Notice the rising and falling of your chest or abdomen as you take each breath, one at a time. Be a relaxed but aware observer of your breathing process as it occurs naturally.

When you become distracted by events other than your breathing, such as thoughts that arise in your mind, sounds in the room, or feelings that occur in your body, first become aware that you are becoming distracted and then gently return your full attention once again to the breath and its rising and falling, in and out. Treat all distractions (external sounds or outside events) in the same gentle manner: First recognize that you are no longer paying attention to your breath and then gently but firmly turn your attention back to your breathing.

After giving the above instructions, continue the meditation practice session for about 10 min in silence. Initially, it maybe useful to briefly repeat the instructions related to becoming distracted and to remind the client that distraction is normal. A small bell or gong can be used to signal the end of the meditation period: "When you hear the sound of the gong ringing, move around gently, bring yourself back into the space of the room, and gently open your eyes whenever you feel ready to do so." Then take a few minutes to discuss the client's reactions and any questions about the experience. It is important to probe whether any particular feelings of uneasiness or discomfort occurred.

For clients who have difficulty maintaining a focus on the breath or for whom intrusive thoughts are a presenting part of their problem, using a mantra-focused concentrative meditation technique is often helpful. The term *mantra* may have undesirable connotations for some clients, either because it implies a "magical" effect or because it connotes an unfamiliar religious practice. Tell such clients that many meditation practices focus awareness on a specific object or event, including sounds, the breath, movement, and visual images, to calm and balance the mind. Rather than providing a specific mantra (a sound, word, or phrase), as is done in some formal meditation practices, we offer clients a range of possible sounds and words, asking them to choose the one that "feels right" or elicits associations of concentration and calmness. We recommend words such as "calm," "peace," "maa," and "alm," noting to the client that this last sound is the word *calm* with the harsh k sound removed, thereby emphasizing the value of the sound itself over the meaning of the word. The only type of word that we discourage is the name of a family member, such as a mother or spouse, explaining that a neutral word or sound might be more useful. For clients with even more difficulty concentrating, the simple counting of breaths (from 1 to 10, and over again) appears to be effective and acceptable.

Some clients may become disconcerted with feelings of dissociation; these are often related to the novel experience of holding the body extremely still, so that the normal proprioceptive feedback from joints does not occur. This sometimes results in a feeling of floating. Although this feeling can be enjoyable and may mark an ability to become more engaged in the meditation task, for others the experience may need to be explained and normalized. The experience of dissociation occasionally appears to be more psychological in nature, in which trancelike feelings are quickly attained or in which disturbing thoughts begin to flood the mind. It is difficult to predict with whom this may occur, although there is limited evidence, consistent with our experience, that individuals with histories of obsessive–compulsive disorder or past trauma may be more susceptible (Carrington, 1998). For example, a 35-year-old woman being seen by J.K. for smoking intervention secondary to debilitating lung disease, who had a history of severe childhood sexual abuse, found that meditating for even a few minutes was accompanied by a flood of unbearable thoughts and images related to this abuse. Although she had had a course of productive therapy earlier in adulthood, this experience with meditation led us to explore whether more therapy work was needed—and led her to realize that one of the ways she kept these thoughts blocked out was by smoking. In this case, she decided to return to her former therapist, with successful results. In another case, a woman with histrionic features appeared to respond well to meditation instruction at first, but after several weeks of practice, it became apparent that she was using meditation techniques to induce a trancelike dissociation that distanced her from dealing with some people and experiences around her. At one point she noted, "It's wonderful! I can be in the room with my husband and he's talking to me—and he doesn't even notice that I'm 'not there'!"

However, meditation can also be used productively by individuals who have histories of severe psychiatric disturbance. A 60-year-old man seen by one of us for debilitating anxiety and depression, with a history of mild obsessive–compulsive disorder, found that using meditation gave him "permission"—and the ability—to engage in "dialogues" between his "wise self" and himself as a 7-year-old boy. Although he did not find formal meditation practice appealing, a growing awareness and the use of these internal dialogues (although his report of them at times appeared somewhat dissociative) led to a growing confidence in himself and ability to resist almost tortuous fears. In another case seen by J.K., a young woman who had recurrent hospitalizations for paranoid schizophrenia was reluctantly allowed to join a stress management group in which meditation was introduced as the primary relaxation technique. She had no problems with dissociative experiences and was able to use the meditation practice to gain awareness of and distance from the paranoid ideas that she frequently experienced, noting that she stopped finding them as compelling and therefore could keep them from escalating as quickly and intruding on her behavior.

Ask clients to practice the meditation between clinical sessions, ideally on a twice-daily basis, once in the morning after arising and again in the late afternoon or early evening, for periods of 10–20 min at a time. Recommend a quiet place to meditate where the client can be relatively free of outside distractions. It is also helpful to begin each clinical session with a brief, 5-min meditation period, followed by a discussion of the client's progress in his or her meditation practice. In more structured group treatment, use of a meditation tape is often valuable and ensures a more uniform experience (Kabat-Zinn, 1990). However, weaning the individual off the tape can be a problem in maintaining practice.

After the client has become comfortable with the basics of concentrative meditation, usually after a week or two of regular practice, we introduce insight meditation as a means of coping with specific stressful events as they occur "on the spot." Here we explain to clients that the practice they have been learning, to focus awareness during concentrative meditation, can also be applied in the "here and now" as a specific coping strategy. As noted in the previous section, the focus of attention in insight meditation is on whatever is happening in the present moment, in the form of cognitive ideation, physical sensations or feelings, or any other event. Instead of attending only to the breath, we describe awareness as being similar to the beam of a flashlight, illuminating whatever exists in its path of light. The object here is to attend to "just what is," to see events clearly without the "excess baggage" of mental judgment or evaluation.

As an example of this insight meditation procedure, Marlatt (1994) developed the technique of "urge surfing" in the treatment of addictive behaviors. Designed as a relapse prevention method, the purpose of urge surfing is to help clients cope with craving or urges that otherwise might trigger a setback or lapse. Ask the client to first self-monitor any urges, cravings, or strong desires to engage in the target behavior (e.g., to ingest a substance or to engage in a high-risk sexual behavior). Encourage clients to identify the specific form that the urge takes when it occurs. Urges often take the form of a verbal intent or command, such as "I must smoke or I will go nuts" or "Just this once won't hurt me" or "Damn it! I OWE myself a drink after this!" Such verbal statements may or may not be accompanied by strong physical sensations or desire cravings. Such urge reactions often appear to take the form of classically conditioned responses, usually triggered by a cue or situation associated with the target behavior (e.g., a recent ex-smoker sees an open pack of cigarettes lying on the table). Contextual and environmental factors such as the client's mood and social environment may also elicit strong urges to indulge.

This method first arose in the course of working with a client who was trying to give up smoking. After he had quit for a week, he reported constant urges to smoke that felt like a growing ball of discomfort that was increasing in intensity to the point that he felt that he would "go crazy" unless he gave in. Recalling a prior account of his reputation as a surfer during his youth, the therapist asked, "What if you could see the craving in the form of a cresting wave instead of a growing ball?" We then discussed his experience as a budding surfer. He described how he learned to keep his balance as the ocean wave swelled up beneath his surfboard and he rode the wave as it finally crested and diminished in size. He learned to keep his balance without being "wiped out" by the wave. He agreed to transfer this surfing metaphor to his meditation practice. As soon as he experienced any indication of a rising urge in his thoughts or feelings, he would direct his full attention to this growing wave while keeping his balance until the wave gradually crested and subsided. Because many urges in fact take the form of conditioned responses elicited by trigger events, their duration and intensity do not necessarily last unless they are reinforced by engaging in a consummatory response (smoking or drinking). The client reported using this meditative urge surfing technique as an effective means of coping with cravings to smoke.

This use of focused but detached awareness can be applied as a means of coping with other cognitive and physiological aspects of behavioral problems. One client seen by J.K. reported successfully coping with compulsive thoughts that would otherwise trigger an episode of binge eating. When she applied the insight meditation technique to observe her own thoughts before a binge, she described them as the thoughts of a "dictator" who ordered her what to do next. The voice dictated to her, "You must eat more cookies until you have finished the entire box!" Instead of just giving in to this dictating thought, she began to label it as "just a thought." By standing back and objectively observing her own thoughts, she found a space in which she did not have to obey the command.

Another characteristic of disordered eating that responds well to insight meditation are experiences of overwhelming hunger, especially those triggered by emotions or situations such as seeing a well-liked food. Again, this is a way in which conditioned response eating can be curtailed by simply noting the feeling, staying aware of it, and keeping in mind that it is "just a feeling." Women with binge eating disorders substantially decreased the frequency and intensity of bingeing while increasing their sense of mindful control around food during a 6-week treatment program that introduced them to meditation and mindful eating (Kristeller & Hallett, in press). Similar successes were reported by clients with panic attacks who participated in the mindfulness meditation program at the University of Massachusetts Medical Center (Kabat-Zinn et al., 1992). They found that over the course of the 8 weeks, mild anxiety reactions that had previously developed into full-blown attacks were curtailed because, by simply noting and watching these milder symptoms rather than "panicking," they were able to keep them at a reduced level and continue with their normal activities.

EVALUATING THE EFFECTIVENESS OF MEDITATION

Understanding the mechanisms related to the clinical application of meditation first began to draw considerable attention in the 1970s, both spurring and being associated with an increasing interest in applying contemporary psychological research methods to understand the relationship between mind and body (Shapiro & Walsh, 1984). The area that has received the most research attention is the impact of meditation practice on stress responses related to anxiety or physiological distress. Systematic study of experienced practitioners documented the hypometabolic effects of meditation practice (Green, Green, & Walters, 1970, Wallace, Benson, & Wilson, 1971); studies of novice meditators using either TM for the Benson-modified version (Benson & Proctor, 1984) suggested that reductions in autonomic nervous system activity could be reliably and easily maintained (Wallace & Benson, 1972). A study carried out by Cuthbert, Kristeller, Simons, and Lang (1981) established that individuals previously unfamiliar with meditation could use it more effectively than biofeedback to lower their heart rates. This area of research therefore successfully demonstrated the value of simple meditation techniques in assisting individuals to gain a state of increased relaxation. However, certain studies that compared meditation techniques with other types of relaxation (Pagano, Rose, Stivers, & Warrenberg, 1976) called into question the uniqueness of these effects.

Researchers also began to explore whether there were unique effects that could be identified at the level of neurological functioning (Delmonte, 1984). Some researchers continued to use a "relaxation" model, measuring shifts in dominant brain wave activity consistent with a more relaxed state, but other researchers began to investigate more sophisticated models exploring laterality effects that were proposed to be related to achieving "altered states of consciousness." Ley and Smylie (1989) provided a critical review of this literature as based on overly simplistic models and understanding of neurological functioning. Given that the understanding and technology of studying brain functioning has improved tremendously in the past 20 years, there may now be more opportunity to gain insight into the specific effects of meditation practice. A detailed review of research findings on the effects of meditation on general metabolic and autonomic functioning has been provided by Shapiro and Walsh (1984).

Meditation has also been applied to the prevention and treatment of addictive behaviors. A recent review of research on the effectiveness of transcendental meditation with alcohol and drug problems documents the overall success of this approach (O'Connell & Alexander, 1994). In a well-compiled meta-analysis of this literature (Alexander, Robinson, & Rainforth, 1994), the authors concluded that use of TM and other meditative methods are highly effective interventions for alcoholism, smoking, and illicit drug use. Although they reviewed a wide range of studies using a variety of research designs, including randomized experimental trials, they also concluded that future researchers need to include more severely addicted users and larger sample sizes.

Mindfulness meditation has also been described as a treatment for alcohol and drug problems. The implications of Buddhist psychology and mindfulness meditation for addiction treatment have been discussed by Groves and Farmer (1994). The effectiveness of this approach, along with a description of various clinical applications of mindfulness and acceptance in addiction treatment, has been discussed by Marlatt (1994). Meditation has also been found to be an effective intervention for reducing excessive drinking and alcohol problems in young-adult drinkers (Marlatt & Marques, 1977).

A group mindfulness meditation course lasting 8 weeks has been shown to be effective in the treatment of chronic pain (Kabat-Zinn, 1982; Kabat-Zinn, Lepworth, & Burney, 1986). The intensive insight meditation training program described by Kabat-Zinn (1990) has also been applied successfully in the treatment of anxiety disorders (Kabat-Zinn et al., 1992). In this study, using an extended baseline design, 20 of 22 participants who met standard diagnostic criteria for panic or anxiety disorders reduced the frequency of panic attacks to minimal levels and their self-reported anxiety into the normal range. These results were sustained after several months' follow-up. Although these results are clinically impressive, a randomized clinical trial testing this type of intervention is still needed.

Substantial research currently in progress may shed more light on the effectiveness of meditation techniques in other populations. Zen meditation and perspectives have influenced the development of dialetical behavior therapy in the treatment of borderline personality disorder (Linehan, 1993). Ongoing studies applying meditation in the treatment of depression (Teasdale, 1997) will provide further information about the effectiveness of this procedure. Another area that is in need of systematic attention from a research perspective is the effect of meditation on spiritual experience. Although innumerable personal accounts exist regarding the positive impact of meditation on the ability to experience meaning, gain a sense of transcendence, and feelings of peace, these dimensions have generally not been systematically measured and evaluated in practicing meditators. Systematically examining the relationship between meditation practice, spirituality, and therapeutic healing therefore remains one of the most significant opportunities in this area. Measures of spirituality are becoming available (e.g., Kass, Friedman, Lesserman, Zuttermeister, & Benson, 1991). This, then, is one of the foremost challenges for future understanding of how meditation as part of the therapeutic process relates to spiritual growth and development.

REFERENCES

Alexander, C. N., Robinson, P., & Rainforth, M. (1994). Treating and preventing alcohol, nicotine, and drug abuse through transcendental meditation: A review and statistical meta-analysis. In D. F. O'Connell & C. N. Alexander (Eds.), *Self recovery: Treating addictions using transcendental meditation and Maharishi Ayur-Veda* (pp. 13–87). New York: Haworth Press.

Beck, A. T., Wright, F. D., Newman, C. F., & Liese, B. S. (1993). *Cognitive therapy of substance abuse.* New York: Guilford Press.

Benson, H., & Proctor, W. (1984). *Beyond the relaxation response*. New York: Putnam/Berkeley.

Bennett, J. E., & Trinder, J. (1984). Hemispheric laterality and cognitive style associated with transcendental meditation. In D. H. Shapiro, Jr., & R. N. Walsh (Eds.), *Meditation: Classic and contemporary perspectives* (pp. 506–509). New York: Aldine.

Carrington, P. (1998). *The book of meditation*. Boston: Element Books.

Carrington, P. (1979). *Clinical standardized meditation*. Kendall Park, NJ: Pace Educational Systems.

Cuthbert, B., Kristeller, J. L., Simons, R., & Lang, P. J. (1981). Strategies of arousal control: Biofeedback, meditation, and motivation. *Journal of Experimental Psychology: General, 110*, 518–546.

Deikman, A. J. (1982). *The observing self*. Boston: Beacon Press.

Delmonte, M. M. (1984). Electrocortical activity and related phenomena associated with meditation practice: A literature review. *International Journal of Neuroscience, 24*(3–4), 581–582.

Epstein, M. (1996). *Thoughts without a thinker: Psychotherapy from a Buddhist perspective*. New York: Basic Books.

Glasser, W. (1976). *Positive addictions*. New York: Harper & Row.

Goldstein, J., & Kornfield, J. (1987). *Seeking the heart of wisdom: The path of insight meditation*. Boston: Shambhala.

Goleman, D. (1971). Meditation as meta-therapy. *Journal of Transpersonal Psychology, 3*, 1–25.

Goleman, D. (1977). *The varieties of meditative experience*. New York: Irvington.

Goleman, D., & Schwartz, G. E. (1984). Meditation as an intervention in stress reactivity. In D. H. Shapiro, Jr., & R. N. Walsh (Eds.), *Meditation: Classic and contemporary perspectives* (pp. 77–88). New York: Aldine.

Glueck, B. C., & Stroebel, C. F. (1984). Psychophysiological correlates of meditation: EEG changes during meditation. In D. H. Shapiro, Jr., & R. N. Walsh (Eds.), *Meditation: Classic and contemporary perspectives* (pp. 519–524). New York: Aldine.

Green, E. E., Green, A. M., & Walters, E. D. (1970). Voluntary control of internatial states: Psychological and physiological. *Journal of Transpersonal Psychology, 9*(1), 1–26.

Groves, P., & Farmer, R. (1994). Buddhism and addiction. *Addiction Research, 2*, 183–194.

Huxley, A. (1944). *Perennial philosophy*. New York: Harper & Row.

Kabat-Zinn, J. (1982). An outpatient program in behavioral medicine for chronic pain patients based on the practice of mindfulness meditation: Theoretical considerations and preliminary results. *General Hospital Psychiatry, 4*, 33–42.

Kabat-Zinn, J. (1990). *Full catastrophe living*. New York: Delacorte.

Kabat-Zinn, J., Lipworth, L., & Burney, R. (1986). The clinical use of mindfulness meditation for the self-regulation of chronic pain. *Journal of Behavioral Medicine, 8*, 163–190.

Kabat-Zinn, J., Massion, A., Kristeller, J., Peterson, L. G., Fletcher, K. E., Pbert, L., Lenderking, W. R., & Santorelli, S. F. (1992). Effectiveness of a meditation-based stress reduction intervention in the treatment of anxiety disorders. *American Journal of Psychiatry, 149*, 936–943.

Kasamatsu, A., & Hirai, T. (1966). An electroencephalographic study of Zen meditation (Zazen). *Folia Psychiataria el Neurologica Japonica, 20*, 315–336.

Kass, J. D., Friedman, R., Lesserman, J., Zuttermeister, P. C., & Benson, H. (1991). Health outcomes and a new index of spiritual experience. *Journal for the Scientific Study of Religion, 30*, 203–211.

Kristeller, J. L., & Hallet, B. (in press). An exploratory study of a meditation-based intervention for binge eating disorder. *Journal of Health Psychology.*

Langer, E. (1989). *Mindfulness.* Reading, MA: Addison-Wesley.

Levine, S. (1979). *A gradual awakening.* Garden City, NY: Anchor/Doubleday.

Ley, R. G., & Smylie, M. (1989). Cerebral laterality: Implications of Eastern and Western therapies. In A. A. Sheikh & K. S. Sheikh (Eds.), *Eastern and Western approaches to healing* (pp. 325–343). New York: Wiley.

Linehan, M. M. (1993). *Cognitive–behavioral treatment of borderline personality disorder.* New York: Guilford Press.

Marlatt, G. A. (1985). Lifestyle modification. In G. A. Marlatt & J. R. Gordon (Eds.), *Relapse prevention: Maintenance strategies in the treatment of addictive behaviors* (pp. 280–349). New York: Guilford Press.

Marlatt, G. A. (1994). Addiction, mindfulness, and acceptance. In S. C. Hayes, N. S. Jacobson, V. M. Follette, & M. J. Dougher (Eds.), *Acceptance and change: content and context in psychotherapy* (pp. 175–197). Reno, NV: Context Press.

Marlatt, G. A., & Marques, J. K. (1977). Meditation, self control, and alcohol use. In R. B. Stuart (Ed.), *Behavioral self-management: Strategies, techniques, and outcomes* (pp. 117–153). New York: Brunner/Mazel.

O'Connell, D. F., & Alexander, C. N. (1994). *Self recovery: Treating addictions using transcendental meditation and Maharishi Ayur-Veda.* New York: Haworth Press.

O'Murchu, D. (1994). Spirituality, recovery and transcendental meditation. In D. F. O'Connell & C. N. Alexander (Eds.), *Self recovery: Treating addictions using transcendental meditation and Maharishi Ayur-Veda* (pp. 169–184). New York: Haworth Press.

Orme-Johnson, D. W. (1984). Autonomic stability and transcendental meditation. In D. H. Shapiro, Jr., & R. N. Walsh (Eds.), *Meditation: Classic and contemporary perspectives* (pp. 432–439). New York: Aldine.

Ornstein, R. E. (1972). *The psychology of consciousness.* NewYork: Viking Press.

Pagano, R. R., & Frumkin, L. R. (1984). The effect of transcendental meditation on right hemispheric functioning. In D. H. Shapiro, Jr., & R. N. Walsh (Eds.), *Meditation: Classic and contemporary perspectives* (pp. 510–518). New York: Aldine.

Pagano, R. R., Rose, R. M., Stivers, R., & Warrenberg, S. (1976). Sleep during transcendental meditation. *Science, 101,* 300–310.

Shapiro, D. H., Jr., & Walsh, R. N. (Eds.). (1984). *Meditation: Classic and contemporary perspectives.* New York: Aldine.

Smith, J. C. (1975). Meditation as psychotherapy: A review of the literature. *Psychological Bulletin, 82,* 558–564.

Snelling, J. (1991). *The Buddhist handbook.* Rochester, VT: Inner Traditions.

Sogyal, S. (1992). *The Tibetan book of living and dying.* New York: Harper & Row.

Teasdale, J. D. (1997, July). *Preventing depressive relapse.* Paper presented at the 25th Annual Conference of the British Association of Behavior and Cognitive Therapy, Canterbury, England.

Teasdale, J. D., Segal, Z., & Williams, J. M. G. (1995). How does cognitive therapy prevent depressive relapse and why should attentional control (mindfulness) training help? *Behavior Research and Therapy, 33,* 25–39.

Wallace, R. K., & Benson, H. (1972). The physiology of meditation. *Scientific American, 226,* 84–90.

Wallace, R. K., Benson, H., & Wilson, A. F. (1971). A wakeful hypometabolic physiological state. *American Journal of Physiology, 221,* 795–799.

Wallace, R. K., Benson, H., & Wilson A. F. (1984). A wakeful hypometabolic physiologic state. In D. H. Shapiro, Jr., & R. N. Walsh (Eds.), *Meditation: Classic and contemporary perspectives* (pp. 417–431). New York: Aldine.

Walsh, R. (1996). Toward a synthesis of Eastern and Western psychologies. In A. A. Sheikh & K. S. Sheikh (Eds.), *Healing East and West* (pp. 542–555). New York: Wiley.

5

PRAYER

MICHAEL E. McCULLOUGH AND DAVID B. LARSON

On one side, prayer is our capacity to enter into that vast community of life in which self and other, human and nonhuman, visible and invisible, are intricately intertwined. While my senses discriminate and my mind dissects, my prayer acknowledges and recreates [sic] the unity of life. In prayer, I no longer set myself apart from others and the world, manipulating them to suit my needs. Instead, I reach for relationship, allow myself to feel the tuggings of mutuality and accountability, take my place in community by knowing the transcendent center that connects it all. On the other side, prayer means opening myself to the fact that as I reach for that connecting center, the center is reaching for me. (Palmer, 1983, p. 11)

Nationally representative surveys have demonstrated that in the United States, most people pray, and many pray frequently. A 1993 Gallup survey (Gallup Organization, 1993) showed that 90% of Americans pray at least occasionally. Of the people who do pray, most people prefer to pray silently rather than aloud and alone rather than with others. A large majority of the population (97%) believe that prayers are heard, believe that their prayers have been answered on occasion, and believe that prayer makes them better people (86%). Furthermore, most people (77%) are satisfied with their prayer life.

Many people use prayer to help them cope with life's problems (Bearon & Koenig, 1990; Ellison & Taylor, 1996; Gurin, Veroff, & Feld, 1960; Neser, Husaini, Linn, & Whitten-Stovall, 1989) and medical problems such as HIV (Kaplan, Marks, & Mertens, 1997), cancer (Potts, 1996; Sodestrom & Martinson, 1987), sickle cell disease (Ohaeri, Shokunbi, Akinlade, & Dare, 1995), cystic fibrosis (Stern, Canda, & Doershuk, 1992), arthritis (Cronan, Kaplan, Posner, Blumberg, & Kozin, 1989), renal transplant surgery (Sutton & Murphy, 1989), and cardiac surgery (Saudia, Kinney, Brown, & Young-Ward, 1991). People frequently use prayer to cope

This chapter was prepared in part through the generosity of the John Templeton Foundation.

with natural (Harvey, Stein, Olsen, & Roberts, 1995) and unnatural (Zeidner, 1993) disasters.

Older adults in particular seem to use prayer regularly as a technique for dealing with many of the concerns that become salient as one ages, such as relocation to nursing facilities (Armer, 1994), fears about death and dying (Fry, 1990), widowhood (Gass, 1987), and health problems (Bearon & Koenig, 1990; Conway, 1985–1986). Indeed, some national surveys suggest that older adults use prayer for coping with life's problems more than do younger adults (Gurin et al., 1960; cf. Ellison & Taylor, 1996).

Prayer is also an important coping resource for caregivers such as nurses (Sodestrom & Martinson, 1987), hospice workers (Schneider & Kastenbaum, 1993), spouses of patients with Alzheimer's disease (Kaye & Robinson, 1994), parents of children with disabilities (Leyser, 1994), and family members of patients with dementia (Segall & Wykle, 1988–1989).

PRAYER IS BOTH RELIGIOUS AND SPIRITUAL

In nearly every religion, prayer is perhaps the most ubiquitous, essential, and personal of religious experiences. Friedrich Heiler, one of the most astute scholars on the psychology of prayer, wrote that it is

> not in dogmas and institutions, not in rites and ethical ideals, but in prayer do we grasp the peculiar quality of the religious life. In the words of a prayer we can penetrate into the deepest and most intimate movements of the religious soul. (Heiler, 1918/1932, p. xv)

Even though prayer is central to religion and religious experience, it is also profoundly spiritual. Even when stripped away from traditional religious frameworks, prayer represents one of the core elements of spirituality—prayer is thoughts, attitudes, and actions designed to express or experience connection to the sacred. Even though Heiler (1918/1932) recognized prayer as a religious phenomenon, he also realized the essentially spiritual functions of prayer, writing that "prayer is the expression of a primitive impulse to a higher, richer, intenser life" (p. 355).

In this chapter we hope to offer clinicians an expanded understanding of this deeply religious, deeply spiritual phenomenon. The chapter is designed to (a) summarize basic social–psychological findings regarding the use of prayer in the general population; (b) review the quantitative empirical research on the relationship between various aspects of prayer (including frequency of prayer, use of prayer for coping with stress, and types of prayer) and various measures of mental health and well-being; and (c) recommend how practitioners might assess, discuss, and possibly encourage prayer in their work with clients. Although the subject of the chapter—prayer—is the means to the ultimate goal of connecting people to something that is transcendent and superempirical, our chapter is, in large part, grounded in the assumption that we can learn much about prayer by examining the quantitative empirical research on how it operates in people's lives.[1]

WHO PRAYS? WHEN DO THEY PRAY?

Although most people pray at least occasionally, not everyone prays with the same frequency. As one might expect, the demographic predictors of prayer behavior are also predictors of general religious involvement. It is well established across many cultures that women are more involved in their religions than are men (Argyle & Beit-Hallami, 1975; P. L. Benson, Donahue, & Erickson, 1989). Similarly, women tend to pray more frequently than do men (Husaini, Moore, & Cain, 1994; Poloma & Gallup, 1991; Taylor & Chatters, 1991; cf. Sered, 1987). Women also report a greater likelihood of praying in a reflective, meditative fashion and experiencing deeper religious experiences during prayer than do men (Gallup Organization, 1993; Poloma & Gallup, 1991).

Racial–ethnic groups also differ on measures of general religiousness and prayer. White people appear to be the least religious demographic group in America (Taylor, Chatters, Jayakody, & Levin, 1996). As one might expect, the percentage of White people who pray is slightly smaller (87%–90%) than the percentage of non-White people who pray (90%–95%; Gallup Organization, 1993; Poloma & Gallup, 1991). In a reanalysis of four nationally representative data sets, Taylor et al. (1996) demonstrated that across several single-item measures of religious involvement (including frequency of church attendance, devotional reading, watching religious TV programming, personal importance of one's religious beliefs, and self-rated closeness to God), Black Americans were much more religious than White Americans. The Black–White differences in the frequency of private prayer followed the same pattern: After adjustments for covariates, the frequency with which Black Americans prayed was slightly higher than the frequency with which White Americans prayed. Non-White Americans also experienced more satisfaction with their prayer lives, more frequently used prayer books when praying, more frequently asked for material things when praying (Gallup Organization, 1993), and

---

[1]There is some apparent irony here. The quotation from Palmer's (1983) book with which we began this article suggests that prayer is essentially about recognition of the unity of life. Scientific research (as usually conducted in the quantitative mode) is about observing regularities in the world with the assumption that the subject and observer are distinct, separate, unrelated. However, science is ultimately about discovering the true nature of things. Science and spirituality both share that goal, even though their methods differ sharply. We do not intend to defend an epistemology here, but to report on what we can learn about prayer from existing empirical research.

reported using prayer as a problem-solving strategy more than did White Americans (Neser et al., 1989).

Older adults also appear to be more generically religious than young adults (Levin, Chatters, & Taylor, 1995). As one might expect, older adults also appear to pray more frequently than do younger people (Chatters & Taylor, 1989; Gallup Organization, 1993; Poloma & Gallup, 1991).

Personality Correlates

In the past few years, researchers have begun to investigate the relationship between prayer and psychological traits, such as locus of control (D. G. Richards, 1990, 1991) and obsessionality (Lewis & Maltby, 1995). Some of the most interesting research on the relationship between personality traits and prayer has related to the extraversion–introversion, neuroticism, and psychoticism factors hypothesized by Eysenck and Eysenck (1976) to be the basic traits intrinsic to the human personality (Francis & Astley, 1996; Francis & Wilcox, 1994, 1996; Lewis & Maltby, 1996; Maltby, 1995; Smith, 1996).

In general, extraversion–introversion and neuroticism appear to be unrelated to the frequency of church attendance or private prayer. However, the results of many studies (Francis & Wilcox, 1994, 1996; Lewis & Maltby, 1996; Maltby, 1995; Smith, 1996) indicate that people lower in psychoticism pray more frequently than do people higher in psychoticism. Psychoticism is a variable that Eysenck associated with impulsivity, egocentricity, and sensation seeking on one hand and lack of empathy and conscience on the other (Eysenck & Gudjonsson, 1989). People who are high in psychoticism are likely to have antisocial characteristics (e.g., cruelty toward others and criminal behavior). Conversely, people who are low in psychoticism (who are generally more religious and more frequently pray) are characterized as thoughtful, empathic, and tender-minded.

Prayer as a Function of Problem Severity

People use prayer as a coping resource more frequently when their problems are more severe, intractable, or unresponsive to conventional interventions (Brown, 1966; Ellison & Taylor, 1996; H. M. Hill, Hawkins, Raposo, & Carr, 1995; Lindenthal, Myers, Pepper, & Stern, 1970). For example, H. M. Hill et al. (1995) found that mothers who lived in areas of high community violence coped differently with community violence than did those mothers who lived in areas with lower levels of community violence. In particular, mothers in low-violence areas used activism to cope more frequently than did mothers in high-violence areas. Conversely, mothers in high-violence areas were more inclined to use prayer to cope than were mothers in low-violence areas.

The relationship between problem severity and prayer seems to extend to health-related stressors as well. In a national sample of African American adults, Neighbors, Jackson, Bowman, and Gurin (1983) surveyed respondents regarding (a) their most stressful life circumstance ever and (b) the strategies that they used to cope with them. Neighbors et al. found that as the severity of the most severe lifetime stressor increased, respondents' self-reported use of prayer for coping with the stressor also increased. Other researchers have found that mothers pray more frequently to cope with more difficult pregnancies than with easier ones (Levin, Lyons, & Larson, 1993) and that people pray more for symptoms that require medication or discussion with physicians than those who do not (Bearon & Koenig, 1990). Thus, the fact that people are most likely to pray when their needs are greatest appears to be a robust human phenomenon that extends across a wide variety of stressful human circumstances.

FREQUENCY OF PRAYER: ASSOCIATIONS WITH WELL-BEING

Some researchers have observed that measures of the frequency with which people pray have had some interesting, but frequently complicated, relationships with measures of health and well-being (McCullough, 1995). For example, frequency of prayer was found to be positively correlated with purpose in life and amount of alcohol consumed among recovering alcoholic individuals (Carroll, 1993; Walker, Tonigan, Miller, Comer, & Kahlich, 1997) but not with purpose in life in a sample of community-dwelling adults (D. G. Richards, 1990). In longitudinal research, the frequency of prayer has been found to be positively correlated with life satisfaction at some time points but not at others (Markides, 1983; Markides, Levin, & Ray, 1987). Frequency of prayer has been positively related to marital adjustment (Gruner, 1985), general life satisfaction, existential well-being, religious satisfaction (Poloma & Pendleton, 1989, 1991), lower delinquency, and more positive attitudes toward school among children and adolescents (Francis, 1992; Long & Boik, 1993; Montgomery & Francis, 1996) as well as reduced fear of death among older adults (Koenig, 1988).

However, frequency of prayer has also been found to be unrelated to negative affect and happiness (Poloma & Pendleton, 1989, 1991), loneliness (D. P. Johnson & Mullins, 1989), rate of anxiety disorders (Koenig, George, Blazer, Pritchett, & Meador, 1993), self-esteem in schoolchildren (Francis & Gibbs, 1996), and depression (Koenig, Hays, George, & Blazer, 1997). Finally, other studies have shown that frequency of prayer was positively related to depression (Ellison, 1995) and poor physical health (Koenig et al., 1997).

The mixed bag of findings regarding the relationship of frequency of prayer to health outcomes is puzzling, but it might be attributable to any of several methodological and substantive explanations. The first set of explanations refers to psychometric artifacts. First, the inconsistency in this group of studies could be (in part) an artifact of sampling error, which depends on the size of the samples in individual studies (Hunter & Schmidt, 1994).

A second artifact that could explain the variation in these findings is that single-item measures, such as those that are almost always used to measure frequency of prayer, are notoriously unreliable. Unreliability of measurement attenuates relationships between two variables (Shadish & Haddock, 1994), and the effects of unreliability of measurement become more complex in multivariate studies. Were the studies on frequency of prayer and health corrected for unreliability of the single-item prayer measures, we might see changes in the pattern of findings, with positive (but nonsignificant) findings becoming more positive and negative (but nonsignificant) findings becoming more negative (Schmidt & Hunter, 1996).

A third artifact that could explain the variation in the findings is the differing degrees of statistical control in these studies. Many of the studies cited above did not control the relationship between health and frequency of prayer for demographic, psychosocial, or other religious variables (e.g., Gruner, 1985; D. G. Richards, 1990). Other studies exerted a high degree of statistical control over the relationship between frequency of prayer and health variables, some even controlling for other measures of religiousness (e.g., Koenig, 1988; Koenig et al., 1997). Differences in the degree of statistical control exerted on the prayer–health relationship might influence the results considerably, as has been found in research on religious involvement and mortality (McCullough, Larson, Hoyt, Koenig, & Thoreson, 1999).

Two other possible explanations for these inconsistencies among the studies of frequency of prayer and health are more substantive in nature. The first and most obvious of these is that frequency of prayer may simply be positively related to certain measures of health and well-being but negatively related or unrelated to others. The research lacks sufficient replications to allow us to know for certain. Second, the studies on frequency of prayer and health have used a variety of populations (e.g., schoolchildren, community-dwelling adults, recovering alcoholic individuals, and older adults). It is also possible that the relationship between frequency of prayer and health changes across the life span and across populations (see McCullough & Larson, 1998).

PRAYER AS A STRESS BUFFER: ASSOCIATIONS WITH WELL-BEING

Along with basic research on the associations of frequency of prayer with various indexes of well-being, several researchers have examined the efficacy of prayer as a coping resource for people who are undergoing stressful life events. Pargament's (1997) excellent review of this literature suggests that frequent prayer (measured with single-item measures of frequency of prayer) appears in some studies to be a stress deterrent (i.e., it averts high levels of stress). In other studies, frequent prayer appears to act as a stress buffer (i.e., it averts the negative effects of stress on measures of physical or mental health). In either case, it appears that people who pray frequently are less likely than people who pray infrequently to encounter psychological or physical illness and impairment in the aftermath of serious life stressors.

However, evidence from Pargament (Brant & Pargament, 1995; Pargament et al., 1990, 1994; Pargament, Smith, & Brant, 1995) suggests that the value of frequent prayer in deterring stress or buffering people against the effects of stress is outstripped by people's more general styles of using their religion to cope with stress (Pargament, 1997). After controlling for people's general styles of religious coping, the effect of frequent prayer on measures of health and well-being for people encountering potentially stressful life events typically disappears.

What seems most important, then, is whether people engage in styles of religious coping (e.g., seeking spiritual support, seeking congregational support, and collaborative religious coping) that have beneficial effects on health and well-being more generally, or potentially harmful styles of religious coping (e.g., discontent with God or one's congregation, viewing one's problems as punishment from God) that have negative effects on health and well-being, rather than the frequency with which they pray. If Pargament is correct, then one must know what type of prayer people use, not simply how frequently they pray, to understand how prayer is linked with indexes of well-being.

TYPES OF PRAYER: ASSOCIATIONS WITH WELL-BEING

Prayer exists in many varieties. D. G. Richards (1991) found that in a group of 345 "spiritual seekers," the most frequent subjects of private prayer were "guidance for self," followed by "healing for others," "thanksgiving," and "protection for others." "Healing for self," "praise of God," and "prayer to be of service" were also frequent themes for both church attenders and nonattenders. To categorize the many different varieties of prayer people use, scholars have developed typologies for the various forms of prayer. For example, Foster (1992) identified 21 types of prayer (including simple prayer, prayer of examen, prayer of relinquishment, covenant prayer, and contemplative prayer) from the Christian tradition. On the other extreme, Heiler (1918/1932) proposed a typology consisting of nine types of prayer, including naïve prayer, ritual prayer, the hymn, and prayer in public worship). In Heider's typology, these nine types could be divided into two classes of prayer. *Primary prayer* is nonrational and emotional. Primary prayer expresses original, profound spiritual experiences. *Secondary prayer* is derivative of spiritual experience but is not authentically spiritual in Heider's view. It is rational, abstract, and highly intellectualized.

In a sort of compromise position between Foster's (1992) 21 types of prayer and Heiler's (1918/1932) two broad classes of prayer, Poloma and Pendleton (1989, 1991) developed a complex but manageable typology of prayer. They developed measures of four basic types of prayer: (a) meditative prayer (e.g., worshiping and adoring God, reflecting on the Bible); (b) ritualistic prayer (e.g., reading from a book of prayers); (c) petitionary prayer (e.g., asking God for things for oneself or others); and (d) colloquial prayer (e.g., thanking God, asking God for guidance, etc.).

Poloma and Pendleton (1989, 1991) administered the multi-item measures of these four types of prayer to a random sample of 560 residents of Akron, Ohio, in the 1985 Akron Area Survey (AAS). Along with the measures of prayer, Poloma and Pendleton collected sociodemographic data, data on other aspects of participants' religious involvement, and measures of subjective well-being. In the following pages, we review the research on types of prayer and measures of well-being using the typology of prayer developed by Poloma and Pendleton (1989, 1991). However, we make one modification: In Poloma and Pendleton's typology, intercessory prayer (or praying for others) is an aspect of petitionary prayer. However, we review research on intercessory prayer on its own terms.

CONTEMPLATIVE-MEDITATIVE PRAYER

What Is It?

As with all of the five types of prayer that we discuss, there is no broadly accepted definition of contemplative-meditative prayer. However, contemplative-meditative prayer generally involves an intimate and personal relationship with the divine and includes components such as "being in the presence of God" (Poloma & Pendleton, 1989). It also typically involves a nonanalytical focus of attention, transcending words and images because of the inadequacy of such cognitions to capture the divine (Finney, 1984). Meditative-contemplative prayer appears to reflect the styles of religious coping (e.g., seeking spiritual support, spiritual support) that Pargament, Koenig, and Perez (1998) found to be positively related to growth in the aftermath of a stressful life event.

Links With Health and Well-Being

In the 1985 AAS, Poloma and Pendleton's (1989, 1991) five-item measure of meditative prayer was positively associated with life satisfaction ($r = .15$), existential well-being ($r = .32$), happiness ($r = .16$), and religious satisfaction ($r = .58$). Meditative prayer was also slightly correlated with negative affect ($r = .07$); however, this correlation was not reliably different from zero. After controlling for a series of demographics and other prayer measures, meditative prayer predicted unique variance in existential well-being ($\beta = .16$) and religious satisfaction ($\beta = .33$). Thus, among measures of prayer, the use of meditative-contemplative practices might be directly related to existential and religious well-being.

When used as an intervention, contemplative-meditative prayer might facilitate positive changes in psychological symptoms. In an uncontrolled study, Finney and Malony (1985a) found that the combination of standard psychotherapy and contemplative prayer outside the sessions produced substantial reductions in target symptoms among seven psychotherapy patients. Griffith, Mahy, and Young (1986) found that an elaborate, 5-day ritual called *mourning* in the Barbadian Spiritual Baptist Church (involving seclusion, limited food intake, and extended periods of prayer and mystical experiences) led to pre–post reductions on every subscale of the SCL-90 except the Somatization subscale. In particular, respondents were more than a 1 SD ($d = 1.16$) lower in depressive symptoms and ($d = .76$) lower in anxiety symptoms after the mourning experience. Carlson, Bacaseta, and Simanton (1988) also found that Christian college students who participated in six sessions of devotional meditative prayer (involving quiet reflective reading of Christian scriptures and responsive prayer) experienced significantly greater reductions in muscle tension, anger, and anxiety than did students who participated in six sessions of progressive relaxation or a control condition.

RITUAL PRAYER

What Is It?

Ritual prayer involves the repetition of prayers from written material or from memory (Poloma & Pendleton, 1989). It is not clear whether ritual prayer reflects a positive or negative style of religious coping using the categories of Pargament et al. (1998). However, preliminary evidence suggests that ritual prayer might be associated with slightly lower well-being.

Links With Health and Well-Being

In the AAS, ritual prayer was measured with a two-item scale. This measure had near-zero correlations with life satisfaction ($r = .05$) and happiness ($r = .02$). It was positively and significantly correlated with existential well-being ($r = .14$), negative affect ($r = .15$), and religious satisfaction ($r = .22$). After controlling for demographics and other measures of prayer, people's use of ritual prayer had near-zero correlations with all five measures of well-being except negative affectivity. The net relationship of ritual prayer and negative affectivity was positive ($\beta = .14$), suggesting that people who engaged in frequent ritual prayer had higher levels of negative affectivity.

PETITIONARY PRAYER

What Is It?

Petitionary prayer involves asking God to meet the specific needs of oneself or one's significant others (Poloma & Pendleton, 1989). Asking God to provide for one's needs is typically identified as one of the most elementary and earliest developed forms of prayer (Paloutzian, 1996). As one element in one's overall prayer life, petitionary prayer is probably indicative of positive religious and spiritual functioning; however, if one relies exclusively on petitionary prayer for coping, it is likely to reflect "pleading for direct intercession," which Pargament et al. (1998) identified as a marker for psychosocial distress in the aftermath of a negative life event.

Links With Well-Being

This appraisal of the links between petitionary prayer and well-being is also supported by the research of Poloma and Pendleton (1989, 1991). In the AAS, petitionary prayer was measured with a two-item scale. The frequency with which people used petitionary prayer was positively related to their life satisfaction ($r = .09$), existential well-being ($r = .12$), negative affect ($r = .09$), and religious satisfaction ($r = .22$). It was positively correlated with happiness ($r = .07$), although this relationship was not significantly different from zero. After controlling for the effects of sociodemographics and all other measures of prayer, the use of petitionary prayer was not uniquely related to any of the five measures of well-being.

Another perspective on the links of petitionary prayer to well-being comes from a series of studies indicating that chronic pain sufferers who pray for relief of their pain actually reported greater pain and poorer adjustment to their pain (see McCullough, 1995, for an earlier review). These findings come from a group of studies that have used the Coping Strategies Questionnaire (CSQ) to evaluate chronic pain patients' self-reported methods for coping with their pain. One of the subscales on the CSQ, Praying and Hoping, is a six-item subscale that includes three religious items, of which two are specifically related to prayer (e.g., "I pray to God [that the pain] won't last long") and three items related to hoping or having faith that doctors or other health care providers will eventually find a remedy for the pain (Rosenstiel & Keefe, 1983). On the basis of factor-analytic investigations of the CSQ, other researchers have combined this subscale with items from other scales to create a 12-item Diverting Attention/Praying and Hoping subscale (e.g., Rosenstiel & Keefe, 1983).

In general, these studies show that scores on the Praying and Hoping subscale or the Diverting Attention/Praying and Hoping subscale are related to increased reports of pain (Ashby & Lenhart, 1994; Estlander, 1989; Keefe, Crisson, Urban, & Williams, 1990; Keefe & Dolan, 1986; Rosenstiel & Keefe, 1983; Turner & Clancy, 1986; Tuttle, Shutty, & DeGood, 1991; however, cf. A. Hill, Niven, & Knussen, 1995) and greater disability from the pain (Ashby & Lenhart, 1994; Rosenstiel & Keefe, 1983).

Although it might indeed be the case that prayer is a maladaptive way to cope with chronic pain, there are several reasons to be wary of such generalizations. First, and most importantly, the data on which these generalizations are based come exclusively from cross-sectional studies. It is just as likely that people with the greatest impairment (and for whom other pain management strategies are not proving effective) turn to petitionary prayer in search of relief. This alternative seems especially plausible given the range of studies reviewed above suggesting that people turn to prayer in times of greatest impairment or when their problems are most severe. In fact, the only longitudinal data that we know of in the prayer–pain area (Turner & Clancy, 1986) suggest that when chronic pain patients actually increase their use of praying and hoping over time, their self-reports of pain intensity in fact decrease.

Second, because a common assumption in the pain management literature is that depression, anxiety, and other forms of psychiatric problems can be major precursors to chronic pain (see Kotarba, 1983, for a review), one would expect that "praying and hoping" would be related to greater levels of psychiatric difficulties if praying actually exacerbated chronic pain. However, the self-reported use of praying seems to be unrelated to anxiety, depression, and general psychological distress (Keefe et al., 1990; Rosenstiel & Keefe, 1983; Turner & Clancy, 1986; Tuttle et al., 1991). Thus, if praying and hoping have a deleterious effect on people's ability to cope with pain, it must be doing so through some route other than increasing psychiatric distress. To date, we know of no one who has proposed an alternative mechanism that does not involve the aggravating effects of prayer on psychiatric symptoms.

Third, researchers have not yet dealt with a basic issue of construct validity. The Praying and Hoping scale consists of two items directly related to prayer, one item related to faith in God and three items that are totally unrelated to prayer (and not explicitly religious). When combined with the items on the six-item Diverting Attention subscale, the resulting 12-item Diverting Attention/Hoping and Praying factor score is composed of only two items (17%) that relate to the use of prayer. The term *construct validity* basically refers to the validity of score meanings (Messick, 1995). It seems questionable that scores on a 12-item scale containing only two prayer-related items could be validly interpreted as "prayer," although Ashby and Lenhart (1994) used this interpretation with little apparent reflection on the limited validity of such a score meaning. Researchers have not yet addressed this construct validity problem empirically through the refinement of better measures of prayer or the isolation of the relationship between the two explicitly prayer-related items and reliable pain assessments.

Finally, the scope of the two prayer items on the CSQ does not take into account the rich variety of ways that people might pray about chronic pain. Both prayer items reflect a petitionary stance (e.g., "I pray that the pain won't last long"), and none have reflected the prayers of relinquishment (e.g., "I pray that God will make me a better person through suffering" or "I pray, 'Thy will be done'") that Kotarba (1983) hypothesized to be a uniquely adaptive function of religion in coping with chronic pain. They also do not reflect the collaborative style of religious coping (e.g., "I talk to God about my pain and together we decide what it means") that Pargament (1997) also has found to be an adaptive form of religious coping in other contexts. Thus, it seems inadequate to make any global generalizations about the prayer–pain relationship based on the two limited items that are included in the CSQ. Future researchers on prayer and adaptation to chronic pain should take these basic methodological concerns into account before attempting to shed any more light on how prayer (especially petitionary prayer) might hinder or facilitate coping with chronic pain.

COLLOQUIAL PRAYER

What Is It?

Colloquial prayer involves conversation with God, and its petitionary elements are less concrete and specific than those of petitionary prayer. In colloquial prayer, people might ask for strength, guidance, or blessings for other people. Colloquial prayer also includes communication of adoration and love for God. It appears that as people progress through adolescence toward adulthood, prayers become progressively less focused on requests for changes in life circumstances and more colloquial in nature, focusing on (a) changing and coping with their own feelings about life circumstances and (b) increasing intimacy with God (Scarlett & Periello, 1991; Tamminen, 1991; see also Finney & Malony, 1985b, for a review of earlier studies). Colloquial prayer seems to reflect the positive forms of religious coping, that is, they seem to reflect the styles of religious coping (such as collaborating with God to solve problems) that Pargament (1997; Pargament et al., 1998) found to be positively related to health and well-being.

Links With Health and Well-Being

In the AAS, Poloma and Pendleton (1989) measured colloquial prayer with a six-item scale. The use of colloquial prayer was positively and significantly associated with life satisfaction ($r = .16$), existential well-being ($r = .29$), happiness ($r = .17$), and religious satisfaction ($r = .48$). After controlling for demographics and other prayer measures, people who engaged in frequent colloquial prayer had higher levels of happiness ($\beta = .14$) than people who engaged in colloquial prayer less frequently.

INTERCESSORY PRAYER

What Is It?

The literature on prayer and health that we have reviewed thus far has examined the role of people's own prayer lives (e.g., the frequency with which they pray, the types of prayer they use, their religious experiences during prayer) on measures of health and well-being. However, many religious traditions, including Christianity, Judaism, and Islam (but probably others as well) have posited that under certain conditions, people's prayers for other people can be efficacious (McCullough, 1995; Spivak, 1917). Not surprisingly, researchers have examined the efficacy of intercessory prayer statistically. Although the first statistical inquiry into the efficacy of intercessory prayer—conducted more than a century ago (Galton, 1872)—was somewhat short on validity, in time it fostered a variety of modern studies on the efficacy of intercessory prayer in facilitating healing in human beings (see Duckro & Magaletta, 1994, and McCullough, 1995, for detailed reviews). Dossey (1993) has also made the case for the efficacy of intercessory prayer from a spiritual, but nonreligious, point of view.[2] Praying for others

[2]Indeed, Dossey (1993) argued that scores of studies have investigated the efficacy of intercessory prayer. He reviewed many experiments—mostly from parapsychology and physics—that have examined the effects of conscious thought and mental effort designed to influence the operation of physical systems (e.g., random number generators) and biological systems (e.g., the growth and function of cells, seeds, plants, and even human thought, physiological activity, or disease processes). Most of these studies used non-theistic or non-religious imagery and visualization or therapeutic touch, or some other healing modality, rather than including "God in the 'loop'" (Dossey, 1993, p. 188). While the paradigms employed in such studies might lack construct validity from a strictly Judeo-Christian view of intercessory prayer, they do seem consistent with a broader, spiritual understanding of prayer as articulated, for example, in our introductory quotation from Palmer (1983).

should also be viewed as a form of coping with one's own stressful life circumstances (Pargament et al., 1998).

Links With Health and Well-Being

Although many researchers have investigated whether intercessory prayer facilitates health and well-being (e.g., Byrd, 1988; Collipp, 1969; Joyce & Welldon, 1965; O'Laoire, 1997; Walker et al., 1997), results are more equivocal than researchers would like. Byrd found that 192 cardiac patients who were prayed for by anonymous intercessors had significantly fewer problems on 6 of 14 recovery-related variables and that they generally had better courses of recovery overall than a matched sample of cardiac patients who received standard medical treatment but no intercessory prayer treatment.

More recently, Walker et al. (1997) investigated the effects of intercessory prayer on the alcohol intake of patients admitted to a treatment program for alcohol abuse and dependence. The patients who were randomly assigned to an experimental condition in which they received intercessory prayer from an anonymous group of intercessors did not consume significantly less alcohol in the 6 months after treatment than did the comparison group of patients who were assigned to a condition in which they received treatment as usual without being prayed for by a group of anonymous intercessors.

We review one final study of intercessory prayer that yielded provocative results about the efficacy of intercessory prayer. O'Laoire (1997) randomly assigned 90 adults (referred to as "agents") to pray for the needs of another 406 people (referred to as "subjects"). Agents were assigned to one of two conditions: a directed prayer group or a nondirected prayer group. Subjects were randomly assigned to either (a) being prayed for with directed prayer; (b) being prayed for with nondirected prayer; or (c) a no-prayer control group. Agents prayed for their subjects for 15 min a day for 12 weeks. Each subject was prayed for by three agents.

Before the beginning of the prayer tasks, the participants in the study completed measures of depression, anxiety, and self-esteem. As is typical in pre–post designs, scores on these well-being variables improved both for the agents and subjects of prayer over the course of the 12-week period. This finding is not surprising. What was surprising, though, was the comparison of agents and subjects on the well-being variables. At the conclusion of the study, it appeared that the agents of prayer actually had improvements in well-being (in particular, self-rated spiritual health and relationships) that were superior to the subjects.

Given the energy that is being devoted to tracking the health benefits of intercessory prayer, the fairly spotty track record of efficacy in such studies, and the metaphysical and theological conundrums raised by putting intercessory prayer "to the test," this creative study turns the literature on intercessory prayer on its head. Its results suggest that, regardless of whether intercessory prayer helps to produce therapeutic change in the person for whom prayer has been offered, intercessory prayer just might also change the agent of prayer for the better.

RESOURCES FOR PRACTITIONERS

Patients and health care providers seem to be increasingly interested in the use of prayer in mental and physical health care. For example, in a survey of 203 family practice adult inpatients, King and Bushwick (1994) found that 48% wanted their physicians to pray with them. Some groups of practitioners are responding to this perceived need of patients by sometimes praying with them (Galanter, Larson, & Rubenstone, 1991; Koenig, Bearon, & Dayringer, 1989; Olive, 1995). Clinicians have also commended prayer as a therapeutic technique for use with recovering substance abusers (Carroll, 1993; Johnsen, 1993; Ranganathan, 1994; Ratner, 1988), HIV-positive clients (Fredrickson, 1993), sufferers of posttraumatic stress syndrome (Jimenez, 1993), and chronically mentally ill patients (Carson & Huss, 1979) as well as in a variety of other explicitly religious approaches to mental health treatment (Abramowitz, 1993; Azhar, Varma, & Dharap, 1994; Holling, 1990; W. B. Johnson & Ridley, 1992; Saucer, 1991; Tan, 1991).

To us, it seems that the literature on prayer suggests five ways that prayer can be used productively in the course of mental health treatment. First, practitioners can assess the types of prayer clients use to understand their overall style of religious coping. Second, practitioners can encourage clients who pray or who express a desire to pray to use various types of prayer outside the therapeutic hour as an adjunct to mental health treatment. Third, practitioners can use prayer to facilitate cognitive–behavioral change with highly religious clients. Fourth, practitioners might, in some circumstances, find it productive to pray with clients in session. Fifth, practitioners can pray about or for their clients.

Assessing Prayer as a Window Into Clients' Religious Coping and Psychosocial Functioning

Clients' preferences for certain types of prayer might reveal much about whether their style of religious coping is positive or negative, active or passive. This information can have implications for how practitioners discuss or intervene in clients' religious lives in general and thus might be relevant for assessing the effects of client's spirituality on their health and well-being (Pargament et al., 1998).

The use of certain forms of prayer might also reveal unique information about clients' psychosocial functioning. Recall that pain patients who use petitionary prayer to the greatest extent and those who pray about their symptoms or life circumstances most frequently are typically the people with the worst adjustment to their pain and the people with the most stressful life circumstances. Petitionary prayer is a call for divine help. People tend to call on God or a higher power for help when they do not know how to ease their pain or solve their problems on their own. Knowledgeable practitioners might find such information useful in assessing clients' distress about their problems in living and clients' confidence that they possess the resources to solve their own problems.

Encouraging Salutary Types of Prayer

Researchers know from the empirical research that there would be little therapeutic value in directing clients simply to "pray more." Prayer is too diverse and too complex for such directives to have much therapeutic effect. However, clients who are open to using prayer as an adjunct to counseling and psychotherapy might find some benefit from using several forms of prayer, including contemplative-meditative prayer, colloquial prayer, and intercessory prayer. Studies by Finney and Malony (1985a) and Carlson et al. (1988) point to the potential therapeutic benefit to be gained from regular periods of meditative-contemplative prayer. O'Laoire's (1997) study also suggests that the positive mental states associated with intercessory prayer could be as salutary for the agents as for the subjects of intercessory prayer.

Even in the absence of evidence of "therapeutic efficacy" (an increasingly ambiguous term in the field of psychotherapy research; see Wampold, 1997), prayer might have what we refer to (for lack of a better term) as an "emboldening effect." It might boost clients' (a) morale; (b) hope for recovery from and resolution of their problems; (c) comfort with the process of counseling or psychotherapy; and (d) openness to the work of counseling and psychotherapy. Encouraging clients to pray for guidance, wisdom, and strength might help them to obtain such short-range outcomes, helping them become more effective participants in counseling and psychotherapy.

Prayer as a Vehicle for Creating Cognitive Change

Encouraging clients to use prayer for coping or encouraging them, if appropriate, to pray in session might help to incorporate therapy into their worldview. Prayers also might productively be viewed as an important source of material about clients' schemas and beliefs about themselves, others, and the world. Moreover, redirecting clients into more hopeful styles of prayer might be an important vehicle for facilitating changes in clients' self-talk and beliefs. Some scholars (e.g., Propst, 1996) have proposed that prayer might be a particularly effective modality, for example, in which cognitive–behavioral interventions can be delivered to religious clients. Indeed, several researchers who have investigated the differential efficacy of religious approaches to cognitive and cognitive–behavioral therapies with religious clients (e.g., Azhar et al., 1994; W. B. Johnson & Ridley, 1992; Propst, Ostrom, Watkins, Dean, & Mashburn, 1992) have used prayer as one element of religious psychotherapy. A recent meta-analysis of outcome studies that compared religious approaches and standard approaches to psychotherapy suggests that such approaches might indeed be as effective as standard psychotherapies for reducing depressive symptoms (McCullough, 1999).

Interesting anecdotal evidence for the efficacy of using prayer to deliver interventions comes from Kiesling and Harris's (1989) detailed description of H. Benson's (1973, 1984, 1996) program of research on the relaxation response. Apparently, when H. Benson began to teach clients to achieve the relaxation response through meditation, he found that religious clients were more apt to stay with the method if they were encouraged to use short prayers from their faith traditions as the focus of meditation rather than meaningless phrases such as "one." By praying and meditating on symbols from their own traditions, rather than strange or meaningless phrases, religiously committed patients were able to achieve the same relaxation effects as others. As an added benefit, they did not become as easily bored and drop out of treatment.

Praying With Clients in Session

Clients and therapists should probably pray together only when three circumstances converge: (a) The client requests in-session prayer; (b) a thorough spiritual and religious assessment and psychological assessment have convinced the therapist that engaging in such explicitly spiritual and religious activities would not lead to the confusion of therapeutic role boundaries; and (c) competent psychological care is being delivered. Obviously, in-session prayer is no substitute for competent psychological practice (P. S. Richards & Bergin, 1997).

With these cautions, there may be times when in-session prayer would be appropriate and potentially helpful. Tan (1996), for instance, discussed several forms of collaborative, in-session prayer designed to accomplish specific therapeutic goals. Practitioners should use such methods only when the client and therapist endorse highly similar religious and spiritual worldviews (P. S. Richards & Bergin, 1997). Even then, such interventions still have the potential to be ethically problematic.

Praying for Clients

Although praying with clients is probably wise only in limited cases, it is not unethical, inappropriate, or therapeutically counterproductive for practitioners to pray for their clients in session (briefly) or out of session. This is true even if (and perhaps especially if) practitioners do not let their clients know that they are praying for them. If one believes in this power of intercessory prayer to effect positive outcomes for clients at a distance, this is all to the good (P. S. Richards & Bergin, 1997).

Even if a practitioner feels certain that intercessory prayer does not directly alter reality, it still could be worthwhile to pray for clients. Short periods of intense prayer may open practitioners' minds and yield insights about clients' lives that they might not have gained while they are in the business-as-usual, professional mode of relating to clients in session or in the left-brained, highly analytical mode required to conceptualize clients and design treatment plans. These intuitions and insights might prove valuable for guiding clients through critical moments in psychotherapy (P. S. Richards & Bergin, 1997). Furthermore, it is difficult to feel resentment or dislike for someone for whom one prays. Practitioners might do well to pray in particular for their most unlikable clients or clients for whom they lack empathy or respect. (We have found no research on this topic but think that such client–therapist dyads do occur from time to time.) Such prayers might not be designed so much to change the client; rather, they might be intended to create in the therapist a transcendent view of things—a transformed, empathic perception of the client and the needs that led that client into counseling or psychotherapy in the first place.

CONCLUSION

Prayer is a quantifiable phenomenon that is central to most people's spiritual and religious lives. Most people pray at least occasionally, many use it frequently for coping with life's difficulties, and it is likely that some clients would be favorably disposed to assessment and discussion of their prayer lives in the context of psychological treatment.

Prayer serves as a marker for many other events in clients' spiritual lives, particularly among clients for whom spirituality and religion are important. For that reason alone, prayer merits the understanding and respect of practitioners. Mental health practitioners should continue to maintain a respect for the centrality of prayer in clients' lives. Furthermore, it might be beneficial for practitioners to take advantage of clinical opportunities to use patients' prayer lives as a potential window into their spiritual and psychosocial functioning, to use prayer as a vehicle for creating cognitive–behavioral change, and to encourage clients to pray in ways that will be salutary and emboldening. Therapists may sometimes pray with clients in session and may choose to pray for clients privately. Through a combination of psychological interpersonal pathways (in addition, possibly, to metaphysical ones), prayer can be a resource for helping clients and therapists to reach for a relationship—(re)connecting them to themselves, each other, their worlds, and the transcendent.

REFERENCES

Abramowitz, L. (1993). Prayer as therapy among the frail Jewish elderly. *Journal of Gerontological Social Work, 19*, 69–75.

Argyle, M., & Beit–Hallami, B. (1975). *The social psychology of religion*. London: Routledge & Kegan Paul.

Armer, J. M. (1994). Coping strategies identified as "utilized" and "helpful" by relocated rural elders. *Clinical Gerontologist, 14*, 55–60.

Ashby, J. S., & Lenhart, R. S. (1994). Prayer as a coping strategy for chronic pain patients. *Rehabilitation Psychology, 39*, 205–209.

Azhar, M. Z., Varma, S. L., & Dharap, A. S. (1994). Religious psychotherapy in anxiety disorder patients. *Acta Psychiatrica Scandinavica, 90*, 1–3.

Bearon, L. B., & Koenig, H. G. (1990). Religious cognitions and use of prayer in health and illness. *The Gerontologist, 30*, 249–253.

Benson, H. (1973). *The relaxation response*. New York: Morrow.

Benson, H. (1984). *Beyond the relaxation response*. New York: Berkley.

Benson, H. (1996). *Timeless healing*. New York: Fireside.

Benson, P. L., Donahue, M. J., & Erickson, J. A. (1989). Adolescence and religion: A review of the literature from 1970 to 1986. In M. Lynn & D. Moberg (Eds.), *Research in the social scientific study of religion* (Vol. 1, pp. 153–181). Greenwich, CT: JAI Press.

Brant, C. R., & Pargament, K. I. (1995, August). *Religious coping with racist and other negative life events among African-Americans*. Paper presented at the 103rd Annual Convention of the American Psychological Association, New York.

Brown, L. B. (1966). Egocentric thought in petitionary prayer: A cross-cultural study. *Journal of Social Psychology, 68*, 197–210.

Byrd, R. C. (1988). Positive therapeutic effects of intercessory prayer in a coronary care unit population. *Southern Medical Journal, 81*, 826–829.

Carlson, C. R., Bacaseta, P. E., & Simanton, D. A. (1988). A controlled evaluation of devotional meditation and progressive relaxation. *Journal of Psychology and Theology, 16*, 362–368.

Carroll, S. (1993). Spirituality and purpose in life in alcoholism recovery. *Journal of Studies on Alcohol, 54*, 297–301.

Carson, V., & Huss, K. (1979). Prayer: An effective therapeutic and teaching tool. *Journal of Psychiatric Nursing, 17*, 34–37.

Chatters, L. M., & Taylor, R. J. (1989). Age differences in religious participation among black adults. *Journals of Gerontology, 11*, S183–S189.

Collipp, P. J. (1969). The efficacy of prayer: A triple-blind study. *Medical Times, 97*, 201–206.

Conway, K. (1985–1986). Coping with the stress of medical problems among black and white elderly. *International Journal of Aging and Human Development, 21*, 39–48.

Cronan, T. A., Kaplan, R. M., Posner, L., Blumberg, E., & Kozin, F. (1989). Prevalence of the use of unconventional remedies for arthritis in a metropolitan community. *Arthritis and Rheumatism, 32*, 1604–1607.

Dossey, L. (1993). *Healing words.* New York: HarperCollins.

Duckro, P. N., & Magaletta, P. R. (1994). The effect of prayer on physical health: Experimental evidence. *Journal of Religion and Health, 33*, 211–219.

Ellison, C. G. (1995). Race, religious involvement and depressive symptomatology in a southeastern U.S. community. *Social Science and Medicine, 40*, 1561–1572.

Ellison, C. G., & Taylor, L. M. (1996). Turning to prayer: Social and situational antecedents of religious coping among African-Americans. *Review of Religious Research, 38*, 111–131.

Estlander, A. (1989). Coping strategies in low back pain: Effects of severity of pain, situation, gender, and duration of pain. *Scandinavian Journal of Behavior Therapy, 18*, 21–29.

Eysenck, H. J., & Eysenck, S. B. G. (1976). *Psychoticism as a dimension of personality.* New York: Crane, Russak.

Eysenck, H. J., & Gudjonsson, G. H. (1989). *The causes and cures of criminality.* New York: Plenum.

Finney, J. R. (1984). *Contemplative prayer and its use in psychotherapy.* Unpublished doctoral dissertation, Fuller Graduate School of Psychology, Pasadena, CA.

Finney, J. R., & Malony, H. N. (1985a). An empirical study of contemplative prayer as an adjunct to psychotherapy. *Journal of Psychology and Theology, 13*, 284–290.

Finney, J. R., & Malony, H. N. (1985b). Empirical studies of Christian prayer: A review of the literature. *Journal of Psychology and Theology, 13*, 104–114.

Foster, R. J. (1992). *Prayer: Finding the heart's true home.* New York: HarperCollins.

Francis, L. J. (1992). The influence of religion, gender, and social class on attitudes toward school among 11-year-olds in England. *Journal of Experimental Education, 60*, 339–348.

Francis, L. J., & Astley, J. (1996). Personality and prayer among adult churchgoers: A replication. *Journal of Social Behavior and Personality, 24*, 405–408.

Francis, L. J., & Gibbs, D. (1996). Prayer and self-esteem among 8- to 11-year-olds in the United Kingdom. *Journal of Social Psychology, 136*, 791–793.

Francis, L. J., & Wilcox, C. (1994). Personality, prayer, and church attendance among 16- to 18-year-old girls in England. *Journal of Social Psychology, 134,* 243–246.

Francis, L. J., & Wilcox, C. (1996). Prayer, church attendance, and personality revisited: A study among 16- to 19-year-olds. *Psychological Reports, 79,* 1266.

Fredrickson, W. C. (1993). *A program of teaching the practice of Christian meditation/ contemplative prayer to HIV positive clients.* Unpublished doctoral dissertation, Drew University, Madison, NJ.

Fry, P. S. (1990). A factor analytic investigation of home-bound elderly individuals' concerns about death and dying, and their coping responses. *Journal of Clinical Psychology, 46,* 737–748.

Galanter, M., Larson, D. B., & Rubenstone, E. (1991). Christian psychiatry: The impact of evangelical belief on clinical practice. *American Journal of Psychiatry, 148,* 90–95.

Gallup Organization. (1993). *GO LIFE Survey on Prayer.* Princeton, NJ: Author.

Galton, F. (1872). Statistical inquiries into the efficacy of prayer. *Fortnightly Review, 18,* 125–135.

Gass, K. A. (1987). Coping strategies of widows. *Journal of Gerontological Nursing, 13,* 29–33.

Griffith, E. E. H., Mahy, G. E., & Young, J. L. (1986). Psychological benefits of spiritual Baptist "mournings" II. An empirical assessment. *American Journal of Psychiatry, 143,* 226–229.

Gruner, L. (1985). The correlation of private, religious devotional practices and marital adjustment. *Journal of Comparative Family Studies, 16,* 47–59.

Gurin, G., Veroff, J., & Feld, S. (1960). *Americans view their mental health: A nationwide interview survey.* New York: Basic Books.

Harvey, J. H., Stein, S. K., Olsen, N., & Roberts, R. J. (1995). Narratives of loss and recovery from a natural disaster. *Journal of Social Behavior and Personality, 10,* 313–330.

Heiler, F. (1932). *Prayer* (S. McComb, Ed. and Trans.). New York: Oxford University Press. (Original work published 1918)

Hill, A., Niven, C. A., & Knussen, C. (1995). The role of coping in adjustment to phantom limb pain. *Pain, 62,* 79–86.

Hill, H. M., Hawkins, S. R., Raposo, M., & Carr, P. (1995). Relationship between multiple exposures to violence and coping strategies among African-American mothers. *Violence and Victims, 10,* 55–71.

Holling, D. W. (1990). Pastoral psychotherapy: Is it unique? *Counseling and Values, 34,* 96–102.

Hunter, J. E., & Schmidt, F. L. (1994). Correcting for sources of artificial variation across studies. In H. Cooper & L. V. Hedges (Eds.), *Handbook of research synthesis* (pp. 323–336). New York: Russell Sage Foundation.

Husaini, B. A., Moore, S. T., & Cain, V. A. (1994). Psychiatric symptoms and help-seeking behavior among the elderly: An analysis of racial and gender differences. *Journal of Gerontological Social Work, 21,* 177–195.

Jimenez, M. J. (1993). The spiritual healing of post-traumatic stress disorder at the Menlo Park Veteran's Hospital. *Studies in Formative Spirituality, 14,* 175–187.

Johnsen, E. (1993). The role of spirituality in recovery from chemical dependency. *Journal of Addictions and Offender Counseling, 13,* 58–61.

Johnson, D. P., & Mullins, L. C. (1989). Religiosity and loneliness among the elderly. *Journal of Applied Gerontology, 8,* 110–131.

Johnson, W. B., & Ridley, C. R. (1992). Brief Christian and non-Christian rational-emotive therapy with depressed Christian clients: An exploratory study. *Counseling and Values, 36,* 220–229.

Joyce, C. R. B., & Welldon, R. M. C. (1965). The objective efficacy of prayer: A double-blind clinical trial. *Journal of Chronic Disease, 18,* 367–377.

Kaplan, M. S., Marks, G., & Mertens, S. B. (1997). Distress and coping among women with HIV infection: Preliminary findings from a multiethnic sample. *American Journal of Orthopsychiatry, 67,* 80–91.

Kaye, J., & Robinson, K. M. (1994). Spirituality among caregivers. *IMAGE: Journal of Nursing Scholarship, 26,* 218–221.

Keefe, F. J., Crisson, J., Urban, B. J., & Williams, D. A. (1990). Analyzing chronic low back pain: The relatively contribution of pain coping strategies. *Pain, 40,* 293–301.

Keefe, F. J., & Dolan, E. (1986). Pain behavior and pain coping strategies in low back pain and myofacial pain dysfunction syndrome patients. *Pain, 24,* 49–56.

Kiesling, S., & Harris, T. G. (1989, October). The prayer war. *Psychology Today,* pp. 65–66.

King, D. E., & Bushwick, B. (1994). Beliefs and attitudes of hospital patients about faith healing and prayer. *Journal of Family Medicine, 39,* 349–352.

Koenig, H. G. (1988). Religious behaviors and death anxiety in later life. *Hospice Journal, 4,* 3–24.

Koenig, H. G., Bearon, L. B., & Dayringer, R. (1989). Physician perspectives on the role of religion in the physician-older patient relationship. *Journal of Family Practice, 28,* 441–448.

Koenig, H. G., George, L. K., Blazer, D. G., Pritchett, J. T., & Meador, K. G. (1993). The relationship between religion and anxiety in a sample of community-dwelling older adults. *Journal of Geriatric Psychiatry, 26,* 65–93.

Koenig, H. G., Hays, J. C., George, L. K., & Blazer, D. G. (1997). Modeling the cross-sectional relationships between religion, physical health, social support, and depressive symptoms. *American Journal of Geriatric Psychiatry, 5,* 131–144.

Kotarba, J. A. (1983). Perceptions of death, belief systems and the process of coping with chronic pain. *Social Science and Medicine, 17,* 681–689.

Levin, J. S., Chatters, L. M., & Taylor, R. J. (1995). Religious effects on health status and life satisfaction among Black Americans. *Journal of Gerontology: Social Sciences, 50B,* 5154–5163.

Levin, J. S., Lyons, J. S., & Larson, D. B. (1993). Prayer and health during pregnancy: Findings from the Galveston Low Birthweight Survey. *Southern Medical Journal, 86,* 1022–1027.

Lewis, C. A., & Maltby, J. (1995). Religious attitude and practice: The relationship with obsessionality. *Personality and Individual Differences, 19,* 105–108.

Lewis, C. A., & Maltby, J. (1996). Personality, prayer, and church attendance in a sample of male college students in the USA. *Psychological Reports, 78,* 976–978.

Leyser, Y. (1994). Stress and adaptation in orthodox Jewish families with a disabled child. *American Journal of Orthopsychiatry, 64,* 376–385.

Lindenthal, J. J., Myers, J. K., Pepper, M. P., & Stern, M. S. (1970). Mental status and religious behavior. *Journal for the Scientific Study of Religion, 9,* 143–149.

Long, K. A., & Boik, R. J. (1993). Predicting alcohol use in rural children: A longitudinal study. *Nursing Research, 42,* 79–86.

Maltby, J. (1995). Personality, prayer, and church attendance among U.S. female adults. *Journal of Social Psychology, 135,* 529–531.

Manfredi, C., & Pickett, M. (1987). Perceived stressful situations and coping strategies utilized by the elderly. *Journal of Community Health Nursing, 4,* 99–100.

Markides, K. S. (1983). Aging, religiosity, and adjustment: A longitudinal analysis. *Journal of Gerontology, 38,* 621–625.

Markides, K. S., Levin, J. S., & Ray, L. A. (1987). Religion, aging, and life satisfaction: An eight-year, three-wave longitudinal study. *The Gerontologist, 27,* 660–665.

McCullough, M. E. (1995). Prayer and health: Conceptual issues, research review, and research agenda. *Journal of Psychology and Theology, 23,* 15–29.

McCullough, M. E. (1999). Research on religion-accommodative counseling: Review and meta-analysis. *Journal of Counseling Psychology, 46,* 92–98.

McCullough, M. E., & Larson, D. B. (1998). Future directions in research. In H. G. Koenig (Ed.), *Handbook of religion and mental health* (pp. 95–107). San Diego, CA: Academic Press.

McCullough, M. E., Larson, D. B., Hoyt, W. T., Koenig, H. G., & Thoresen, C. (1999). *A meta-analytic review of research on religious involvement and mortality.* Manuscript submitted for publication.

Messick, S. (1995). Validity of psychological assessment: Validation of inferences from person's responses and performances as scientific inquiry into score meaning. *American Psychologist, 50,* 741–749.

Montgomery, A., & Francis, L. J. (1996). Relationship between personal prayer and school-related attitudes among 16-year-old girls. *Psychological Reports, 78,* 787–793.

Neighbors, H. W., Jackson, J. S., Bowman, P. J., & Gurin, G. (1983). Stress, coping, and Black mental health: Preliminary findings from a national survey. *Prevention in Human Services, 2,* 5–29.

Neser, W. B., Husaini, B. A., Linn, J. G., & Whitten-Stovall, R. (1989). Health care behavior among Black and White women. *Journal of Health and Social Policy, 1,* 75–89.

Ohaeri, J. U., Shokunbi, W. A., Akinlade, K. S., & Dare, L. O. (1995). The psychosocial problems of sickle cell disease sufferers and their methods of coping. *Social Science and Medicine, 40,* 955–960.

O'Laoire, S. (1997). An experimental study of the effects of distant, intercessory prayer on self-esteem, anxiety, and depression. *Alternative Therapies in Health and Medicine, 3,* 38–53.

Olive, K. E. (1995). Physician religious beliefs and the physician-patient relationship: A study of devout physicians. *Southern Medical Journal, 88,* 1249–1255.

Palmer, P. J. (1983). *To know as we are known.* New York: HarperCollins.

Paloutzian, R. F. (1996). *Invitation to the psychology of religion* (2nd ed.). Boston: Allyn & Bacon.

Pargament, K. I. (1997). *The psychology of religion and coping.* New York: Guilford Press.

Pargament, K. I., Ensing, D. S., Falgout, K., Olsen, H., Reilly, B., Van Haitsma, K., & Warren, R. (1990). God help me: I. Religious coping efforts as predictors of the outcomes to significant life events. *American Journal of Community Psychology, 18,* 793–824.

Pargament, K. I., Ishler, K., Dubow, E., Stanik, P., Rouiller, R., Crowe, P., Cullman, E., Albert, M., & Royster, B. J. (1994). Methods of religious coping with the gulf war: Cross-sectional and longitudinal analyses. *Journal for the Scientific Study of Religion, 33,* 347–361.

Pargament, K. I., Koenig, H. G., & Perez, L. M. (1998, August). *The many methods of religious coping: Development and initial validation of the RCOPE.* Paper presented at the 106th Annual Convention of the American Psychological Association, San Francisco.

Pargament, K. I., Smith, B., & Brant, C. (1995, November). *Religious and nonreligious coping methods with the 1993 Midwest flood.* Paper presented at the meeting of the Society for the Scientific Study of Religion, St. Louis, MO.

Poloma, M. M., & Gallup, G. H., Jr. (1991). *Varieties of prayer.* Philadelphia: Trinity Press International.

Poloma, M. M., & Pendleton, B. F. (1989). Exploring types of prayer and quality of life: A research note. *Review of Religious Research, 31,* 46–53.

Poloma, M. M., & Pendleton, B. F. (1991). The effects of prayer and prayer experiences on measures of general well-being. *Journal of Psychology and Theology, 19,* 71–83.

Potts, R. G. (1996). Spirituality and the experience of cancer in an African-American community: Implications for psychosocial oncology. *Journal of Psychosocial Oncology, 14,* 1–19.

Propst, L. R. (1996). Cognitive-behavioral therapy and the religious person. In E. P. Shafranske (Ed.), *Religion and the clinical practice of psychology* (pp. 391–408). Washington, DC: American Psychological Association.

Propst, L. R., Ostrom, R., Watkins, P., Dean, T., & Mashburn, D. (1992). Comparative efficacy of religious and nonreligious cognitive–behavioral therapy for the treatment of clinical depression in religious individuals. *Journal of Consulting and Clinical Psychology, 60,* 94–103.

Ranganathan, S. (1994). The Manjakkudi experience: A camp approach towards treating alcoholics. *Addiction, 89,* 1071–1075.

Ratner, E. (1988). A model for the treatment of lesbian and gay alcohol abusers. *Alcoholism Treatment Quarterly, 5,* 25–46.

Richards, D. G. (1990). A "universal forces" dimension of locus control in a population of spiritual seekers. *Psychological Reports, 67,* 847–850.

Richards, D. G. (1991). The phenomenology and psychological correlates of verbal prayer. *Journal of Psychology and Theology, 19,* 354–363.

Richards, P. S., & Bergin, A. E. (Eds.). (1997). *A spiritual strategy for counseling and psychotherapy.* Washington, DC: American Psychological Association.

Rosenstiel, A. K., & Keefe, F. J. (1983). The use of coping strategies in chronic low back pain patients: Relationship to patient characteristics and current adjustment. *Pain, 17,* 33–44.

Saucer, P. R. (1991). Evangelical renewal therapy: A proposal for the integration of religious values into psychotherapy. *Psychological Reports, 69,* 1099–1106.

Saudia, T. L., Kinney, M. R., Brown, K. C., & Young-Ward, K. (1991). Health locus of control and helpfulness of prayer. *Heart and Lung, 20,* 60–65.

Scarlett, W. G., & Periello, L. (1991). The development of prayer in adolescence. *New Directions for Child Development, 52,* 63–76.

Schmidt, F. L., & Hunter, J. E. (1996). Measurement error in psychological research: Lessons from 26 research scenarios. *Psychological Methods, 1,* 199–223.

Schneider, S., & Kastenbaum, R. (1993). Patterns and meanings of prayer in hospice caregivers: An exploratory study. *Death Studies, 17,* 471–485.

Segall, M., & Wykle, M. (1988–1989). The black family's experience with dementia. *Journal of Applied Social Sciences, 13,* 170–191.

Sered, S. S. (1987). Ritual, morality, and gender: The religious lives of oriental Jewish women in Jerusalem. *Israel Social Science Research, 5,* 87–96.

Shadish, W. R., & Haddock, C. K. (1994). Combining estimates of effect size. In H. Cooper & L. V. Hedges (Eds.), *Handbook of research synthesis* (pp. 261–281). New York: Russell Sage Foundation.

Smith, D. L. (1996). Private prayer, public worship and personality among 11–15-year-old adolescents. *Personality and Individual Differences, 21,* 1063–1065.

Sodestrom, K. E., & Martinson, I. M. (1987). Patients' spiritual coping strategies: A study of nurse and patient perspectives. *Oncology Nursing Forum, 14,* 41–46.

Spivak, C. D. (1917). Hebrew prayers for the sick. *Annals of Medical History, 1,* 83–85.

Stern, R. C., Canda, E. R., & Doershuk, C. F. (1992). Use of nonmedical treatment by cystic fibrosis patients. *Journal of Adolescent Health, 13,* 612–615.

Surwillo, W. W., & Hobson, D. P. (1978). Brain electrical activity during prayer. *Psychological Reports, 43,* 135–143.

Sutton, T. D., & Murphy, S. P. (1989). Stressors and patterns of coping in renal transplant patients. *Nursing Research, 38,* 16–19.

Tamminen, K. (1991). *Religious development in childhood and youth: An empirical study.* Helsinki, Finland: Suomen Tiedeakatemia.

Tan, S. (1991). Religious values and interventions in lay Christian counseling. *Journal of Psychology and Christianity, 10,* 173–182.

Tan, S. (1996). Religion in clinical practice: Implicit and explicit integration. In E. P. Shafranske (Ed.), *Religion and the clinical practice of psychology* (pp. 365–390). Washington, DC: American Psychological Association.

Taylor, R. J., & Chatters, L. M. (1991). Nonorganizational religious participation among elderly black adults. *Journals of Gerontology, 46,* S103–S111.

Taylor, R. J., Chatters, L. M., Jayakody, R., & Levin, J. S. (1996). Black and white differences in religious participation: A multisample comparison. *Journal for the Scientific Study of Religion, 35,* 403–410.

Turner, J. A., & Clancy, S. (1986). Strategies for coping with chronic low back pain: Relationship to pain and disability. *Pain, 24,* 355–364.

Tuttle, D. H., Shutty, M. S., & DeGood, D. E. (1991). Empirical dimensions of coping in chronic pain patients: A factorial analysis. *Rehabilitation Psychology, 36,* 179–187.

Walker, S. R., Tonigan, J. S., Miller, W. R., Comer, S., & Kahlich, L. (1997). Intercessory prayer in the treatment of alcohol abuse and dependence: A pilot investigation. *Alternative Therapies, 3,* 79–86.

Wampold, B. E. (1997). Methodological problems in identifying efficacious psychotherapies. *Psychotherapy Research, 7,* 21–43.

Zeidner, M. (1993). Coping with disaster: The case of Israeli adolescents under threat of missile attack. *Journal of Youth and Adolescence, 22,* 89–108.

6

SPIRITUALITY AND THE 12-STEP PROGRAMS: A GUIDE FOR CLINICIANS

J. SCOTT TONIGAN, RADKA T. TOSCOVA,
AND GERARD J. CONNORS

WHY 12-STEP GROUPS?

Twelve-step programs are the most popular mutual-help organizations for individuals seeking relief from a common problem. It is estimated that 3.5 million individuals attend 12-step programs annually (Room, 1993) and that 1 in 10 Americans will attend an Alcoholics Anonymous (AA) meeting, the largest of the 12-step programs, in their lifetime (McCrady & Miller, 1993). Among individuals seeking professional treatment, prior 12-step involvement is relatively common (especially in substance abuse; Burton & Williamson, 1995), at rates that are certainly higher than for the general population. For example, in a national study of alcohol treatment–client matching (Project MATCH Research Group, 1997), a majority of clients seeking professional treatment for alcohol problems had already attended AA (Tonigan, Connors, & Miller, 1996), and clinical experience suggests that many successful AA members seek professional counseling after achieving abstinence. Similarly, since its emergence in

1960, Overeaters Anonymous (OA) has grown to the point where more than 9,000 meetings are offered in more than 50 countries.

There are several reasons why clinicians should be familiar with the ideology and practice of 12-step programs. First, client beliefs about the nature of therapeutic change are important considerations in treatment planning and processes. Twelve-step programs offer a distinct spiritual perspective on the etiology and pathway to recovery, and it is likely that a significant proportion of clients presenting for treatment will endorse prescribed 12-step beliefs, values, and practices. Second, correlational research suggests that 12-step participation is associated with reductions in targeted behavior, such as drinking, illicit drug use, or overeating (Emrick, Tonigan, Montgomery, & Little, 1993; Tonigan, Connors, & Miller, 1996). Likewise, membership in 12-step programs has been associated with improved psychosocial functioning (Emrick et al., 1993; Tonigan, Connors, & Miller, 1996) and increased commitment to change, and it may offset the influence of unsupportive social networks (Longabaugh, Wirtz, Zweben, & Stout, 1998). Therefore, for some clients, you may wish to facilitate affiliation and involvement in 12-step programs.

PURPOSE OF THIS CHAPTER

The purpose of this chapter is to acquaint practitioners with several key aspects of 12-step programs. After a brief review of the history of 12-step programs, in the first section of this chapter we highlight distinctions between the 12-step *program* and *fellowship*. Relationships between these constructs and core 12-step literature are also described. Substantial variability can be found in how 12-step groups function and are structured. The more salient features of different kinds of 12-step meetings are also described. It will become apparent that the 12-step program is fundamentally a spiritual plan for recovery. In the second section of this chapter we thus examine spirituality as it is prescribed and practiced in 12-step groups. In the first part of this section we identify core beliefs and values of spirituality in 12-step programs. Next, we focus on the practice of spirituality in 12-step groups. Emphasis is placed on the practice and behaviors associated with "working" the Twelve Steps. The final part of this section describes the subjective experience of spirituality in 12-step groups. Finally, although Gorsuch and Miller described measurement issues and assessment tools related to spiritual and religious constructs and dimensions in chapter 3, in the third section of this chapter we review specific assessment tools for measurement of 12-step involvement and spirituality.

BRIEF HISTORY OF 12-STEP ORGANIZATIONS

The founding and largest 12-step organization, AA, originated in Akron, Ohio, in the spring of 1935. Strongly influenced by the principles of the Oxford group, AA membership had grown to 100 by 1939. The first edition of the basic text of AA, *Alcoholics Anonymous* (known in AA as "the Big Book"), appeared in 1939, and it was soon followed by favorable media attention in periodicals such as *Liberty* and the *Saturday Evening Post*. By 1941, membership had expanded dramatically to 8,000, and AA was self-described as having attained the status of an "American institution" (forward to the second edition, *Alcoholics Anonymous*, 1955). The second core text of AA, *Twelve Steps and Twelve Traditions* (1981), was approved in 1950 at the first international AA conference. Today, the worldwide AA membership is estimated to be 2,000,000, with about 97,000 groups scattered across 100 countries (Emrick, in press). Kurtz (1988) prepared an engaging and detailed account of the history of AA's beliefs, practices, and personalities, and interested readers are urged to study this text.

Other 12-step programs emerged in the 1950s and flourished in the 1960s. These programs are categorized as 12-step programs because they endorse a spiritual path to recovery, amending in only minor ways the Twelve Steps of AA to conform to problems other than alcoholism and viewing, like AA, characterological flaws as the major obstruction to recovery. Al-Anon, a 12-step organization for people who have significant others with past or current alcohol problems, was formed in 1951 and printed its first hardcover text in 1955. Today, Al-Anon is estimated to have 600,000 active members worldwide attending more than 33,000 groups in 112 countries (according to the Al-Anon Web site). Gamblers Anonymous (GA) began in 1957 and now boasts 1,200 chapters in 23 countries. Narcotics Anonymous (NA) grew slowly from its inception in the early 1950s to 200 registered groups in 1978. With publication of core NA literature in 1983, however, NA experienced rapid growth such that in 1994 NA reported 19,822 registered meetings in 70 countries.

More broad-focused 12-step programs took root in the 1970s and 1980s. Adult Children of Alcoholics, for example, relies on 12-step practice for life coping for individuals raised in an alcoholic household. Broader yet, Emotions Anonymous (EA) addresses 21 emotional complaints by application of the 12-step program. Among many other emotional problems, potential EA affiliates may seek relief in EA for problems with anxiety, depression, guilt, and obsessive and negative thinking. Although precise figures are not available, it is estimated that there are 1,200 EA chapters in 39 countries.

A few historical eddies are noteworthy. First, changes in the core 12-step literature are made only after lengthy debate and considerable deliberation (Miller & Kurtz, 1994; Montgomery, Miller, & Tonigan, 1993). Therefore, it is understandable that much of this literature, including the Twelve Steps, which were written in the late 1930s, are male dominant in the use of pronouns, and subsequent editions have maintained this tone. We decided not to modify the language of the core 12-step literature quoted in this chapter.

Second, migration across 12-step programs is common. Some migration is explained by polysubstance abuse itself, in which members address specific substance addictions in separate 12-step contexts. Migration also occurs because of the greater availability of AA meetings relative to alternative 12-step programs. Finally, it is noteworthy that members in non–12-step mutual-help groups (e.g., Rational Recovery and Secular Organization for Sobriety) also attend 12-step meetings because of the limited availability of desired mutual-help programs (Connors & Dermen, 1996).

12-STEP PROGRAMS AND FELLOWSHIP

A fundamental distinction to be understood is the difference between the 12-step program and fellowship. The "program" consists of the stated prescribed beliefs, values, and behaviors of a 12-step organization. In essence, the program is the sequential plan for recovery, and it is most succinctly stated in the Twelve Steps.

Traditionally, working the steps is done sequentially with the aid of a sponsor who also is a member who has already worked the Twelve Steps. Furthermore, step work is felt to be a lifelong process, and members often have more than one sponsor after months or years of 12-step affiliation (7% of one AA sample reported having multiple sponsors at the same time; Brown & Peterson, 1991). It is estimated that a majority of members have sponsors, and an integration of findings from four studies indicates that having a sponsor is positively related to abstinence (Tonigan & Toscova, in press). There is also limited evidence that older individuals are more likely to acquire sponsors than younger affiliates and that men are more likely to have sponsors than women (Kingree, 1997).

The "fellowship" of the 12-step program, on the other hand, refers to the practice or activities of a 12-step organization. Nearly all social interactions related to 12-step group membership can be categorized as aspects of the fellowship. Helping others, building relationships among other members, and the sharing of joys and hardships all belong to what is described as the fellowship. In short, the fellowship refers to the *experiencing* of a 12-step program. The guiding principles for fellowship are stated in the Twelve Traditions (Alcoholics Anonymous, 1981).

What does research have to say about 12-step programs and fellowship? Restricted largely to the study of AA, one consistent finding is that increased meeting attendance is associated with greater involvement in program and fellowship dimensions (e.g., Caldwell & Cutter, in press; Montgomery et al., 1993; Snow, Prochaska, & Rossi, 1994; Tonigan, Connors, & Miller, 1996). It is probably a mistake, however, to equate higher levels of attendance with greater engagement in all prescribed mutual-help activities. Caldwell and Cutter (in press), for example, reported that "mid-level" attendees (20–60 meetings in 90 days) adopted program activities as often as "high-level" attendees (90 meetings in 90 days) but were less likely than high-level attendees to endorse fellowship activities requiring trust and intimacy. In addition, Tonigan, Connors, and Miller (1996) have found that attendance is positively related to engagement activities to a threshold level of about two thirds of the available days. Thereafter, increased attendance is not associated with increased involvement. It therefore appears that although the relationship between 12-step group attendance and the practicing of the program and fellowship is positive in nature, the relationship is complex and becomes manifest at different rates across program and fellowship dimensions.

Research suggests that AA groups differ in perceived fellowship dimensions and that the extent of discussion of the Twelve Steps is associated with these differences. Specifically, Montgomery et al. (1993) reported that among four AA groups, the extent of perceived group cohesion and aggressiveness differed significantly across groups such that the group with the highest perceived aggressiveness also had the lowest perceived cohesiveness. In a follow-up study of the same AA groups, Tonigan, Ashcroft, and Miller (1995) replicated the same group social climate differences and found that the most cohesive group also tended to discuss the Twelve Steps most frequently in typical meetings. Whether these findings apply to 12-step groups in general is unclear, but the seeking of more cohesive groups may be advisable when the objective is to maximize exposure and involvement in the Twelve Steps.

TYPES OF 12-STEP MEETINGS

Important commonalities can be identified across different types of 12-step programs. As a rule, meetings are held in a rented building called a "club" or in places of religious worship. Meetings tend to last 1 hr. Meetings usually begin with the members reciting the Serenity Prayer (see chap. 12 in this book), followed by a reading from the Big Book of "How It Works" and the "Twelve Traditions." Generally, each meeting is guided by a chairperson, a role that typically rotates among group members on a daily or weekly basis. Announcements relevant to the mission of the 12-step group are then made. Visitors and newcomers are asked to introduce themselves only by their first name; some will choose to self-label themselves as "alcoholic," "addict," "compulsive overeater," or "gambler" depending on the exact purpose of the 12-step group. During the course of a meeting, a basket is passed among members to collect donations. Twelve-step groups are completely self supporting, although members can give or not give as they wish with little or no stigma. Cross-talk (i.e., commenting on others' experiences) is highly discouraged during a meeting. The meeting generally closes with group members holding hands in a circle while saying the Lord's Prayer. Afterward, newcomers are often approached by group members in what is called by members "the meeting after the meeting."

A wide variety of 12-step meetings are available within this structured format. Meetings are offered, for example, in "open" and "closed" formats. Open meetings can be attended by any interested person regardless of whether he or she shares or suspects that he or she shares the common problem. In contrast, closed meetings are reserved only for members of a 12-step program, with the only requirement for membership being a sincere desire to change the target behavior. Offered in both open and closed meeting formats, 12-step meetings also may cater to demographic subsets of a 12-step program, such as men, women, adolescents, gays, and lesbians. Times, locations, and designations (e.g., open or closed) of 12-step meetings can most easily be obtained in printed schedules available for most metropolitan areas. More recently, meeting schedules for selected areas in the United States have been posted on the Internet.

There are at least five common meeting formats. In "open discussion meetings," individuals are asked to share by the chairperson or by the preceding person who shared (tag meeting). Here, a general topic may be provided at the onset of the meeting, most often a reading from the core 12-step literature, but individuals are free to share any feelings or thoughts related to the shared problem. In "speaker meetings," one to three members talk for the entire meeting. Generally, the recommended format for sharing in speaker meetings is to describe what life was like before membership, what happened to facilitate membership, and what life is now like as a result of membership. Meetings can also be focused studies of the core 12-step literature and in this regard are offered as "Big Book" and "Twelve by Twelve meetings." In these meetings, core literature is read, one or two paragraphs at a time, by different members. These meetings are often collectively referred to as "step meetings" because a primary focus is on the meaning and practice of the Twelve Steps. Finally, most groups that meet regularly offer "birthday meetings." These meetings, generally occurring once a month, are intended to recognize specified periods of continuous abstinence from a targeted behavior. Most 12-step groups recognize 30-, 60-, and 90-day intervals as well as 6-, 9-, and 12-month birthdays. Thereafter, members typically celebrate birthdays annually.

SPIRITUAL BELIEFS IN 12-STEP PROGRAMS

Higher Power

The first spiritual belief is in a transcendental being, or *higher power*. The nature of a higher power, or God to other people, is intentionally ill-defined in the core literature. Kurtz (1988) has detailed the sociopolitical and religious considerations of the AA founders in choosing a broad definition of God, much of which can be summarized as the wish of the AA founders for a God concept that would be acceptable to newcomers and would not alienate Judeo-Christian denominations. Written in the Big Book of AA (1976), for example, is the following:

> Much to our relief, we discovered we did not need to consider another's conception of God. Our own conception, however inadequate, was sufficient to make the approach and to effect a contact with Him. As soon as we admitted the possible existence of a creative intelligence, a Spirit of the Universe underlying the totality of things, we began to be possessed of a new sense of power and direction. ... To us, the Realm of the Spirit is broad, roomy, all inclusive; never exclusive or forbidding to those who earnestly seek. (p. 46)
>
> The basic AA text proposes that all persons have an innate sense or awareness of a Higher Power. In the chapter, *We agnostics* [*sic*], it is stated that a God concept resides "deep down in every man" (p. 55), and it is from within that God is to be found. While tolerance is prescribed regarding different conceptions of a Higher Power, there is a single mindedness in AA that a Higher Power is external to the individual. Consistent with the great religions, 12 step programs also assert that a Higher Power is greater than the individual, is all knowing, and that there is a larger purpose to life than simple daily activities.

Personal Relationship

The second spiritual axiom in 12-step programs is that one must develop a personal relationship with a higher power. In fact, development of a personal relationship with God is one of the primary objectives in the practice of the Twelve Steps. Prayer and meditation, for example, are two methods to enhance this relationship, and these practices are directly endorsed in several of the steps (Steps 3 and 11).

What is the nature of a personal relationship with God in the view of members? Clearly, spirituality is viewed as a protective mechanism against relapse, and in this capacity, it serves as a template for conducting daily life. Social interactions, employment and financial decisions, parenting, and family and love relationships are all viewed as areas in which spiritual beliefs and practices are required for proper living. Early members often describe their discoveries of spiritual principles as means to more satisfying and useful lives (Alcoholics Anonymous, 1976)

The pragmatic application of spirituality to daily situations is a hallmark of 12-step beliefs, and it is fitting to define the nature of a relationship with a higher power in the context of coping with daily situations. Not specific to 12-step programs, Pargament et al. (1988) defined three styles of spiritual coping differentiated on the basis of communication patterns with a transcendent power. The first style, collaborative, emphasizes the exchange between the individual and God. In contrast, a deferring style is one in which the individual is passive and answers to life problems are received from God. Finally, a self-directing style of coping capitalizes on free will, emphasizing personal responsibility, and seeks little support in the form of answers from a transcendent power. References and endorsements to each of these coping styles can be found in the AA literature (e.g., pp. 13 and 62 of the Big Book).

We suspect that AA members use multiple spiritual coping styles but that preference in styles may change with membership length. For example, Steps 1–3 are often described as the "surrender steps" in which newcomers admit powerlessness over alcohol, derive hope in the ability of a higher power to restore health, and acknowledge submission to God's will. In large part, these steps may be interpreted as fostering a deferring relationship with a higher power. In contrast, Steps 4–10 involve self-examination, disclosure, and making amends to harmed persons, and Steps 11 and 12 call for deepened commitment to prayer and meditation and to service work. Here, emphasis is placed on listening and speaking with a higher power. These latter steps are indicative of a collaborative relationship with a higher power. Accepting personal responsibility is highly valued in 12-step philosophy, and in this regard a self-directing coping strategy is evidenced in the 12-step literature. The merits of free will, however, tend not to be stressed in 12-step beliefs and practices.

Mysticism

The third axiom of spirituality in AA is a belief in the mystical. Belief in mysticism or miracles should not be mistaken for a belief in magic (Kurtz, 1988). Rather, mysticism in AA underscores the belief that transcendental intervention can and does occur. What should follow laws of physics may not, and what seems impossible may occur. Transcendental intervention, however, is not a random event in the view of AA members. Rather, such intervention represents an unfolding of a larger purpose or reality that may (or may not) become clear. The cornerstone miracle for members of AA is the achievement of sobriety. Whether divine intervention is sudden, powerful, and dramatic as experienced by founder Bill Wilson or experienced more slowly as described in the Spiritual Experience

Appendix to the Big Book, a period of abstinence after years of alcohol abuse is attributed to a power greater than oneself. In the words of founder Bill Wilson, "the central fact of our lives today is the absolute certainty that our Creator has entered into our hearts. . . . He has commenced to accomplish those things for us which we could never do by ourselves" (Alcoholics Anonymous, 1976, p. 25).

As important as abstinence is, the realm of divine intervention extends well beyond a reprieve from alcohol consumption. In the course of sequentially working the Twelve Steps, the basic text of AA predicts that a "sense of uselessness, self-pity, fear of people and economic insecurity and self-seeking will vanish," and that the AA member will "suddenly realize that God is doing for us what we could not do for ourselves" (Alcoholics Anonymous, 1976, p. 84). Described as the promises of AA, divine intervention is credited with the alleviation of numerous psychological problems.

Renewal

A fourth spiritual axiom in AA is that spirituality must recapitulate itself. Here, faith in a higher power should begin anew and should be restored each day. Implied is that a conscious decision is required to lead a spiritual life. This spiritual precept focuses member attention on the present and promotes what Kus (1992) referred to as "leading the examined life." A profound implication is that spirituality has neither a past nor a future for AA members. In essence, spirituality is only experienced in present tense and may evaporate at any moment yet be restored as quickly. Reference to the fragility of spirituality is frequently voiced in the Big Book, and little doubt is left for the reader regarding the consequence of ignoring spiritual growth:

> It is easy to let up on the spiritual program of action and rest on our laurels. We are headed for trouble if we do, for alcohol is a subtle foe. We are not cured of alcoholism. What we have is a daily reprieve contingent on the maintenance of our spiritual condition. (Alcoholics Anonymous, 1976, p. 85)

Discord

The final spiritual truth in 12-step programs is that every time a person is disturbed, no matter what the cause, there is something wrong with that person (Twelve Steps and Twelve Traditions, 1981). Distress, then, is identified as a signal of one's incongruency with the plan of a higher power. Discord and conflict may arise in the course of social interactions because of self-serving motives, but it also may arise because of lack of acceptance of current circumstances. Can 12-step members be entirely free of such discord, and what state describes accord? Detailed later in this chapter, the subjective experience of being free of distress and conflict is serenity (see chap. 12 in this book). To the first question, the expectation is that few if any members of 12-step groups can sustain harmony with the purposes of the universe for any extended period of time. Rather, the intent of this axiom is to direct spiritual growth to an ideal realizing that, in fact, the ideal is not achievable. Approximations to the ideal can be achieved through consistent and incremental striving of group members to work the steps.

THE PRACTICE OF SPIRITUALITY

The practice of 12-step programs is exemplified in working the Twelve Steps. The focus of this section is to highlight concordance between spiritual behaviors associated with working the steps and core spiritual beliefs of 12-step programs. We see merit in the popular classification scheme that groups Steps 1–3 into acceptance or surrender-based steps, Steps 4–10 as action-focused steps, and Steps 11–12 as maintenance steps. This scheme is a useful means to evaluate how spiritual beliefs correspond with behavior, and research suggests that some forms of spiritual behavior (e.g., surrender-based steps) receive more attention in AA meetings than others (e.g., action-focused steps; Tonigan et al., 1995). A significant limitation of this scheme, however, is that it blurs the distinction between the practice of AA (behavior) and the subjective experience of AA.

Prayer and Meditation

To begin, Steps 2, 3, and 11 acknowledge and affirm the existence and power of God, and they solicit prayer and meditation on the part of AA members. Evidence suggests that members of AA and 12-step programs believe that this behavior is extremely important. Brown and Peterson (1991), for example, surveyed members of several types of 12-step programs and found that all respondents reported contact with a higher power on a daily basis, with respondents (mean years of recovery = 3.13) reporting some form of prayer on awakening (57%), on retiring (74%), or during a typical day (35%). Likewise, and in spite of some significant group differences in social functioning, different AA groups uniformly endorsed the importance of a personal contact with God (Montgomery et al., 1993; Tonigan et al., 1995).

The belief in miracles has a prominent role in AA spirituality, and Steps 2, 7, and 12 make direct reference to divine intervention in the lives of members. Except for Step 12, behaviors associated with miracles rely mostly on prayer and meditation. Step 2, for example, asks members to believe that a higher power can restore health and sanity. Step 7 requests that a higher power remove shortcomings, and Step 12 asks members to carry the message to suffering alcoholic individuals, thus reenacting the miracle of arresting alcoholism. Ninety-five percent of one AA sample reported that they had faith in recovery with the help of a higher power (Brown & Peterson, 1991).

What is the result of this emphasis on prayer and mediation? On one hand, such behavior seems to result in greater "God consciousness" (i.e., an awareness of transcendent power) and to a lesser extent the adoption of formal religious practices. In Project MATCH, for example, clients with greater exposure to AA before study recruitment reported significantly more God consciousness than did clients having little or no prior AA exposure. Clients with prior AA exposure, however, were about equally divided on whether they adopted religious practices (e.g., attended worship services; Connors, Tonigan, & Miller, 1996). On the other hand, few positive findings have been reported suggesting that prayer is directly related to abstinence in AA (Tonigan & Toscova, in press), and the more general relationship between prayer and reductions in substance abuse are complex and not easily understood (Walker, Tonigan, Miller, & Kahlich, 1997).

Amends

Several of the Twelve Steps require identification of wrongdoing and personal disclosure to another about past misdeeds (Steps 4, 5, and 10) as well as a willingness and action to make amends for misdeeds (Steps 8–10). Putting aside the subjective experience of these behaviors (e.g., humility), most readers would agree that these behaviors promote healthy social interactions and relations. Valued in these steps is the development of social relationships based on honesty, mutual respect, trust, and the ability to admit past wrongdoings. These are the same qualities that ultimately characterize a personal relationship with a higher power. This is especially true for those 12-step members whose personal relationship with God is characterized by a collaborative coping style.

Relationships

How important is it for 12-step members to develop personal relationships as prescribed in Steps 9 and 10? Kingree (1997) reported that the "sharing of experiences" among AA members was significantly and positively related to commitment to AA. More directly, Brown and Peterson (1991) found that 43% of AA members said they promptly admitted when they were wrong, 50% treated others as they wanted to be treated, 45% tried to forgive others, 74% listened carefully when others were talking, and 53% reported listening even when disagreeing with others. Although future work needs to be done to confirm the findings of this study, it seems that 12-step members focus substantial energy on developing helping relationships as they are prescribed.

Service

Steps 1, 10, 11, and 12 are prescribed to be done on a daily basis (conventional wisdom also recommends Steps 1–3 on a daily basis). Behavioral aspects of these steps include admission of powerlessness, personal inventory and subsequent amends if necessary, prayer and mediation, service work, and practice of the 12-step principles in all affairs. In cognitive–behavioral terms, this is indeed a tall order. The implications are that one is required to vigilantly self-monitor behavior and to lead an examined life (Kus, 1992). These behaviors appear to exemplify and reinforce the core belief that spirituality must renew itself on a daily basis.

SUBJECTIVE EXPERIENCE OF SPIRITUALITY

In this section we identify and briefly review some of the key subjective experiences related to the practice of AA. To this end, we review the subjective experiences of humility, serenity, and gratitude. Our primary objective in this regard is to identify key subjective experiences as they are defined in the spiritual program of AA, connecting these experiences to AA-related spiritual behaviors.

Humility

Humility implies an accurate sense of proportion about self-importance. Described in the Big Book (Alcoholics Anonymous, 1976), the affiliate is an extreme example of "self-will run riot" and much of the 12-step spiritual experience is intended to deflate ego. The Big Book (Alcoholics Anonymous, 1976) stresses that "our troubles, we think, are basically of our own making. . . . Above everything, we *alcoholics must* be rid of this selfishness. . . . We must or it kills us! . . . First of all, we had to quit playing God. It didn't work" (p. 62). Humility is thus most clearly experienced in relation to core spiritual belief in an external transcendent power who is all knowing and powerful.

How is humility associated with step work? Steps 1 and 3 emphasize the powerlessness of the individual to overcome undesirable behavior and the desirability of turning one's life over to the care of God. The sharing of a written personal inventory (Step 5) that lays bare—without excuses—lifelong misdeeds and wrongdoing to another person is yet another means by which the member experiences humility (i.e., guilt and shame are acknowledged and processed). Finally, the practice of Step 10 with daily amends for oversights and misdeeds is a behavioral means to elicit, with some frequency, a sense of humility.

Serenity

The term *serenity* refers to a sense of completeness in being one with a transcendent power and feeling at ease with (not in spite of) personal limitations and weaknesses (see chap. 12 in this book). Being one with a higher power implies heightened wisdom, the wisdom required to make the decision asked for in the Serenity Prayer: "God grant me the serenity to accept the things I cannot change, the courage to change the things I can, and the wisdom to know the difference."

The practice of Steps 3 and 11 evokes feelings of release that may precede a sense of serenity. Furthermore, Step 11 includes dialogue with a higher power through prayer (speaking to) and meditation (listening to).

Gratitude

In spiritual terms, the term *gratitude* refers to awareness or recognition of God's grace. Grace may take the form of a gift or, alternatively, may be seen as the provision of strength to accomplish a difficult task. Cessation of problematic behavior is generally interpreted by members as divine intervention, and in this light abstinence itself is a gift from God. Self-labeling and the daily admission of powerlessness over the problematic behavior or substances are two behavioral methods in which members renew their sense of gratitude. The practice of the steps can evoke gratitude at many points, some obvious ones including the working of Step 2 and coming to believe in the restoration of physical, spiritual, and mental health; completing amends in Step 9 and feeling release from past debt and wrongdoing; and, finally, in helping other suffering people (Step 12), the reminder of past problems removed.

MEASURES OF SPIRITUALITY IN 12-STEP PROGRAMS

In this section we introduce some assessment tools that will be useful in the measurement of spirituality in 12-step programs. For inclusion in this review, assessment tools had to have been already used in 12-step settings and had to have published psychometric data documenting their reliability, validity, or both. Eight assessment tools are presented, seven of which are self-report questionnaires and one of which is a semistructured interview. A majority of the tools covered in this review have been recently developed, and we anticipate continued growth in the number and kind of assessment tools available to those interested in studying 12-step spirituality, affiliation, and involvement.

Table 6.1 shows the characteristics of the assessment instruments selected for inclusion. These instruments canvassed an array of behaviors, practices, and beliefs specifically related to 12-step programs. A majority of the assessments use Likert-scaled items and are self-report questionnaires with fewer than 15 items. All provide a total score and some yield subscale scores. Notably, none of the tools infers spirituality on the sole basis of the frequency of meeting attendance.

The Alcoholics Anonymous Inventory (AAI; Tonigan, Connors, & Miller, 1996) and the Alcoholics Anonymous Affiliation Scale (AAAS; Humphreys, Kaskutas, & Weisner, 1998) are examples of self-administered brief inventories of AA activities, including items directly assessing spirituality (e.g., "Have you had a spiritual awakening or conversion experience through your involvement in AA?") and the indirect measurement of spirituality (e.g., the reading of AA literature and the working of steps). Both the AAAS and the AAI provide normative data. The Recovery Interview (Morgenstern, Kahler, Frey, & Labouvie, 1996) is similar in content to the AAI and AAAS, but it differs from these tools in being a fully structured interview. When questions arise about the literacy or validity of self-report, the Recovery Inventory has distinct advantages.

The Brown–Peterson Recovery Progress Inventory (Brown & Peterson, 1990) and the Composite AA Index (Kingree, 1997) are more exhaustive inventories of AA-related behaviors, practices, and beliefs. As such, these assessments provide a detailed assessment of respondent values and beliefs associated with recovery in 12-step programs, facilitating more reliable separation of respondent beliefs, practices, and perceived benefits.

TABLE 6.1
Summary of Assessment Instruments Used to Measure Spirituality in
12-Step Programs

Inventories	Author	Items	Scales
AAAS	Humphreys et al. (1998)	9	AA affiliation
12-Step affiliation	Kingree (1997)	22	AA affiliation
B-PRPI	Brown and Peterson (1991)	53	Spiritual practice
RI	Morgenstern et al. (1996)	9	AA involvement
SQ	Gilbert (1991)	15	Working Steps 1–3
SBS	Schaler (1996)	8	Tolerance Release–gratitude
AAI	Tonigan, Connors, and Miller (1996)	13	AA involvement AA attendance
MMSS	Mathew et al. (1995)		Six subscales

Note. Alcoholics Anonymous Affiliation Scale (AAAS); Alcoholics Anonymous Inventory (AAI); Brown-Peterson Recovery Progress Inventory (B-PRPI); Mathew Materialism Spiritualism Scale (MMSS); Recovery Interview (RI); Spiritual Belief Scale (SBS); Step Questionnaire (SQ).

Unfortunately, both instruments have been used only in small samples and lack normative data.

The Spiritual Belief Scale (SBS; Schaler, 1996) is an eight-item assessment tool that measures the extent to which 12-step participants believe in and experience tolerance and release–gratitude–humility. The item content of the SBS is specific to the core AA literature, and the questionnaire has been used in measuring the beliefs of treatment providers in recovery and participating in AA. Convergent and divergent validity analyses suggest that SBS scores increase with length of time in AA and that abstinence and SBS scores are positively related.

The Step Questionnaire (Gilbert, 1991) is a 15-item self-report questionnaire that measures AA member beliefs and practices related to Steps 1–3. The Step 1 (Powerlessness) scale solicits information about the extent of perceived powerlessness over alcohol and alcoholic self-labeling. The second and third scales measure the extent to which AA members adopt prescriptions about a higher power and acknowledge surrender to alcoholism. Normative data are available for the instrument and the author provides alternative scoring methods.

Finally, the Mathew Materialism Spiritualism Scale (MMSS; Mathew, Georgi, Wilson, & Mathew, 1996; Mathew, Mathew, Wilson, & Georgi, 1995) consists of six scales measuring belief in God, religious practices, mystical experiences, existence of the soul after death, value of altruism and unselfishness, and belief in paranormal phenomena. The MMSS has been used with recovering members of 12-step programs and normal controls. Significant increases on the six scales have been observed among recovering 12-step members.

LEARNING MORE ABOUT 12-STEP PROGRAMS

The objective of this chapter has been to introduce readers to some of the basic spiritual aspects and practices of 12-step programs. In this section, we outline strategies for gaining a deeper understanding of 12-step programs, dividing these strategies according to whether they are experiential or instructional in nature. Ideally, we believe that the two strategies should be pursued jointly to fully understand and appreciate the 12-step experience.

Experiential

First, we encourage you to attend some 12-step meetings. There is no substitute for this experience. In fact, because of differences in how the fellowship is perceived, we recommend that you sample various meetings to adequately sample a particular kind of 12-step program. Described earlier, 12-step meetings are offered in open and closed formats, and some meetings are smoke free. All interested individuals can attend an open 12-step meeting regardless of whether they share the common problem. It is customary at the beginning of a meeting for newcomers and visitors to introduce themselves by their first name. Although it is appropriate to remain silent, it is suggested that visitors introduce themselves by first name, saying, "My name is _____, and I'm a visitor interesting in learning about _____" (AA, NA, OA, etc.). Anonymity is a cornerstone of 12-step groups, and occupational status is rarely if ever discussed. We strongly counsel against the introduction, "My name is _____ and I'm a therapist interested in _____" (AA, NA, OA etc.).

Recently, most 12-step programs have developed and maintain home pages on the Internet. Void of human interaction, which is the essence of 12-step programs, these home pages nevertheless provide important information on program history, meeting locations, chat rooms, approved and recommended literature, regional and national conference schedules, listing of the Twelve Steps as adapted to a particular program, screening questions for prospective members, and statements of the program's philosophy. It is our experience that Internet home pages are most useful in small community settings where access and availability to 12-step meetings are limited.

Finally, the experience of 12-step programs is perhaps best reflected in the lives of their members. Be sensitive to the importance of these experiences and beliefs to some clients and in so doing learn of the 12-step program and fellowship. With appropriate client populations (e.g., those presenting for the treatment of addictive behaviors), the assessment of prior and current affiliation and involvement in 12-step programs should be routine. Become aware of different dimensions of the 12-step experience and recommend to clients who express an interest in 12-step affiliation that they sample a number of different meetings, finding the group that best meets their needs.

Some writers have pointed to potentially harmful effects of 12-step ideology and practice. For example, there are high attrition rates from 12-step programs that suggest that they often fail to provide perceived benefits even when formal treatment is specifically intended to facilitate 12-step involvement (Tonigan, Connors, & Miller, in press). Bufe (1998) argued that the practice of the Twelve Steps can actually foster learned helplessness and low self-esteem by admissions of powerlessness and reliance on a higher power. Clients seeking the social support of mutual-help groups without the spiritual aspects of 12-step ideology can sample a number of other programs, including Rational Recovery, Secular Organization for Sobriety, and Women for Sobriety.

Nevertheless, decades of correlational research point to the advantages of 12-step participation for some individuals. Recent clinical trials with substance abusers have demonstrated that a 12-step treatment model is as effective as cognitive–behavioral approaches (Ouimette et al., 1997; Project MATCH Research Group, 1997). In the context of managed care and with accumulating evidence for the effectiveness of 12-step approaches, we anticipate greater reliance on mutual-help programs to sustain client gains made in psychotherapy. It is helpful to understand the principles and practices of 12-step programs to facilitate, as warranted, your clients' engagement in 12-step programs.

The 12-step program is a spiritual plan for recovery. In this chapter, this spiritual plan was judged to consist of five core spiritual beliefs. Combined, these beliefs suggest that there is a transcendent power in the universe that is external to the individual. Development of a personal relationship with a higher power is a major objective for 12-step membership, with strong prescriptions for daily renewal of a commitment to God. In the 12-step view, God's purpose is often mysterious, leading to a belief in mysticism and acceptance of present circumstances regardless of how unpleasant. Distress and conflict are interpreted as signals of disharmony with one's higher power. Members are therefore encouraged to vigilantly monitor negative mood states. Evidence suggests that many 12-step members adhere to these spiritual precepts, as do many people with a family history of addiction disorders.

Instructional

Keep abreast of emerging research. Health professionals may be understandably cautious about conclusions drawn from 12-step research. Historically, this research has been of fair-to-poor quality (Tonigan, Toscova, & Miller, 1996), and, equally important, past research has not been focused on issues immediately relevant to practitioners. However, this situation is changing. Foremost, an emergent research base is developing that examines the curative processes and change mechanisms associated with 12-step participation. Limited mostly to AA, findings in this area suggest clear advantages to some prescribed 12-step behaviors and practices.

It is also important to study the 12-step literature. The founding 12-step program, AA, has both the Big Book and Twelve Traditions text, and many of the offshoot programs have adopted this two-book format. These texts are considered the approved literature and thus have the endorsement of the 12-step organization's governing board. It is worthwhile to read the founding AA texts as a backdrop to interpreting alternative versions associated with non-AA 12-step groups and to see how the program has been modified.

CONCLUSIONS

Most practitioners see clients with prior or current 12-step experience. Twelve-step mutual-help programs are popular in the United States, and individuals affiliated with these organizations are more likely to receive formal treatment than are non–12-step members. Important distinctions were identified between the 12-step program and fellowship. Although the 12-step program remains relatively stable across both time and different types of 12-step organizations, there seems to be substantial variation in perceptions about and the practice of the program's prescriptions. Prayer and meditation are practiced by a majority of members on a daily basis. Members also report expending substantial energy on the making of amends and the development of healthy social relationships.

Self-examination is required to practice the 12-step program. The process of self-monitoring can, in itself, be an important therapeutic asset. Clients actively engaged in 12-step programs may be amenable to insight-oriented therapies. Similarly, clients preferring self-examination in therapy may be well suited to the focus of 12-step programs.

Many questions remain about spirituality as it is practiced in 12-step programs. Little is known, for example, about the relationship between membership attrition and spirituality. Estimates of dropout rates among 12-step organizations vary considerably, but most agree that they are high. Nearly all 12-step researchers have studied AA. In question is whether the proposed curative mechanisms in AA transfer readily to other 12-step organizations. The development of spiritual beliefs and practices in 12-step groups is poorly understood. Spirituality in 12-step organizations is, in practice, highly pragmatic and therefore serves as a coping mechanism for members. Working the steps, a primary activity of 12-step members, can thus be seen as fostering different coping orientations. Finally, the role of spiritual beliefs and practices in relief from problems is unclear, with studies providing mixed findings (see, e.g., Brown & Peterson, 1991; Sebenick, 1997; Tonigan & Toscova, in press). Theory-driven prospective research is needed to clarify how spirituality may predict or mediate mutual-help group participation.

We believe that a renaissance in thinking about 12-step organizations is afoot, evidenced in statements of what researchers do not know but want to understand. At the heart of this research is the study of spirituality. This chapter was intended to introduce you to the key aspects of 12-step spirituality as it is now understood. Clearly, all who become better acquainted with the 12-step movement develop their own conceptions of the meaning and benefits of spirituality in 12-step programs.

REFERENCES

Alcoholics Anonymous. (1955). *Alcoholics Anonymous* (2nd ed.). New York: Alcoholics Anonymous World Services, Inc.

Alcoholics Anonymous. (1976). *Alcoholics Anonymous* (3rd ed.). New York: Alcoholics Anonymous World Services.

Alcoholics Anonymous. (1981). *Twelve steps and twelve traditions.* New York: Alcoholics Anonymous World Services.

Brown, H. P., & Peterson, J. H. (1991). Assessing spirituality in addiction treatment and follow-up: Development of the Brown-Peterson Recovery Progress Inventory (BPRPI). *Alcoholism Treatment Quarterly, 8,* 21–50.

Bufe, C. (1998). *Alcoholics Anonymous: Cult or cure* (2nd ed.). San Francisco: Sharp Press.

Burton, T. L., & Williamson, D. L. (1995). Harmful effects of drinking and the use and perceived effectiveness of treatment. *Journal of Studies on Alcohol, 56,* 611–615.

Caldwell, P. E., & Cutter, H. S. G. (in press). Alcoholics Anonymous during early recovery. *Journal of Substance Abuse Treatment.*

Connors, G. J., & Dermen, K. H. (1996). Characteristics of participants in Secular Organizations for Sobriety (SOS). *American Journal of Drug Alcohol Abuse, 22*(2), 281–295.

Connors, G., Tonigan, J. S., & Miller, W. R. (1996). The Religious Background and Behavior Instrument: Psychometric and normed findings. *Psychology of Addictive Behaviors, 10,* 90–96.

Emrick, C. D. (in press). Alcoholics Anonymous and other 12 step groups. In M. Galanter & H. Kleber (Eds.), *Textbook of substance abuse treatment.* Washington, DC: American Psychiatric Press.

Emrick, C. D., Tonigan, J. S., Montgomery, H., & Little, L. (1993). Alcoholics Anonymous: What is currently known? In B. S. McCrady & W. R. Miller (Eds.), *Research on Alcoholics Anonymous: Opportunities and alternatives* (pp. 41–76). New Brunswick, NJ: Rutgers Center of Alcohol Studies.

Gilbert, F. S. (1991). Development of a "Steps Questionnaire." *Journal of Studies on Alcohol, 52,* 353–360.

Humphreys, K., Kaskutas, L. A., & Weisner, C. (1998). The Alcoholics Anonymous Affiliation Scale: Development, reliability, and norms for diverse treated and untreated populations. *Alcoholism: Clinical and Experimental Research, 22,* 974–978.

Kingree, J. B. (1997). Measuring affiliation with 12-step groups. *Substance Use and Misuse, 32,* 181–194.

Kurtz, L. F. (1988). Mutual aid for affective disorders: The manic depressive and depressive association. *American Journal of Orthopsychiatry, 58,* 152–155.

Kus, R. J. (1992). Spirituality in everyday life: Experiences of gay men of Alcoholics Anonymous. *Journal of Chemical Dependency Treatment, 5*(1), 49–66.

Longabaugh, R., Wirtz, P. W., Zweben, A., & Stout, R. L. (1998). Network support for drinking, Alcoholics Anonymous, and long-term matching effects. *Addiction, 93,* 1313–1333.

Mathew, R. J., Georgi, J., Wilson, W. H., & Mathew, G. (1996). A retrospective study of the concept of spirituality as understood by recovering individuals. *Journal of Substance Abuse Treatment, 13,* 67–73.

Mathew, R. J., Mathew, G., Wilson, W. H., & Georgi, J. M. (1995). Measurement of materialism and spiritualism in substance abuse research. *Journal of Studies on Alcohol, 56,* 470–475.

McCrady, B. S., & Miller, W. R. (1993). The importance of research on Alcoholics Anonymous. In B. S. McCrady & W. R. Miller (Eds.), *Research on Alcoholics Anonymous: Opportunities and alternatives* (pp. 3–12). New Brunswick, NJ: Rutgers Center of Alcohol Studies.

Miller, W. R., & Kurtz, E. (1994). Models of alcoholism used in treatment: Contrasting AA and other perspectives with which it is often confused. *Journal of Studies on Alcohol, 55,* 159–166.

Montgomery, H. A., Miller, W. R., & Tonigan, J. S. (1993). Differences among AA groups: Implications for research. *Journal of Studies on Alcohol, 54,* 502–504.

Morgenstern, J., Kahler, C., Frey, R., & Labouvie, E. (1996). Modeling therapeutic responses to 12 step treatment: Optimal responders, non-responders and partial responders. *Journal of Substance Abuse, 8,* 45–59.

Ouimette, P. C., Finney, J. W., & Moos, R. H. (1997). Twelve-Step and cognitive-behavioral treatment for substance abuse: A comparison of treatment effectiveness, *Journal of Consulting and Clinical Psychology, 65*(2), 230–240.

Pargament, K. I., Kennell, J., Hathaway, W., Grevengoes, N., Newman, J., & Jones, W. (1988). Religion and the problem-solving process: Three styles of coping. *Journal for the Scientific Study of Religion, 27,* 90–104.

Project MATCH Research Group. (1997). Matching alcoholism treatments to client heterogeneity: Project MATCH posttreatment drinking outcome. *Journal of Studies on Alcohol, 58,* 7–29.

Room, R. (1993). Alcoholics Anonymous as a social movement. In B. S. McCrady & W. R. Miller (Eds.), *Research on Alcoholics Anonymous: Opportunities and alternatives* (pp. 167–188). New Brunswick, NJ: Rutgers Center of Alcohol Studies.

Schaler, J. A. (1996). Spiritual thinking in addiction-treatment providers: The Spiritual Belief Scale (SBQ). *Alcoholism Treatment Quarterly, 14,* 7–33.

Sebenick, C. W. (1997, January–February). Spirituality and AA recovery. *The Counselor,* pp. 14–17.

Snow, M. G., Prochaska, J. O., & Rossi, J. S. (1994). Processes of change in Alcoholics Anonymous: Maintenance factors in long-term sobriety. *Journal of Studies on Alcohol, 55,* 362–371.

Tonigan, J. S., Ashcroft, F., & Miller, W. R. (1995). AA group dynamics and 12 step activity. *Journal of Studies on Alcohol, 56,* 616–621.

Tonigan, J. S., Connors, G. J., & Miller, W. R., (1996). The Alcoholics Anonymous Involvement Scale (AAI): Reliability and norms. *Psychology of Addictive Behaviors, 10,* 75–80.

Tonigan, J. S., Miller, W. R., & Connors, G. J. (in press). Prior Alcoholics Anonymous involvement and treatment outcome: Matching findings and causal chain analyses. In R. H. Longabaugh & R. W. Wirtz (Eds.), *Project MATCH: A priori matching hypotheses, results, and mediating mechanisms* (NIAAA Project MATCH Monograph Series). Rockville, MD: U.S. Government Printing Office.

Tonigan, J. S., & Toscova, R. (in press). Mutual-help groups: Research and clinical implications. In W. R. Miller & N. Heather (Eds.), *Treating addictive behaviors* (2nd ed.). New York: Plenum.

Tonigan, J. S., Toscova, R., & Miller, W. R. (1996). Meta-analysis of the Alcoholics Anonymous literature: Sample and study characteristics moderate findings. *Journal of Studies on Alcohol, 57*, 65–72.

Walker, S. R., Tonigan, J. S., Miller, W. R., & Kahlich, L. (1997). Intercessory prayer in the treatment of alcohol dependence. *Alternative Therapies, 3*, 79–86.

7

VALUES, SPIRITUALITY, AND PSYCHOTHERAPY

P. SCOTT RICHARDS, JOHN M. RECTOR, AND ALAN C. TJELTVEIT

There is growing empirical evidence that people's spiritual values and behaviors can promote physical and psychological coping, healing, and well-being (Benson, 1996; Borysenko & Borysenko, 1994; Gartner, Larson, & Allen, 1996; Pargament, 1997; Payne, Bergin, Bielema, & Jenkins, 1991; Richards & Bergin, 1997). This finding has led many mental health professionals to conclude that clients' spiritual values should be viewed as a potential resource in psychotherapy rather than as something to be ignored (Bergin, 1980a; Richards & Bergin, 1997; Shafranske, 1996; Worthington, Kurusu, McCullough, & Sanders, 1996). The purpose of this chapter is to discuss how psychotherapists can bring values, particularly spiritual ones, to the foreground of therapy to facilitate clients' healing and growth. We first review some historical perspectives about values, spirituality, and psychotherapy to lay the groundwork for our approach. We then describe a spiritual approach to working with values in therapy.

HISTORICAL AND PHILOSOPHICAL BACKGROUND

Modern psychology and psychotherapy began late in the 19th century, during the coming of age of modern science. To escape religion's influence, some early scientists, including behavioral scientists, adopted a number of assumptions about reality that directly conflicted with religious views of the world (Richards & Bergin, 1997). Several of these assumptions, particularly naturalism, ethical relativism, ethical hedonism, and positivism, had a profound influence on the way therapists came to view the role of values in psychotherapy.

Some Early Assumptions About Values

Naturalism is the belief that "the universe is self-sufficient, without supernatural cause or control" (Honer & Hunt, 1987, p. 225). Naturalists assume that human beings and the universe can be understood without resorting to religious or spiritual explanations and that "the explanation of the world given by the sciences is the only satisfactory explanation of reality" (Honer & Hunt, 1987, p. 225). Naturalism led some behavioral scientists to conclude that all moral values are ephemeral and of human origin.

Having accepted naturalism, some behavioral scientists also endorsed ethical relativism. Ethical relativism is the belief that "there are no universally valid principles, since all moral principles are valid relative to cultural or individual choice" (Percesepe, 1991, p. 572). Thus, "whatever a culture or society holds to be right is therefore right or, at least, 'right for them'" (Solomon, 1990, p. 235). Ethical relativism led some behavioral scientists to conclude that if all values are relative, therapists should not question their clients' values. Values, they also assumed, were irrelevant to mental health and therapeutic change.

Although ethical relativism implies that the values of all cultures and individuals are equally valid and good (Kitchener, 1980; Percesepe, 1991), some behavioral scientists contradicted this assumption by endorsing hedonistic ethical views. Ethical hedonism is the belief that "we always ought to seek our own pleasure and that the highest good for us is the most pleasure together with the least pain" (Honer & Hunt, 1987, p. 222). Relying in part on the influence of the Darwinian view that human beings are highly similar to the rest of the animal kingdom, some early behavioral scientists theorized that human beings are basically hedonistic and reward seeking (Hillner, 1984; Lundin, 1985; Watson, 1924/1983). As a result, many psychotherapists encouraged their clients to "throw off the shackles" of religion and be more accepting of their hedonistic tendencies (Bergin, 1980a; Campbell, 1975; Ellis, 1980, Watson, 1924/1983).

Many early behavioral scientists also adopted positivism, holding that "knowledge is limited to observable facts and their interrelations" (Honer & Hunt, 1987, p. 226) and that scientific theories can be "shown to be true on the basis of evidence" (Bechtel, 1988, p. 18). Positivists assume that it is possible for scientists to be objective, impartial observers and that their empirical observations will eventually lead to a complete understanding of reality. This assumption led behavioral scientists to conclude that psychotherapy, an applied "science," could also be conducted in an objective, impartial, value-free manner. Furthermore, logical positivists sharply distinguished facts and values. Because only scientific thinking and logical assertions were held to be cognitively meaningful (Toulmin & Leary, 1992), values (understood in ethical terms) were regarded as intellectually meaningless (O'Donahue, 1989; Putnam, 1993).

The assumptions discussed above had a major influence on psychotherapists' beliefs about how values should be handled. During the first half of the 20th century, most therapists believed that they could keep their values out of psychotherapy (Kessell & McBrearty, 1967; Patterson, 1958). Psychoanalysts thought they could be "blank slates," behaviorists claimed to be "objective, scientific technicians," and client-centered therapists were "nonjudgmental, unconditional listeners." Many therapists also thought clients' religious and spiritual values were irrelevant or damaging to mental health, interpersonal relationships, and therapeutic growth (Bergin, 1980a, 1983; Bergin, Payne, & Richards, 1996; Ellis, 1980; Freud, 1927). Although claiming that they could be "value free," many therapists did nevertheless often endorse relativistic and hedonistic ethical philosophies in their writings and clinical practice (Bergin, 1980a; Campbell, 1975; Ellis, 1980; Freud, 1927).

Changing Professional Views About Values

The assumptions about values adopted by early behavioral scientists have been vigorously challenged during the past few decades. The belief that therapists can and should keep their values out of therapy has been discredited because of penetrating theoretical critiques and accumulating empirical evidence to the contrary (Bergin, 1980a, 1980b, 1980c; Campbell, 1975; Kitchener, 1980; London, 1964; Lowe, 1976; Tjeltveit, 1986; Woolfolk, 1998). Research has provided evidence that therapists' values influence every phase of psychotherapy, including the theories of personality and therapeutic change, assessment strategies, goals of treatment, the design and selection of interventions, and evaluations of therapy outcome (Bergin, 1980a; Tjeltveit, 1986). Furthermore, clients are influenced by therapists' values, often adopting their health, moral, and religious values (Bergin et al., 1996; Jensen & Bergin, 1988; Tjeltveit, 1986).

The belief that therapists could be value free was further undermined by the recognition of serious problems with traditional formulations of positivism (Howard, 1986; Jones, 1994; Kuhn, 1970; Lakatos & Musgrave, 1970; Polanyi, 1962). Scientific observations are value and theory laden (Laudan, 1984), for even so-called "objective" scientists have values that limit and bias their observations (Howard, 1986; Jones, 1994). Psychotherapists have been forced to acknowledge that if basic scientific research cannot be value free, neither can an applied discipline such as psychotherapy.

Many professionals also now recognize that the adoption of ethical relativism as an underlying assumption was problematic. Kitchener (1980) and Bergin (1980c) clearly pointed out that ethical relativism is a logically untenable belief for therapists. All therapists advocate (value) and pursue certain therapeutic goals—goals that are based on nonempirical assumptions about human nature and what constitutes mental health (Bergin, 1980a; London, 1986; Lowe, 1976; Szasz, 1960). Bergin (1980c) criticized therapists who profess to be relativists, saying, "It is interesting to observe professional change agents who believe in a relativistic philosophy and simultaneously assert dogmatically the virtue of the therapeutic goals they promote" (p. 11). Thus, although they may profess to believe in relativism, in practice therapists find it extremely difficult to *be* relativists.

Ethical relativism also implies that therapists should accept all of their clients' values as equally good and valid. This creates a dilemma in therapy because it sometimes becomes clear that clients' values and lifestyles have negative emotional, social, or physical consequences (e.g., a married man who values abusing drugs and engaging in promiscuous, unprotected sex increases his and his spouse's risk of contracting AIDS). Ethical relativists cannot logically challenge such values without contradicting the premise that all values are equally good (Richards & Bergin, 1997).

The psychology profession's acceptance and promotion of ethically hedonistic values has also been criticized (Bergin, 1980b; Campbell, 1975; Schwartz, 1986; Wallach & Wallach, 1983). For example, Bergin (1980b) argued that

> it is crucial to identify selfish and hedonistic values as destructive to mental health and societal integrity. By accepting such views without criticism, the psychological sciences are implicitly sanctioning them and colluding in subverting values and traditions that have had a demonstrated, constructive role in the positive achievements of western civilization (Campbell, 1975). . . . I, and scores of other psychologists . . . abhor such uncritical acceptance of divergent standards. (p. 642)

There is evidence that a majority of mental health professionals no longer concur with ethical relativism and hedonism. A national survey of clinical psychologists, psychiatrists, marriage and family therapists, and clinical social workers documented that most of them agreed that certain values are important for mentally healthy lifestyles and that they use these values to guide and evaluate therapy (Jensen & Bergin, 1988). Most of the therapists also rejected ethically hedonistic views by endorsing values such as personal responsibility, family commitment, self-control, humility, self-sacrifice, forgiveness, and honesty (Jensen & Bergin, 1988; see also, Doherty, 1995; Kelly, 1995a).

The demise of the belief that therapy is a relativistic, value-free enterprise and the recognition that certain values are important for mental health has created a great deal of ambiguity and confusion in the profession about how therapists should deal with values (Bergin et al., 1996). Many therapists remain uncertain about how to ethically and effectively address values in therapy. This confusion persists for at least two reasons. First, although the American Psychological Association's (1992) ethical principles say that therapists should "respect the rights of others to hold values, attitudes, and opinions that differ from their own" (p. 1599), there are no clear guidelines about how to apply this during psychotherapy. Second, many therapists lack an awareness of their own values and of the value assumptions that underlie their therapeutic approach. This lack of awareness is rooted in deficiencies in clinical training programs that give too little attention to the value assumptions that the profession and therapy approaches are based on and that do little to help students examine their own worldviews and values (Shafranske & Malony, 1996; Slife & Williams, 1995).

According to Richards and Bergin (1997), because of the ambiguity and confusion about values in the profession, "many therapists continue to implicitly advance their value agendas during treatment" (p. 131). They hypothesized that there are four problematic therapist value styles, all of which tend to impose therapists' values and reduce clients' freedom to make choices about the direction of their lives (Richards & Bergin, 1997). *Deniers* believe in ethical relativism. By accepting all of their clients' values as valid or okay, they believe they can avoid imposing their values on clients. They deny that their ethically relativistic worldview is value laden or that values are embedded in the therapeutic goals they pursue and the interventions they use. *Implicit minimizers* believe that they cannot totally keep their values out of therapy, but they believe they can minimize their influence by not sharing them or revealing them. Implicit minimizers fail to recognize that not openly sharing their values may be more coercive than explicitly sharing them (Frank & Frank, 1991).

Explicit imposers believe that their beliefs and values about certain issues (e.g., gender roles, sexual orientation, religion) are correct. They believe that their clients will be happier and the world would be a better place if they get clients to accept these values. They openly and zealously promote their value agenda and reject and emotionally punish clients who do not agree with them. *Implicit imposers* also believe that their beliefs and values about various issues are correct. Implicit imposers do not openly promote their values but deliberately and covertly attempt to convert clients to their views. A less problematic valuing style, according to Richards and Bergin (1997), is an *explicit minimizing approach*, which we discuss in some detail later in this chapter.

Religious and Spiritual Understandings of Values

Although religious and spiritual views were excluded from mainstream psychology and psychotherapy for nearly a century, this alienation is ending. Many behavioral scientists are now questioning psychology's long-standing adherence to naturalism (Bergin, 1980a; Jones, 1994; Richards & Bergin, 1997) and are incorporating spiritual perspectives and interventions into psychological theory, research, and practice (Kelly, 1995b; Richards & Bergin, 1997; Shafranske, 1996; Worthington et al., 1996).

We believe that religious and spiritual understandings about values could help bring some clarity to the confusion about values that currently exists in the psychotherapy profession. We agree with Campbell (1975, p. 1103) that the moral principles and values taught by the great world religious traditions are "recipes for living that have been evolved, tested, and winnowed through hundreds of generations of human social history" (p. 1103). Perhaps there *is* something psychotherapists can learn from the world's great religions.

There are five major theistic religions (i.e., Judaism, Christianity, Islam, Zoroastrianism, and Sikhism) and six major Eastern spiritual traditions (i.e., Hinduism, Buddhism, Janism, Shinto, Confucianism, and Taoism). Although there is great diversity between and within these traditions regarding their beliefs and practices, they agree that human beings can and should transcend hedonistic and selfish tendencies to grow spiritually and to promote the welfare of others (Richards & Bergin, 1997). There is also general agreement among the world religions about what moral principles and values promote spiritual enlightenment and personal and social harmony.

According to Smart (1983), a respected world religion scholar, "The major faiths have much in common as far as moral conduct goes. Not to steal, not to lie, not to kill, not to have certain kinds of sexual relations—such prescriptions are found across the world" (p. 117). There is, however, considerable variety in the specific interpretations and applications of these general moral principles (Smart, 1983, 1993). Members of the world religions also believe that moral values should be taught and transmitted from one generation to the next (Smart, 1993, 1994).

In Table 7.1 we contrast religious and spiritual teachings about values with the views of some early behavioral scientists and with those of many contemporary social scientists. Although contemporary professional notions about values are more compatible with religious and spiritual views than in the past, contemporary views fail to take full advantage of the benefits to be derived from spiritual and religious perspectives. Accordingly, we now turn to an approach to therapeutic valuing that draws more fully on spiritual and religious values. This approach is respectful of clients'

TABLE 7.1
Some Traditional and Contemporary Psychological Views Compared With Some Spiritual Understandings About Values

Traditional psychology	Contemporary psychology	Spiritual view
Values are of human origin and are ephemeral.	Values are of human origin, but some values have endured for centuries and have played a constructive role in civilization.	God has revealed moral values, or there are values built into the universe, that are eternal and beneficial.
There are no universal values. All values are equally valid and good. Whatever a culture or individual views as right is therefore right for them.	There may be health-related values that promote better physical and mental health and harmonious relationships.	There are moral and ethical values that universally promote growth and well-being. Some values are better than others because they do more to promote spirituality, health, and harmonious relationships.
Human beings should always seek pleasure and avoid pain. They should gratify their biological and psychological impulses and desires.	Humans should seek pleasure and happiness and avoid pain, but they should not do so without considering the long-term consequences and impact of their behaviors on others. Responsibility, self-sacrifice, and altruistic service are often desirable.	Humans should "often forego their own rewards (pleasure) for the welfare of others. Responsibility, self-sacrifice, suffering, love, and altruistic service are valued above personal gratification" (Richards & Bergin, 1997, p. 30).
Therapists can and should keep their values out of therapy. Clients' values, especially spiritual ones, are irrelevant to therapy.	Therapists cannot totally keep their values out of therapy, but they should avoid "imposing" them on clients. The best way to not impose one's values on clients is to not disclose them. Therapists should not challenge or try to influence clients' values.	Therapist cannot keep their values out of therapy, nor should they always try. When appropriate, therapists should explicitly endorse and respectfully teach healthy values. It is often important for therapists to explore clients' values, especially spiritual values, to promote growth.

spiritual values, and it offers therapists greater clarity and direction when they deal with such issues during the course of treatment.

A SPIRITUAL THERAPEUTIC VALUING APPROACH

According to Richards and Bergin (1997), the most ethical and effective manner for therapists to deal with values is to adopt an *explicit minimizing valuing style*. The words *explicit* and *minimizing* are used to describe this spiritual valuing style because they communicate the belief that the best way for therapists to *minimize* the likelihood that they will impose their values on clients is to be *explicit* about them at appropriate times during therapy. An explicit minimizing valuing approach is grounded in religious and spiritual views about values, but it is also consistent with current theory and research about values and psychotherapy. Many scholars have laid the foundation for this approach (e.g., Kitchener, 1980; London, 1986; Lowe, 1976; Maslow, 1971; Tjeltveit, 1986, 1989), but Bergin's pioneering writings about values, religion, and psychotherapy have been most influential (Bergin, 1980a, 1980b, 1980c, 1985, 1991; Jensen & Bergin, 1988).

An explicit minimizing therapeutic valuing approach is based on the following assumptions (Richards & Bergin, 1997):

1. Psychotherapists' metaphysical worldviews and values have a major influence on how they conduct therapy. Therapists' theoretical orientations, treatment goals, assessment methods, interventions, and evaluations of therapy outcome are all ultimately grounded in and influenced by nonempirical assumptions and values about the nature of the universe and deity, human beings, ethics, death and suffering, spirituality, and the purpose of life (Browning, 1987; Jones & Butman, 1991; Tjeltveit, 1989).

2. The most ethical way for therapists to handle values during therapy is often to be explicit about their own values at appropriate times during therapy. Unethical value imposition is least likely to occur when therapists openly and explicitly disclose and own their values while also clearly affirming their clients' right to disagree with them.

3. Metaphysical beliefs and values affect people's goals, lifestyle, and physical and mental health. When appropriate, therapists should let clients know that values have physical, emotional, and spiritual consequences and help them examine the consequences of their value choices.

4. Teaching, endorsing, and modeling healthy values is a desir-

able, ethical, and honorable activity. Therapists should accept the fact that they are value agents and purposely attempt to model and teach consensus health and human welfare values (see below) to their clients.

5. Clients' core spiritual values may be especially influential in promoting clients' coping, healing, and change. When clients wish to do so, therapists should help them access their spiritual values and resources to assist them in their efforts to heal and grow.

We do not think that therapists should attempt to teach their clients specific moral rules or "do's" and "don'ts" because this would not be respectful of clients' diversity and would prevent clients' from growing by making their own value and lifestyle choices (Richards & Bergin, 1997). However, we believe that there are some general values or principles that can promote health and that should be used to guide and evaluate therapy. Therapists can appeal to both the psychotherapy profession and the world's great religious traditions for insight into these health-related values.

Jensen and Bergin's (1988) national interdisciplinary survey gives insight into mental health values that the majority of psychotherapists believed at that time were important for mentally healthy lifestyles and for guiding and evaluating therapy. They found that most therapists believe they should endorse and promote (a) competent perception and expression of feelings; (b) freedom, autonomy, and responsibility; (c) integration, coping, and work; (d) self-awareness and growth; (e) human relatedness and interpersonal and family commitment; (f) self-maintenance and physical fitness; (g) mature values; and (h) forgiveness. More details about each of these themes is provided in Table 7.2, which is reprinted from their article.

Therapists could use such consensus mental health values and principles to guide their work with clients. At appropriate times during therapy, they may find it helpful to let their clients know how they feel about such behaviors or values as they relate to clients' goals for improving their mental health. At times, it may be equally appropriate to note that there is professional disagreement about the health effects of certain sexual mores (e.g., having sexual relations exclusively within marriage) and religious behaviors (e.g., actively participating in a religious group; Jensen & Bergin, 1988).

When working with clients who are spiritually or religiously inclined (which appears to be a majority), therapists may promote better functioning by appealing to more spiritually oriented health values to guide their work. Richards and Bergin (1997) described a variety of spiritual values and lifestyles that they believe, based on theory and growing empirical evidence, are associated with, or characteristic of, better mental and physical health and harmonious interpersonal relationships. These spiritual

TABLE 7.2
Responses by Mental Health Professionals to 10 Value Themes

Theme/sample items	Important for a positive, mentally healthy lifestyle		Important in guiding and evaluating psychotherapy in all or many clients
	Total % agree[a]	% agree[b]	% agree
Theme 1 (5 items): Competent perception and expression of feelings	97	87	87
29. Increase sensitivity to others' feelings	98	93	92
30. Be open, genuine, and honest with others	96	86	87
Theme 2 (10 items): Freedom/autonomy/responsibility	96	88	85
7. Assume responsibility for one's actions	99	98	98
5. Increase one's alternatives at a choice point	100	96	96
11. Increase one's capacity for self-control	99	86	89
10. Experience appropriate feelings of guilt	88	70	65
Theme 3 (9 items): Integration, coping, and work	95	81	81
50. Develop effective strategies to cope with stress	99	97	97
49. Develop appropriate methods to satisfy needs	99	95	94
53. Find fulfillment and satisfaction in work	97	86	82
54. Strive for achievement	83	52	58
Theme 4 (5 items): Self-awareness/growth	92	74	77
37. Become aware of inner potential and ability to grow	96	89	90
42. Discipline oneself for the sake of growth	82	54	59
Theme 5 (12 items): Human relatedness/interpersonal and family commitment	91	77	73
12. Develop ability to give and receive affection	97	94	95
35. Increase respect for human value and worth	98	88	79
17. Be faithful to one's marriage partner[c]	91	78	70
19. Be committed to family needs and childrearing	90	80	76
41. Become self-sacrificing and unselfish	52	26	30

Table continues

TABLE 7.2 *Continued*

| Theme/sample items | Important for a positive, mentally healthy lifestyle | | Important in guiding and evaluating psychotherapy in all or many clients |
	Total % agree[a]	% agree[b]	% agree
Theme 6 (3 items): Self-maintenance/physical fitness	91	78	71
45. Practice habits of physical health	94	77	69
46. Apply self-discipline in use of alcohol, tobacco, and drugs	95	83	75
Theme 7 (6 items): Mature values	84	66	68
56. Have a sense of purpose for living	97	87	85
14. Regulate behavior by applying principles and ideals	96	81	78
55. Adhere to universal principles governing mental health	67	47	55
Theme 8 (4 items): Forgiveness	85	64	62
60. Forgive others who have inflicted disturbance in oneself	93	77	78
62. Make restitution for one's negative influence	79	54	51
Theme 9 (9 items): Regulated sexual fulfillment	63	51	49
27. Understand that sexual impulses are a natural part of oneself	97	94	85
24. Have sexual relations exclusively within marriage	63	49	49
25. Prefer a heterosexual sex relationship	57	43	39
17. Be faithful to one's marriage partner	91	78	70
Theme 10 (6 items): Spirituality/ religiosity	49	34	29
69. Seek spiritual understanding of one's place in the universe	68	53	41
68. Seek strength through communion with a higher power	50	34	31
67. Actively participate in a religious affiliation	44	28	25

Note. N = 425. The Mentally Healthy Lifestyle Scale provided for seven possible ratings: *Hi, Med,* and *Lo Agree; Uncertain;* and *Lo, Med,* and *Hi Disagree.* The Guiding and Evaluating Psychotherapy Scale provided for four categories: Applicable to *All, Many, Few,* or *No Clients.* [a]*Hi, Med,* and *Lo.* [b]*Hi* and *Med* only. [c]This item appears under two themes (5 and 9). The full scale included 69 items. From "Mental Health Values of Professional Therapists: A National Interdisciplinary Survey," by J. P. Jensen & A. E. Bergin, 1988, *Professional Psychology: Research and Practice, 19,* p. 290. Copyright 1988 by the American Psychological Association. Adapted with permission.

health values are summarized in Table 7.3. In the left column of the table, terms that describe healthy, mature, spiritually oriented values and lifestyles are listed, and in the right column are unhealthy ones. With religious and spiritually oriented clients, these values can provide therapists with another framework for evaluating whether their clients' values and lifestyles are healthy and mature and for deciding what therapeutic goals to endorse. By grounding their therapy in such values, therapists can avoid lapsing into ethical relativism, or the belief that "anything goes."

Cautions and Caveats

We recognize that there are dangers in deliberately endorsing and promoting even those values and principles that have widespread professional and spiritual support. We agree with Bergin (1991), who cautioned that

> a strong interest in value discussions ... can be problematic if it is overemphasized. It would be unethical to trample on the values of clients, and it would be unwise to focus on value issues when other issues may be at the nucleus of the disorder, which is frequently the case in the early stages of treatment. It is vital to be open about values but not coercive, to be a competent professional and not a missionary for a particular belief, and at the same time to be honest enough to recognize how one's value commitments may or may not promote health. (p. 399)

We agree that value themes should not usually be the central focus of therapy. We recommend that techniques for working with values should be part of a multidimensional, integrative approach to therapy in which many other techniques may be used (Richards & Bergin, 1997). We also acknowledge that therapists of different theoretical orientations (e.g., cognitive–behavioral, psychodynamic) may address value issues somewhat differently. It is also important to keep in mind that value discussions and interventions are at times contraindicated. Some clients may have such severe pathology or acute symptoms that they are not capable of rationally understanding and responding to value issues. Discussing value issues with them may lead into cul-de-sacs, or it may provoke unnecessary (or premature) transference reactions (e.g., hostility, confusion, dependency, etc.).

In criticizing ethical relativism as we have done, we also want to make it clear that we do not endorse ethical absolutism or, in other words, the belief that there is a set hierarchy of values that never change regardless of time, context, or other values. Although we do believe that there are certain values that are more moral and that do more to promote mental and physical health, harmonious relationships, and spiritual growth than other values, the application and prioritization of these values may vary somewhat depending on the time, context, and other competing values.

TABLE 7.3
Healthy and Unhealthy Religious and Spiritual Values and Lifestyles

Adaptive and healthy values and lifestyles	Maladaptive and unhealthy values and lifestyles

1A. Intrinsic
    Sincere
    Congruent
    Lives religion
    Personal faith
	1B. Extrinsic
	    Role playing
	    Incongruent
	    Uses religion
	    Normative faith

2A. Actualizing
    Growth oriented
    Self-regulated agency
    Experiential/creative
    Self-renewing/repentant
    Integrates ambiguity and
      paradox
	2B. Perfectionistic
	    Righteous performances
	    Overcontrolled inefficacy
	    Compulsively ritualistic/stagnant
	    Self-punitive/depressed
	    Anxious about the unanticipated

3A. Reforming/renewing
    Change-oriented
    Benevolent/reforming power
    Tolerant
    Egalitarian
	3B. Authoritarian
	    Rigid
	    Dogmatic/absolutistic
	    Intolerant/prejudiced
	    Controlling/dominating

4A. Interpersonal/social orientation
    Networking/familial/kinship
    Cooperative
    Open/authentic/integrity
    Self-sacrificing
	4B. Narcissistic
	    Self-aggrandizing
	    Competitive
	    Manipulation/deception
	    Self-gratifying

5A. Nurturing
    Tender/protective
    Warm/faithful/intimate
    Caring
    Facilitating growth
    Empathic
	5B. Aggressive
	    Angry/abusive/violent
	    Antisocial/unfaithful
	    Sadistic
	    Power seeking
	    Insensitive

6A. Reconciling
    Forgiving
    Humble
    Appropriately direct
    Problem solving
	6B. Dependent
	    Pleasing/submissive
	    Compliant/masochistic
	    Passive–aggressive
	    Conflict avoidant

7A. Inspiring
    Attunement to spirit of truth
    Prophetic
    Mystical—good reality testing
	7B. Hyperspiritual
	    God controlled/externalizing
	    Occult/evil inspired
	    Mystical—poor reality testing

Note. From *A spiritual strategy for counseling and psychotherapy* (p. 189) by P. S. Richards & A. E. Bergin, 1997; Washington, DC: American Psychological Association. Copyright 1982 by the American Psychological Association. Reprinted by permission.

For example, we think that honesty, compared with dishonesty, is a value that if practiced consistently in one's life will lead to better relationships, mental health, and spiritual well-being. Nevertheless, there may be some situations or contexts in which being honest is not the highest value and in which dishonesty may be justified (e.g., a young girl promising her abuser that she will not tell her parents about the abuse when she fully intends to do so once she is safe). Even a seemingly absolute value such as "It is wrong to kill another human being" may depend on the context for its application and validity (e.g., perhaps one is morally justified in killing, if necessary, an attacker who is trying to murder one's spouse or children).

Thus, in endorsing the idea that there are certain values that are more moral and beneficial and that therapists should share their understanding with clients about what these values and principles are, this does not mean that therapists should tell their clients how to apply these values in a given situation. Ultimately, therapists must permit clients to make their own choices about what they value and how they will apply these values in their lives, but it would be irresponsible for therapists not to share what wisdom they can about values when it is relevant to clients' problems.

We also recognize the logical circularity of suggesting that science has and may continue to provide empirical evidence that certain values, compared with other values, may do more to promote health and well-being (Woolfolk, 1998). Science is a value-laden enterprise that makes value-based assumptions about what constitutes health and well-being (Woolfolk, 1998). How, then, can science objectively verify what values promote health and well-being? It cannot. It can verify only what values promote the kinds of health and well-being scientists believe in and value (Woolfolk, 1998). Nevertheless, we agree with Richards and Slife (in press), who suggested that

> as long as behavioral scientists (1) remember the potential problem of circularity, (2) attempt to be explicit about what assumptions and value judgments underlie their definitions of mental health and science, and (3) don't claim that behavioral science offers the only, or necessarily the best, available understanding about values, perhaps research can offer considerable insight into the nature of human values and their potential impact on physical and mental health. (pp. 6–7)

In light of all of these cautions, how can therapists ethically and effectively work with clients' values in therapy? Although values should not be the exclusive focus of therapy, we think there are certain decision points when they should become more central. In the remainder of this chapter, we discuss occasions when it may be the most helpful for therapists to be explicit about values and when and how therapists can help clients explore their values and find optimal solutions to their lifestyle dilemmas.

Making Therapists' Values Explicit

Each psychotherapy orientation is based on certain underlying assumptions about the nature of the world, human beings, healthy functioning, and therapeutic change. For example, Freud assumed that there is no God, that human beings are primarily biological organisms, and that human development and functioning are largely determined by intrapsychic forces and events that occur during the first few years of a child's life (Freud, 1927; Wulff, 1991). The theistic, spiritual strategy described by Richards and Bergin (1997) assumes that God exists, that humans have an eternal spiritual identity, and that human development and functioning, although influenced to some degree by biological, social, and psychological factors, is ultimately a spiritual process in which humans can transcend barriers to actualize their God-given potential. These views, along with the myriad that lie in between, drive therapists' conceptions of what is salient and important in therapy. Because value assumptions play a role at every stage of therapy and influence a variety of dimensions of therapy, we need to make them explicit in a variety of ways and at various times during therapy.

The First Session: Informed Consent

Therapists may find it helpful in the first session to inform clients about the values that underlie and guide their therapy approach, such as their assumptions about the nature of human beings and their beliefs about why certain assessment and intervention techniques are valuable. Therapists may also wish to briefly describe the values that underlie their conceptions of healthy functioning (e.g., Jensen & Bergin, 1988, Table 2). We recommend including this information in a written informed consent document, although some therapists may prefer to do this verbally.

Information about therapists' values will help clients make more informed decisions about whether they wish to use a practitioner's services. In our experience, disclosing values during the first session usually has the effect of quickly facilitating trust and rapport, unless the client seriously disagrees with our values. When clients have a problem with therapists' values, therapists can discuss this openly and nonjudgmentally. If clients or therapists feel that their value systems are too incongruent, therapists should help clients find other therapists whose values are more compatible. Regardless of the outcome, clients' autonomy is promoted by giving them the information that is necessary for them to make choices about which therapy services seem best suited to them. Therapists should use discretion and good clinical judgment about when and how to disclose their values. They do not need to overload clients with value disclosures in the first session. Making values explicit will probably need to be an ongoing process.

Assessment

When therapists make decisions about what assessment methods and instruments to use, they are answering the question, "What do I, as a therapist, believe is valuable to learn about my client?" Therapists' beliefs about this question guide their assessment decisions. For example, psychoanalytically oriented therapists believe that it is good and valuable to understand clients' unconscious processes; thus, they might use the Rorschach Inkblot Test. Each therapy orientation uses different assessment methods and instruments because each values different assessment information. Inasmuch as the choices therapists make about what assessment methods to use are value-based decisions, we believe it is good practice for therapists to let clients know why they think the assessment instruments they recommend are valuable (i.e., what information they provide and why this information is helpful).

Treatment Goals

Generally speaking, every system of psychotherapy values and works toward the same goal: greater psychological health and functioning for the client. Yet, each approach attempts to accomplish this overarching goal in a different fashion because of diverse views about human nature and the mechanisms of therapeutic change (Tjeltveit, 1999). Each therapy orientation makes assumptions about which client system (e.g., physical, cognitive, behavioral, family, spiritual) therapists should intervene in to effect change (Richards & Bergin, 1997). For example, is it most valuable to address the client's unconscious? The client's behavior? The client's family system? Cognitive therapists believe that it is most valuable to intervene in the clients' cognitive system because they assume that cognition causes disturbance and that they can most effectively help clients change by modifying their dysfunctional cognitions. Some spiritually oriented therapists believe it may be valuable to intervene in the spiritual system because they assume that spiritual beliefs and influences can promote healing and growth (Richards & Bergin, 1997). Seen in this light, it is clear that therapists' beliefs and values influence their selection of therapeutic goals.

Another related issue to bear in mind is the cultural boundedness of treatment goals (Marsella & White, 1982; Minsel, Becker, & Korchin, 1991). Levine and Padilla (1980) noted that the goals of therapy in any culture can range from the removal of symptoms to attitude change, behavior change, insight, improved relations with others, social effectiveness, personal adjustment, and preventive health. Which goal to pursue will depend on the cultural and religious values of the client, the host society, and the therapist.

We believe that therapy is generally most effective when the goals of treatment, and the values underlying them, are discussed explicitly in a collaborative way between therapists and clients. When clients are general or vague in stating their goals for treatment, it is important for therapists to assist them in becoming more specific about what they want to change. In doing so, however, we think it is appropriate for therapists to be explicit about their reasons for valuing certain treatment goals, so that clients can make informed decisions about which ones they wish to pursue.

Therapeutic Interventions

Seen from a values perspective, when therapists make any intervention, they are implicitly answering the questions, "What types of changes in clients do I value?" and "What interventions are valuable for facilitating these changes?" In light of this, we think it is appropriate for therapists to explicitly discuss with clients why they believe certain interventions or classes of interventions are valuable or helpful (e.g., hypnosis, gestalt techniques, cognitive restructuring, behavioral techniques, spiritual interventions, etc.). For example, when first introducing gestalt techniques, therapists could explain to their clients that such techniques are helpful for promoting an increased awareness of one's immediate, "here-and-now," emotional experiencing and that they believe such experiencing is valuable because it can promote insight and better psychological and social functioning. Such an explanation would help clients better understand the potential effects and value of gestalt techniques, which would maximize their ability to participate willingly or to decline.

We are not saying that therapists should discuss the underlying values for each and every intervention they make in therapy. This would be awkward and time-consuming, and it would probably not be in clients' best interest. Moreover, some interventions would lose their effectiveness and would be undermined by being more explicitly discussed (e.g., paradoxical techniques). In general, however, our experience is that when therapists explicitly discuss why a certain class of techniques is valuable, this increases clients' willingness to participate in these interventions and safeguards their autonomy.

Value Conflicts

Clients and therapists may disagree about a variety of values. For example, questions about the right to die (including physician-assisted suicide), abortion, religion, drug use, and various types of sexual behavior are controversial social and moral issues that may lead to serious value disagreements (Corey, Corey, & Callanan, 1993). Value conflicts about such issues can threaten the therapeutic relationship by undermining trust, liking, and credibility. However, value conflicts are not necessarily problematic: What is critical is *how* these delicate situations are handled. Genuine interpersonal interaction, connection, understanding, and ultimate appreciation permit people holding differing values to transcend conflict.

When therapists recognize that a serious value conflict exists between them and their clients, we recommend that they openly acknowledge this while also affirming their clients' right to disagree with them. Therapists can explore with their clients whether the value difference will undermine trust or otherwise prevent them from helping the clients pursue their therapeutic goals. If it does, they can refer their clients to a therapist whose values are more compatible. Naturally, this approach will not be enough to transcend all value conflicts, nor do therapists need to use it in every instance of conflict, as value conflicts come in varying degrees of severity. Also, clients will sometimes be irrational or otherwise lacking in the personal resources to understand and resolve such issues. In many cases, such matters will have to be delayed until the immediate distress is reduced or the client's legal agent or guardian will have to be consulted. However, whenever therapists recognize that a core value conflict may prevent them from fully supporting or helping clients who are capable of making reasonable decisions in their self-interest, we think it is appropriate for therapists to openly and respectfully discuss the conflict so that their clients' autonomy can be protected (e.g., an atheistic, socially liberal therapist and a religiously devout, social conservative client).

Evaluating Therapy Outcome and Termination

Decisions about when therapy has been successful and should be terminated are influenced to some degree by the outcomes therapists and clients value (e.g., do they value extinguishing symptomatic behaviors, realigning unhealthy systemic triangles, modifying irrational thoughts, or facilitating spiritual healing?). Ideally, therapy is terminated when the desired outcomes have been achieved, although in today's managed care environment, therapy is all too often terminated because clients' insurance coverage has ended. Nevertheless, keeping in mind the time limitations often imposed by managed care, it may be helpful for therapists and clients to mutually decide, preferably when treatment goals are set, what criteria or values will be used to judge when success has been achieved. Therapists may need to revise such criteria as therapy progresses, of course, but they can promote their clients' autonomy by being explicit about what outcomes they value and wish to work toward.

Making Clients' Values Explicit

In addition to disclosing their own values, therapists must also promote clients' healing and growth by assessing, exploring, and helping clients modify their values. Below we describe four occasions when we think it may be helpful for therapists to purposely make clients' values a therapeutic focus. We then describe several values assessment and intervention techniques that may prove useful for helping them do so and discuss how clients' core spiritual values can be used to promote healing and growth.

Assessing Clients' Values

Depending on the nature of clients' presenting problems, it may be appropriate early in therapy to assess clients' core values. During the past two decades, many professionals have written about the importance of therapists gaining an understanding of their clients' worldviews and core values (e.g., Ibrahim, 1985, 1991; Kluckhohn, 1951; Richards & Bergin, 1997; Speight, Myers, Cox, & Highlen, 1991; Sue, 1978; Sue & Sue, 1990). Gaining an understanding of their clients' worldviews and values provides therapists with valuable contextual information and is essential for conducting culturally sensitive therapy. In addition, people's spiritual worldviews and values can have a significant impact on their mental and physical health and interpersonal relationships (Richards & Bergin, 1997). Emotional and interpersonal difficulties may be caused by people's failure to live in harmony with healthy values, and therapists need to be alert to this possibility. Once therapists have assessed their clients' worldview, values, and lifestyles, they are better able to decide whether further values interventions are needed.

Exploring Value–Behavior Incongruencies

A second occasion when it may be helpful to make clients' values a therapeutic focus is when therapists recognize that there is a conflict between their clients' values and behaviors. Value–behavior incongruencies may be one of the defining characteristics of humankind in that all human beings experience conflict between their behavior and their expressed values from time to time in their lives. However, for some clients, these conflicts may lie at the heart of their emotional problems (Mowrer, 1961, 1967).

Value–behavior conflicts can be problematic for all people, but it can be especially salient for individuals belonging to certain religious groups that profess explicit codes of conduct or ideals for living. For example, most religions teach that value–behavior conflicts reflect sin. The member understands and professes a value or belief but then behaves in a contrary fashion.

Guilt and shame, low self-esteem, depression, anxiety, and relational distress are common consequences of value–behavior discrepancies (Mowrer, 1961, 1967). Although some therapists have regarded all guilt and associated symptoms as pathological, we think that when such symptoms are caused by value–behavior discrepancies they can be useful if they help clients recognize the need to achieve more congruence (Bergin, 1980a, 1980b; Mowrer, 1961, 1967; Richards, 1991). When clients manifest discrepancies between their professed values and behavior, therapists may find it useful to help them explicitly examine and explore their incongruencies and to assist them in becoming more congruent. Of course, incongruence can also be modified by softening rigid, self-punitive ideals. In either case, this may help free clients of guilt and other unpleasant emotional symptoms that have resulted from their incongruencies.

Correcting Value Deficiencies and Confusion

A third occasion when making clients' values a therapeutic focus may be helpful is when clients are confused or unclear about what their values are. Some people seek psychological help because they feel ungrounded, normless, and without specific purpose or meaning. When pressed, these clients will acknowledge that they are confused about what their personal values really are or realize that they have never explicitly articulated what they deem as being good and desirable for their lives. When clients lack an understanding of health values and how they might use and internalize these values in their lives, therapists might find it helpful to explicitly teach clients what psychotherapists tend to regard as healthy values and encourage their exploration and implementation. They should, however, acknowledge that therapists disagree to some extent, that different intellectual bases for these values exist, and that clients are free to accept or reject these values.

Therapists may also find it useful to encourage clients to explore and identify the values that they believe are most significant and meaningful to them. It is likely that clients, to some degree, have lived their lives in accord with some unarticulated values. Becoming more aware of their own values can help clients better self-monitor their behavior, be more responsible for their actions, and better evaluate the direction and quality of their lives. Moreover, a heightened awareness of one's own values, including being able to explicitly express or state one's values, may be an important component of healthy psychological functioning (Richards & Bergin, 1997).

Confronting Unhealthy Client Values

Finally, another occasion when it may be helpful to make clients' values a therapeutic focus is when they have adopted unhealthy lifestyle values and behaviors (e.g., engaging in unprotected sex, stealing, drug abuse, crime or violence, spouse or child abuse). Individuals with unhealthy values often come into conflict with others, both in their personal and communal relationships. They may also experience unpleasant symptoms such as depression, low self-esteem, guilt and shame, and anxiety. The reasons for these conflicts and symptoms may often seem incomprehensible to clients, but they are likely to persist as long as the unhealthy values are endorsed and operative in the person's life. As a result, many clients ultimately will seek psychological services because of the pain caused by their unhealthy values, and the behaviors and negative consequences that stem from their value choices, or because their familial or subcultural group negatively reinforces their maladaptive values.

When therapists perceive that clients' value choices are contributing to their problems, therapists can help clients understand the conflict and pain in their lives by pointing out the behaviors or social conditions that seem to be contributing to their conflicts and the attitudes and values that are implied by such behaviors. Therapists may find it useful to help clients explicitly examine their value choices, identify those that appear to be problematic, and suggest more healthy alternatives. This is by no means necessarily an easy therapeutic task. Confronting clients about unhealthy values can sometimes upset them and threaten the therapeutic relationship (Richards & Potts, 1995). A caring and trusting therapeutic relationship, honesty, patience, and considerable therapeutic skill may all be needed when teaching clients healthier value alternatives.

Values Assessment and Intervention Techniques

Therapists can use numerous techniques to assess, explore, and modify their clients' values and lifestyles. For example, in their initial interviews with clients, therapists can simply ask them value-related questions such as the following: "Do you believe in God or a supreme being?" "Are you religious or spiritually oriented?" "What do you believe is the purpose of life?" "What gives your life meaning?" "What is most important to you in life?" "What moral, ethical, or spiritual values, if any, do you use to guide your life?" "What are your goals and dreams?" "Do you feel that your behavior and lifestyle are consistent with the values you profess?" These questions can give therapists considerable insight into their clients' world-views and core values, whether their values are healthy, and the degree to which their values and behavior are congruent.

Therapists can also ask clients to rank order their value priorities. The Rokeach Value Survey (Rokeach, 1967) has been used for this purpose, but we prefer a more contemporary list of values published by Miller and C'deBaca (1994). Miller and C'deBaca's list includes a sizable number of spiritually oriented values that we think makes it more suitable for religious and spiritual clients. Examples of values included on Miller and C'deBaca's list are as follows: achivement, attractiveness, career, caring for others, equality for all, fame, family, forgiveness, fun, God's will, growth, happiness, health, honesty, intimacy, justice, knowledge, loving, pleasure, popularity, power, rationality, romance, self-control, self-esteem, spirituality, and wealth.

After clients finish ranking the values, therapists can review their rankings with them and encourage them to explain and elaborate on why they ranked the values the way they did. Therapists can also ask clients to explore how these values are expressed or manifested in their lives and to examine whether their behavior and lifestyle choices are consistent with their professed values. Miller and C'deBaca (1994) also published data showing the value rankings of people who feel that they have experienced lasting, spiritually oriented changes in their values and lifestyles. Therapists could compare their clients' value priorities with the rankings of these people, although in light of the small size of Miller and C'deBaca's (1994) sample, such comparisons should be made tentatively and only for client self-exploration purposes.

Another technique is to ask clients to think and write about what they would do with their time if they found out they were terminally ill and had only 1 year of good health left to enjoy before they would deteriorate quickly and die (Corey & Corey, 1986). After clients have completed the exercise, therapists can help them process what they felt and learned from it. This is a potentially powerful technique for helping clients identify and affirm their core values and recognize any discrepancies that may exist between these values and their current lifestyle. A sizable literature on values clarification has been published and a variety of techniques have been described that can help people explore, clarify, and recommit to their core values (e.g., Corey, 1986; Corey & Corey, 1986; Kirschenbaum, 1977; Raths, Harmin, & Simon, 1966), including writing one's philosophy of life and preparing one's "tombstone inscription." Many of these techniques can be used in either group or individual therapy.

Therapists may also ask clients to write a *personal mission statement* (Covey, 1989). When writing a personal mission statement or philosophy, clients should focus on what they want to be and do. According to Covey (1989),

> a personal mission statement based on correct principles becomes . . . [a] standard for an individual. It becomes a personal constitution, the basis for making major, life-directing decisions, the basis for making daily decisions in the midst of the circumstances and emotions that affect our lives. (p. 108)

Once clients have identified their core values, it then becomes more feasible for them to set long- and short-term goals that will help them regulate their behavior and lifestyle in harmony with their values. Several books and systems for helping people do this have been published (e.g., Covey, 1989; Franklin International Institute, 1989).

Therapists may also ask questions or make statements that bring to light the value implications and health consequences of behaviors and choices that clients report during therapy sessions. For example, if a religious client told her therapist that she was trying to decide whether to move in with her boyfriend, the therapist could invite her to examine the implications and discuss the "pros and cons" of doing so. Examples of value-related questions the therapist might ask during such a discussion include "Do you think moving in with your boyfriend would be a healthy choice for you (emotionally, spirituality, physically)?" "Would there be any negative consequences if you moved in with your boyfriend and are you willing to live with those consequences?" "Would moving in with your boyfriend be in harmony with your religious and spiritual values?" "What are your values about marriage and would this decision be in harmony with those values?" "If you move in with your boyfriend, is this a decision that will feel congruent with who you are and what you value?" Therapists can entertain such queries from either a spiritual and theistic perspective or a philosophically pragmatic one depending on the client. Many other questions could potentially be asked depending on the situation to help clients examine the value implications and health consequences of their behaviors and lifestyle choices.

Another technique, useful for correcting value deficiencies and for challenging unhealthy values, is to share with clients what mental health professionals (see Table 7.2) regard as healthy values (Jensen & Bergin, 1988) and with religious and spiritually oriented clients what the world religious traditions generally agree are mature values (see Table 7.3). Therapists can prepare written descriptions of these values or describe them verbally at appropriate times during therapy. Therapists can discuss with clients whether they agree with these values and incorporate them as values in their lives. When teaching clients what mental health professionals and the spiritual traditions generally agree are healthy values, we recommend that therapists point out that not all therapists or spiritual leaders necessarily agree with the values and that their clients certainly also have the right to disagree.

Spiritual practices such as praying, meditating, reading sacred writings, and seeking spiritual direction from religious and spiritual leaders can also be valuable interventions for helping religious and spiritually oriented clients clarify and affirm their core values. It is beyond the scope of this chapter to describe these practices in detail, but several recent publications and other chapters in this book have done so (e.g., Ball & Goodyear, 1991; Benson, 1996; Richards & Bergin, 1997; Richards & Potts, 1995; Shafranske, 1996). When clients are struggling with difficult lifestyle choices, encouraging them to seek spiritual enlightenment by engaging in one or more of these spiritual practices can potentially help them spiritually focus and center on those values that are most important to them. Transcendent spiritual enlightenment about the meaning and purpose of their lives, and what values are most important, may at times come to clients as they seek such guidance (Richards & Bergin, 1997).

CONCLUSION

When clients explore and identify their values during therapy, many of them will affirm that their most important, core values are spiritual in nature. Gallup Organization polls during the past two decades have revealed that approximately 95% of people in the United States profess to believe in God, 70% belong to a church or synagogue, 72% say that their religious faith is the most important influence in their life, and 84% say that they try hard to put their religious beliefs into practice in their relations with all people (Bergin & Jensen, 1990; Gallup Organization, 1985; Richards & Bergin, 1997; cf. Hoge, 1996). In light of this, and given the empirical evidence that spiritual beliefs and values may promote physical and psychological healing and adjustment (Benson, 1996; Borysenko, 1993; Koenig, 1997; Miller & C'deBaca, 1994; Richards & Bergin, 1997), we recommend that therapists make greater efforts to use such values to facilitate therapeutic change.

Therapists can facilitate the integration of spirituality into treatment by asking clients whether they can think of ways that their spiritual beliefs and values might help them cope with their problems. By helping clients affirm their core spiritual values, live congruently with these values, and access the spiritual resources in their lives (i.e., their spiritual beliefs, values, practices, and community), therapists can more effectively assist clients in their efforts to cope, heal, and grow.

REFERENCES

American Psychological Association. (1992). Ethical principles of psychologists and code of conduct. *American Psychologist, 47*, 1597–1611.

Ball, R. A., & Goodyear, R. K. (1991). Self-reported professional practices of Christian psychologists. *Journal of Psychology and Christianity, 10*, 144–153.

Bechtel, W. (1988). *Philosophy of science: An overview for cognitive science.* Hillsdale, NJ: Erlbaum.

Benson, H. (1996). *Timeless healing: The power and biology of belief.* New York: Scribner.

Bergin, A. E. (1980a). Psychotherapy and religious values. *Journal of Consulting and Clinical Psychology, 48*, 75–105.

Bergin, A. E. (1980b). Religious and humanistic values: A reply to Ellis and Walls. *Journal of Consulting and Clinical Psychology, 48*, 642–645.

Bergin, A. E. (1980c). Behavior therapy and ethical relativism: Time for clarity. *Journal of Consulting and Clinical Psychology, 48*, 11–13.

Bergin, A. E. (1983). Religiosity and mental health: A critical reevaluation and meta-analysis. *Professional Psychology: Research and Practice, 14*, 170–184.

Bergin, A. E. (1985). Proposed values for guiding and evaluating counseling and psychotherapy. *Counseling and Values, 29*, 99–116.

Bergin, A. E. (1991). Values and religious issues in psychotherapy and mental health. *American Psychologist, 46*, 394–403.

Bergin, A. E., & Jensen, J. P. (1990). Religiosity of psychotherapists: A national survey. *Psychotherapy, 27*, 3–7.

Bergin, A. E., Payne, I. R., & Richards, P. S. (1996). Values in psychotherapy. In

E. Shafranske (Ed.), *Religion and the clinical practice of psychology* (pp. 297–323). Washington, DC: American Psychological Association.

Borysenko, J. (1993). *Fire in the soul: A new psychology of spiritual optimism.* New York: Warner Books.

Borysenko, J., & Borysenko, M. (1994). *The power of the mind to heal.* Carson, CA: Hay House.

Browning, D. S. (1987). *Religious thought and the modern psychologies: A critical conversation in the theology of culture.* Philadelphia: Fortress.

Campbell, D. T. (1975). On the conflicts between biological and social evolution and between psychology and moral tradition. *American Psychologist, 30,* 1103–1126.

Corey, G. (1986). *I never knew I had a choice* (3rd ed.). Monterey, CA: Brooks/Cole.

Corey, G., & Corey, M. S. (1986). *Instructor's resource manual for "I never knew I had a choice"* (3rd ed.). Monterey, CA: Brooks/Cole.

Corey, G., Corey, M.S., & Callanan, P. (1993). *Issues and ethics in the helping professions* (4th ed.). Monterey, CA: Brooks/Cole.

Covey, S. R. (1989). *The 7 habits of highly effective people.* New York: Fireside.

Doherty, W. J. (1995). *Soul searching: Why psychotherapy must promote moral responsibility.* New York: Basic Books.

Ellis, A. (1980). Psychotherapy and atheistic values: A response to A. E. Bergin's "Psychotherapy and religious values." *Journal of Consulting and Clinical Psychology, 48,* 635–639.

Frank, J. D., & Frank, J. B. (1991). *Persuasion and healing: A comparative study of psychotherapy* (3rd ed.). Baltimore: Johns Hopkins University Press.

Franklin International Institute. (1989). *Franklin day planner system.* Salt Lake City, UT: Author.

Freud, S. (1927). *The future of an illusion.* Garden City, NY: Doubleday.

Gallup Organization. (1985). *Religion in America* (Gallup Rep. No. 236). Princeton, NJ: Author.

Gartner, J., Larson, D. B., & Allen, G. D. (1996). Religious commitment, mental health, and prosocial behavior: A review of the empirical literature. In E. Shafranske (Ed.), *Religion and the clinical practice of psychology* (pp. 187–214). Washington, DC: American Psychological Association.

Hillner, K. P. (1984). *History and systems of modern psychology: A conceptual approach.* New York: Gardner Press.

Hoge, D. R. (1996). Religion in America: The demographics of belief and affiliation. In E. P. Shafranske (Ed.), *Religion and the clinical practice of psychology* (pp. 21–41). Washington, DC: American Psychological Association.

Honer, S. M., & Hunt, T. C. (1987). *Invitation to philosophy: Issues and options* (5th ed.). Belmont, CA: Wadsworth.

Howard, G. S. (1986). *Dare we develop a human science?* Notre Dame, IN: Academic Publications.

Ibrahim, F. A. (1985). Effective cross-cultural counseling and psychotherapy: A framework. *The Counseling Psychologist, 13,* 625–683.

Ibrahim, F. A. (1991). Contribution of cultural worldview to generic counseling and development. *Journal of Counseling and Development, 70,* 13–19.

Jensen, J. P., & Bergin, A. E. (1988). Mental health values of professional therapists: A national interdisciplinary survey. *Professional Psychology: Research and Practice, 19,* 290–297.

Jones, S. L. (1994). A constructive relationship for religion with the science and profession of psychology: Perhaps the boldest model yet. *American Psychologist, 49,* 184–199.

Jones, S. L., & Butman, R. E. (1991). *Modern psychotherapies: A comprehensive Christian appraisal.* Downers Grove, IL: InterVarsity.

Kelly, E. W., Jr. (1995a). Counselor values: A national survey. *Journal of Counseling and Development, 73,* 648–653.

Kelly, E. W. (1995b). *Religion and spirituality in counseling and psychotherapy.* Richmond, VA: American Counseling Association.

Kessell, P., & McBrearty, J. F. (1967). Values and psychotherapy: A review of the literature [Monograph]. *Perceptual and Motor Skills, 25,* 669–690.

Kirschenbaum, H. (1977). *Advanced values clarification.* La Jolla, CA: University Associates.

Kitchener, R. F. (1980). Ethical relativism and behavior therapy. *Journal of Consulting and Clinical Psychology, 48,* 1–7.

Kluckhohn, C. (1951). Values and value orientations in the theory of action. In T. Parsons & F. A. Shields (Eds.), *Toward a general theory of action* (pp. 388–433). Cambridge, MA: Harvard University Press.

Koenig, H. G. (1997). *Is religion good for your health? The effects of religion on physical and mental health.* New York: Haworth Press.

Kuhn, T. (1970). *The structure of scientific revolutions* (2nd ed.). Chicago: University of Chicago Press.

Lakatos, I., & Musgrave, A. (Eds.). (1970). *Criticism and the growth of knowledge.* New York: Cambridge University Press.

Laudan, L. (1984). *Science and values: The aims of science and their role in scientific debate.* Berkeley: University of California Press.

Levine, E. S., & Padilla, A. M. (1980). *Crossing cultures in therapy: Pluralistic counseling for the Hispanic.* Pacific Grove, CA: Brooks/Cole.

London, P. (1964). *Modes and morals of psychotherapy.* New York: Holt, Rinehart & Winston.

London, P. (1986). *The modes and morals of psychotherapy* (2nd ed.). New York: McGraw-Hill.

Lowe, C. M. (1976). *Value orientations in counseling and psychotherapy: The meanings of mental health* (2nd ed.). Cranston, RI: Carroll Press.

Lundin, R. W. (1985). *Theories and systems of psychology* (3rd ed.). Lexington, MA: Heath.

Marsella, A. J., & White, G. M. (Eds.). (1982). *Cultural conceptions of mental health and therapy*. Dordrecht, The Netherlands. Reidel.

Maslow, A. H. (1971). *The farther reaches of human nature*. New York: Viking Press.

Miller, W. R., & C'deBaca, J. (1994). Quantum change: Toward a psychology of transformation. In T. Heatherton & J. Weinberger (Eds.), *Can personality change?* (pp. 253–280). Washington, DC: American Psychological Association.

Minsel, B., Becker, P., & Korchin, S. (1991). A cross-cultural view of positive mental health. *Journal of Cross-Cultural Psychology, 22*, 157–181.

Mowrer, O. H. (1961). *The crisis in psychiatry and religion*. Princeton, NJ: Van Nostrand.

Mowrer, O. H. (Ed.). (1967). *Morality and mental health*. Chicago: Rand McNally.

O'Donohue, W. (1989). The (even) bolder model: The clinical psychologist as metaphysician-scientist-practitioner. *American Psychologist, 44*, 1460–1468.

Pargament, K. I. (1997). *The psychology of religion and coping*. New York: Guilford Press.

Patterson, C. H. (1958). The place of values in counseling and psychotherapy. *Journal of Counseling Psychology, 5*, 216–223.

Payne, I. R., Bergin, A. E., Bielema, K. A., & Jenkins, P. H. (1991). Review of religion and mental health: Prevention and the enhancement of psychosocial functioning. *Prevention in Human Services, 9*, 11–40.

Percesepe, G. (1991). *Philosophy: An introduction to the labor of reason*. New York: Macmillan.

Polanyi, M. (1962). *Personal knowledge: Towards a post-critical philosophy*. Chicago: The University of Chicago Press.

Putnam, H. (1993). Objectivity and the science-ethics distinction. In M. Nussbaum & A. Sen (Eds.), *The quality of life* (pp. 143–157). Oxford, England: Oxford University Press.

Raths, L., Harmin, M., & Simon, S. B. (1966). *Values and teaching*. Columbus, OH: Charles E. Merrill.

Richards, P. S. (1991). Religious devoutness in college students: Relations with emotional adjustment and psychological separation from parents. *Journal of Counseling Psychology, 38*, 189–196.

Richards, P. S., & Bergin, A. E. (1997). *A spiritual strategy for counseling and psychotherapy*. Washington, DC: American Psychological Association.

Richards, P. S. & Potts, R. W. (1995). Using spiritual interventions in psychotherapy: Practices, successes, failures, and ethical concerns of Mormon psychotherapists. *Professional Psychology: Research and Practice, 26*, 163–170.

Richards, P. S., & Slife, B. D. (in press). Curing souls: A philosophical analysis of psychotherapy's functions, assumptions, and values [Review of the book *The cure of souls: Science, values, and psychotherapy*]. *Contemporary Psychology*.

Rokeach, M. (1967). *Value Survey*. Lansing, MI: Jenca Associates Testing Division.

Schwartz, B. (1986). *The battle for human nature: Science, morality and modern life*. New York: Norton.

Shafranske, E. P. (Ed.). (1996). *Religion and the clinical practice of psychology*. Washington, DC: American Psychological Association.

Shafranske, E. P., & Malony, H. N. (1996). Religion and the clinical practice of psychology: A case for inclusion. In E. P. Shafranske (Ed.), *Religion and the clinical practice of psychology* (pp. 561–586). Washington, DC: American Psychological Association.

Slife, B. D., & Williams, R. N. (1995). *What's behind the research? Discovering hidden assumptions in the behavioral sciences*. Thousand Oaks, CA: Sage.

Smart, N. (1983). *Worldviews: Crosscultural explorations of human beliefs*. New York: Scribner.

Smart, N. (1993). *Religions of Asia*. Englewood Cliffs, NJ: Prentice Hall.

Smart, N. (1994). *Religions of the West*. Englewood Cliffs, NJ: Prentice Hall.

Solomon, R. C. (1990). *The big questions: A short introduction to philosophy* (3rd ed.). San Diego, CA: Harcourt Brace Jovanovich.

Speight, S. L., Myers, L. J., Cox, C. I., & Highlen, P. S. (1991). A redefinition of multicultural counseling. *Journal of Counseling and Development, 70,* 29–36.

Sue, D. W. (1978). Eliminating cultural oppression in counseling: A conceptual analysis. *Personnel and Guidance Journal, 55,* 422–424.

Sue, D. W., & Sue, D. (1990). *Counseling the culturally different: Theory and practice* (2nd ed.). New York: Wiley.

Szasz, T. S. (1960). The myth of mental illness. *American Psychologist, 15,* 113–118.

Tjeltveit, A. C. (1986). The ethics of value conversion in psychotherapy: Appropriate and inappropriate therapist influence on client values. *Clinical Psychology Review, 6,* 515–537.

Tjeltveit, A. C. (1989). The ubiquity of models of human beings in psychotherapy: The need for rigorous reflection. *Psychotherapy, 26,* 1–10.

Tjeltveit, A. C. (1999). *Ethics and values in psychotherapy*. London: Routledge.

Toulmin, S., & Leary, D. E. (1992). The cult of empiricism, and beyond. In S. Koch & D. E. Leary (Eds.), *A century of psychology as science* (pp. 594–617). Washington, DC: American Psychological Association.

Wallach, M. A., & Wallach, L. (1983). *Psychology's sanction for selfishness: The error of egoism in theory and therapy*. New York: Freeman.

Watson, J. B. (1983). *Psychology from the standpoint of a behaviorist*. Dover, NH: Frances Pinter. (Original work published 1924)

Woolfolk, R. L. (1998). *The cure of souls: Science, values, and psychotherapy*. San Francisco: Jossey-Bass.

Worthington, E. L., Jr., Kurusu, T. A., McCullough, M. E., & Sanders, S. J. (1996). Empirical research on religion and psychotherapeutic processes and outcomes: A ten-year review and research prospectus. *Psychological Bulletin, 119,* 448–487.

Wulff, D. M. (1991). *Psychology of religion: Classic and contemporary views*. New York: Wiley.

8

BEHAVIORAL APPROACHES TO ENHANCE SPIRITUALITY

JOHN E. MARTIN AND JENNIFER BOOTH

In this chapter we address the enhancement of spirituality from a practical standpoint. Our primary focus is on applying behavioral methods to strengthen spiritual and religious practices, which in turn may be efficacious in enhancing one's physical health, mental health, and overall quality of life (Levin & Vanderpool, 1991; Larson, 1994; Larson & Larson, 1994; Larson, Swyers, & McCullough, 1998).

THE BEHAVIORAL IN SPIRITUALITY

Spirituality, whether religious or nonreligious, can be a difficult concept for the behavioral scientist, as has been noted in the previous chapters in this book. The definition of spirituality tendered in chapter 1 is useful here: as occupying a multidimensional "space" and including the three components of spiritual behavior, spiritual beliefs, and personal experience. For the purposes of the present chapter, we treat spiritual and religious *practices* uniformly, without seeking to differentiate between the two. Our focus is on how to develop or enhance behaviors that are important to spirituality and religiousness, and thus, overall physical and psychological health.

Although spiritual belief and faith practices vary considerably from one context to another, there are some common behaviors found in many spiritual traditions that we use for illustrative purposes. These include practices such as prayer, fasting, meditation, reading and studying faith literature, practicing particular rituals (e.g., sacraments, holy days, dances), and compassionate sacrificial service (Foster, 1988). Inasmuch as they involve specific actions, it is possible to explore well-established behavioral methods to increase and strengthen such spiritual practices (W. Miller & Martin, 1988). Indeed, people often express a desire to be more "faithful" (health professionals might say "compliant") in their spiritual practices. To a behavioral scientist, this sounds like a familiar problem to which well-established methods can be applied.

APPROACHES TO ENHANCING SPIRITUALITY

Behavioral science has much to offer those who would like to strengthen their spiritual and religious life. Spiritual and religious practices are subject to the fundamental principles of learning and other processes of behavioral and cognitive science. As with other behavior, these principles can be applied to enhance a person's spiritual and religious practices. The generic methods discussed here could be applied to many of the components of spirituality discussed in other chapters in this book, including meditation and prayer; following the Twelve Steps; surrendering control; practicing acceptance and forgiveness; developing mindfulness; and manifesting values, hope, and serenity. We use some of these as examples along the way.

Is it possible to develop and promote spirituality through distinctly earthly, even seemingly artificial, means? We believe that the answer is yes, providing that the interventions that follow are offered respectfully, sensitively, and lovingly. They can be made free of jargon and explained in spiritually compatible contexts and terminologies. Certain behavioral methods may not be appropriate within certain spiritual contexts, and one must also be mindful of its content. One example is the paradox of using popular TV or movies to reinforce spiritual behavior that represents opposite values. Clearly, when venturing into this territory, it is wise to understand and pay particular attention to the client's spiritual goals, background, orientation, motivation, and environmental and personal constraints before launching into behavioral interventions to enhance spiritual behavior. The client-centered motivational approach described by W. R. Miller and Rollnick (1991) is an excellent resource for the clinician wishing to venture caringly and effectively into this tender area of a client's life and experience.

This chapter is divided into three major sections based on different directions of change. Simply put, these can be stated as doing more, being more, and doing less. In the following three sections we present these general goal directions in the context of how they may be initiated (behavioral acquisition) and maintained. We focus primarily on traditional cognitive–behavioral approaches to spiritual enhancement, although principles of behavioral science more generally could be applied similarly.

Doing More: Increasing Spiritual and Religious Behavior

Many of the spiritually oriented practices highlighted in this book fit readily into the "do more" category: meditation (chap. 4), prayer (chap. 5), exercising forgiveness (chap. 10), and following the 12-step program (e.g., Alcoholics Anonymous, 1976; see also chap. 6 in this book). Such spiritually motivated behaviors do not just appear spontaneously or occur randomly. Developing and maintaining a lifestyle of regular spiritual discipline require committed efforts over a period of time. It is also the case that the real fruits of such practices ("being more") are usually not immediate but occur over long spans of time. Some spiritual practices (such as fasting) must be maintained in the face of aversive immediate consequences. This delayed-reinforcement problem (i.e., short-term pain, long-term gain) is by no means unique to spiritual behavior. Shaping, prompting, reinforcing, generalizing, and maintaining such behavior are commonly (and successfully) addressed challenges in cognitive and behavioral science (Chance, 1994; Martin & Dubbert, 1984; Miller, 1980; Salkovskis, 1996; Sulzer-Azaroff & Reese, 1982).

Behavior Management of Spiritual Practices

Principles of behavior management are directly applicable in strengthening spiritual practices. *Goal setting* is one important aspect of effective behavior change. Setting appropriate goals and systematically tracking and monitoring them may be equally critical to the acquisition of spiritual behavior and its maintenance within lifestyle patterns. For example, prayer and meditation goals could be specified in terms of frequency, duration, time and place, and type (see chaps. 4 and 5 in this book), all of which make it possible to define progress toward goals.

Because progress toward goals is often a matter of successive approximations, it can be beneficial to teach *self-monitoring*. Daily diary forms can be developed, specifying the particular spiritual behaviors to be recorded. Self-monitoring is a common component of behavioral management programs whether secular (Martin & Dubbert, 1984; Miller, 1975; Moss, Prue,

Lomax, & Martin, 1982) or religion based (Shamblin, 1997). We have had encouraging experience in applying this method with African American church members (Martin, Ameika, & Lydston, 1999) in dietary practices and exercise participation.

With a goal and regular monitoring, it is a minor step to specify an oral or written *agreement* or *contract*. Such a contract involves a public commitment, at least to the therapist and preferably to significant others as well (perhaps those within a client's own spiritual community). Written agreements help to ensure common understanding of the client's goals and specify positive reinforcement to occur as goals are met.

The *shaping* of spiritual practices such as prayer and meditation is typically more realistic than sudden adherence. Although some people do "get" spiritual insight and change suddenly (W. R. Miller & C'de Baca, 1994), for many the process of growing spiritually is a gradual, successive one punctuated by some backsliding. The "Big Book" of Alcoholics Anonymous (AA, 1976) relates some stories of sudden transformation (including that of cofounder Bill W.) but acknowledges that alcoholic individuals are more likely to experience a "gradual (spiritual) awakening."

Shaping prayer and meditation, then, might begin from a first approximation (e.g., 2 min of prayer) toward the person's target goal (e.g., perhaps an hour of prayer or meditation at the start of each day). First steps are best kept simple, brief, and highly achievable. This may be followed by gradual progressive increases toward the behavioral goals (e.g., adding 1 min per day or 5 min per week). This commonsense approach is not alien to religious contexts. Virkler (1986) described a method of gradually learning the process of seeking spiritual awareness. He suggested spending a gradually increasing amount of time alone, with paper-and-pencil or computer handy for recording one's questions and emerging answers or wisdom, a regular time of "seeking God's voice." Virkler stressed that it takes time and considerable practice to learn to discern this "voice." Again, the challenge is to establish and sustain a valued practice that may not yield immediate salient positive reinforcement.

As it is with other behaviors of this kind, attempting too much too soon is a commonly reported reason for failure in the building up of spiritual habits such as prayer, study, and meditation. The therapeutic concept of "relapse" mirrors what has been bemoaned in spiritual and religious circles for many centuries: "That which I would, I do not; and that which I would not, I do." A variety of cognitive–behavioral relapse prevention strategies have been developed (Brownell, Marlatt, Lichtenstein, & Wilson, 1986) that could be applied in combination with gradual and appropriate shaping of spiritual habits and goals.

Especially at earlier approximations, more liberal amounts of positive *reinforcement* may be helpful to enhance acquisition of a newer or less established spiritual behavior. Many worthy prayer and meditation resolutions (like countless New Year's resolutions) have been defeated not only by too ambitious a progression or lack of a systematic shaping plan but also by failure to include richer sources of effective reinforcement in the early stages of development of the fledgling practices. A practical *contingency management approach* is the Premack principle, also known as "grandma's rule" because of its commonsense face validity. This sequencing principle suggests that a favorite well-established (higher probability) activity (e.g., exercising, relaxing with an engaging book, enjoying a special treat, or talking on the telephone with a friend) is contingent or conditional on completing a goal level of a less established behavior. That is, the higher probability activity occurs only after the target (lower probability) behavior is done. This works well in combination with clear and specific goals, self-monitoring, and contracting to specify the agreed-on system of reinforcement. Other forms of contracting have also been used. The *deposit-return contract* has been applied particularly with difficult-to-change behavior where the client's motivation is high. In this method the individual provides a monetary deposit that is returned either weekly, in apportioned amounts, or in full at the end of the contract period, contingent on successful changes in the target behavior. This procedure, however, has the disadvantage of being aversive (possibly losing rather than gaining something), and more positive contingencies are generally much more effective over the long run.

For various reasons, material reinforcers may not be the best choice for establishing and maintaining spiritual behaviors. A more creative approach is to link the desired behavior to a higher probability "reward" that is also highly consistent with the client's spiritual values. Sometimes it is as simple as powerful positive social reinforcers such as smiles, praise, pats on the back, and hugs. It is also wise to keep in mind what is known about schedules of reinforcement—that consistent positive reinforcement works best when establishing a new behavior and that maintenance is improved by fading to a thin schedule of partial and secondary reinforcement.

Spiritual disciplines such as prayer, meditation, and study may also be promoted through *stimulus control* or contextual prompting techniques in which certain places, people, or events are reliably associated with the spiritual practice. The desired behavior may be generally or always engaged in at a particular place (e.g., favorite chair, "prayer closet," mosque, etc.) and a regular time. It follows that merely entering into this stimulus setting eventually tends to elicit the behavior automatically depending on the strength of the association. Through such associative learning, an individual might literally stimulate the positive urge to perform the spiritual behavior merely by going to the appointed place where it has commonly been practiced. Voorhees et al. (1996) incorporated stimulus control procedures effectively in a smoking cessation intervention across 22 African American churches in Baltimore using a variety of religious settings (e.g., church, small groups, prayer groups) and stimuli (e.g., live and audiotaped testimonial, preaching, written spiritual materials). Stimulus prompts can also be provided by other means (e.g., an alarm watch, carrying a prayer book in one's briefcase) to initiate particular spiritual practices. Creativity is needed to find applications of such principles that are appropriate to the client's own circumstances and spirituality.

Social learning theory (Bandura, 1986) has amply demonstrated the value of observing others engaging in the desired behavior. Such *social modeling*, particularly from valued or similar people, can have a significant positive impact on the initiation and maintenance of spiritual practices. Role models, mentors, or sponsors can be found in individuals or groups with more established spiritual practices. Good modeling may be particularly helpful for those who have been attempting to engage in these spiritual practices alone and are having trouble initiating or maintaining them. Positive role models of spiritual practices may also be particularly helpful for people who have previously been in an aversive, abusive, or punishing religious environment.

Spiritual practices occur in behavioral as well as social and environmental contexts. The *chaining* of stimuli and responses is another principle by which spiritual practices can be strengthened. For instance, to establish and maintain early morning prayer on waking, one might develop the following chain: (a) wake up; (b) lie still and breathe slowly and deeply, anticipating a time of prayer; (c) wash face; (d) go straight to a comfortable location, perhaps a recliner, where any needed materials (incense, prayer shawl, meditation book, Bible, etc.) are within reach; (e) again breathe slowly and deeply for a minute, read a meditation or scripture, or both; and (f) enter into prayer. Such links are reliably connected through repeated practice, with no interrupting behaviors, until the sequence is overlearned and well established. With time, it becomes an automatic process requiring little prior thought or planning. Prior elements in the chair (such as periods of deep breathing in this example) begin to anticipate and induce a state of prayer. Similar stimulus control and chaining methods are commonly recommended in learning transcendental meditation.

Spiritual behavior, like other behavior, may not naturally transfer or generalize to different settings. A spiritual example of a *stimulus generalization problem* occurs when an individual has learned to meditate in one setting (at home in a particular "meditation place") and wants to expand the practice to his or her work setting as well as to hotel rooms when traveling. Common mistakes in developing and maintaining behavioral repertoires include premature or failed generalization (Martin & Dubbert, 1994). In the former case, attempts are made to transfer or generalize the behavior before it has been solidly established in one setting, which may result in the breakdown of the whole behavior. Once good stimulus control of the practice is established in one setting, the person can begin to meditate at work until it becomes a regular, if not automatic, habit and then expand to other settings such as hotel rooms. Anticipatory cues that have been incorporated into the initial behavior chain (like deep breathing or accessing meditative or religious scripture in the example above) can help to transfer the practice to new contexts.

Response generalization is the opposite process—engaging in different forms of the desired response while in the same setting. For example, a person may want to practice various forms of meditation (chap. 4) and prayer (chap. 5) during a daily time of spiritual focus. In this case, the new less established response is gradually faded in, usually in brief periods at first, followed by a higher probability, well-established practice. The new response may be progressively increased until it can remain independently or be generalized to other stimulus settings.

Overlearning is valuable here. There is a reason why monastic discipline often includes highly repetitive practice. With overlearning, the response pattern becomes able to withstand significant disruptive influences (e.g., schedule changes, travel, high stress levels, etc.) before generalization is attempted. The overlearned response pattern is developed through many repeated pairings of the behavior with the specific stimulus and response chains, progressively persisting through changes that would disrupt a weaker habit. Caution is warranted to avoid pressing the limits too quickly. If the person is not ready to practice under more difficult circumstances (premature stimulus generalization), it is best to continue practicing and strengthening the spiritual habit in less difficult situations. This is no different than for strengthening other types of behavior.

Cognitive Approaches to Spirituality Enhancement

The principles of cognitive therapy are also highly applicable in helping people establish and maintain spiritual practices. Several clinical researchers have presented methods of using cognitive approaches in addressing or enhancing spirituality (Propst, Ostrom, Watkins, Dean, & Mashburn, 1992; Richards & Bergin, 1997). As pointed out in other chapters in this book, the overall effectiveness of cognitive therapy for depression can be significantly improved for religiously oriented clients by incorporating their spiritual perspectives. The theory and methodology of cognitive science (e.g., Salkovskis, 1996) are readily adaptable to spiritual development. The cognitive aspects of appraisal, belief, attribution, and expectancy are all important components of spirituality (see chap. 11 in this book) and can be addressed through cognitive approaches. Addressing faulty beliefs and attributions (e.g., Beck, Rush, Shaw, & Emery, 1979) may significantly enhance a client's ability and motivation to overcome barriers to spiritual practice, one of which may be depressive affect that decreases the motivation to engage in spiritual practice. Cognitive science principles can be applied in facilitating spiritual development. The principle of variable encoding, for example, suggests that spiritual material would be best retained when it has been learned from a variety of standpoints, contexts, and processes. Variable encoding not only facilitates recall but it also allows for more flexible and generalizable application of learned concepts.

Although cognitive principles and therapy are appropriately discussed here in the context of "doing more," they also overlap importantly with the next section on "being more" because of the critical role of thought and belief in the "state of the heart." An interesting spiritual "do more'" practice that is also a "be more" phenomenon is forgiveness for perceived and actual offenses (see chap. 10 in this book). Although it may be defined as an overt act of the will (rather than action or feeling), a decision and commitment to forgive and cease to hold onto bitterness and blame, forgiveness can also be understood as a behavioral process subject to the principles described above. The seeking of forgiveness may also be combined with overt behaviors such as confession and restitution. For example, the 12-step program incorporates the goal of listing all those one has harmed (i.e., those from whom one needs to seek forgiveness; Step 8) and to whom restitution may be warranted (Step 9), whereas Steps 4 and 5 address the confession of shortcomings through the development of a "fearless and searching" personal inventory (see chap. 6).

The 12-step program (Alcoholics Anonymous, 1976) is also an excellent model for the cognitive–behavioral shaping of spiritual practices, in that adherents learn not to attempt to race through those progressive steps of spiritual development. The AA principles of "easy does it" and "keep it simple" are good reminders of sound behavioral shaping principles. In addition, the stimulus control and social modeling and reinforcement characteristics of 12-step meetings represent powerful supports for spiritual development. Effective therapeutic procedures have been developed and tested for facilitating clients' involvement in 12-step programs (cf. Nowinski, Baker, & Carroll, 1992; Project MATCH Research Group, 1997).

Being More: Enhancing Inward Spirituality

Spiritual enhancement includes not only the stimulation and maintenance of overt spiritual practices as presented in the previous section, but also the strengthening of spirituality as an inward state of being. Foster (1988) addressed the phenomenology of spiritual "being" in his seminal work *Celebration of Discipline*, presenting both the historical as well as the philosophical and religious roots of various spiritual disciplines. In a cardiovascular rehabilitation program described in chapter 1 (Powell, Friedman, Thoresen, Gill, & Ulmer, 1984), patients were encouraged to listen to their (spiritual) heart for broader life directions as well as immediate decisions about how to react in certain situations.

From a strictly behavioral standpoint, the promotion of "being more" presents somewhat of a dilemma: How does one target and enhance a state of mind, heart, and being—of *having* rather than doing, so to speak? One value of a behavioral approach is to think of somewhat abstract spiritual virtues (e.g., mindfulness, lovingness, acceptance, humility, hope, and serenity) as being partly comprised of certain behaviors and cognitions. One need not adopt naturalism's "nothing but" view to find useful a behavioral analysis of complex traits one wishes to acquire.

The importance of including these more inward spiritual attributes is evident throughout the various chapters in this book. Although the focus of this chapter thus far has been on the application of behavioral principles to increasing specific spiritual behaviors, there are also important character components of becoming more loving, honest, accepting, hopeful, faithful, humble, and serene. Furthermore, focusing on the development and enhancement of such broader attributes may in turn facilitate successful application of "outward" spiritual practices (e.g., prayer, meditation, study, etc.). The more spiritual ideals and values are internalized (and practiced) by the individual, the more resilient (i.e., resistant to extinction and reversal) these spiritual practices will be.

A cognitive–behavioral approach seems well suited to the task of enhancing spiritual values, beliefs, and ideals. In a practical sense, a therapist might use familiar cognitive therapy methods (Beck et al., 1979; Persons, 1989) to help clients evaluate their thoughts and behaviors in relation to core belief systems. The goal here is an integral spirituality, a spiritual identity with daily thoughts and actions based on and consistent with core beliefs and values. This would be expected to engender greater strength of both the "doing" and "being" aspects of spirituality. As thought patterns and behaviors are found to be incongruent with the client's identified core spiritual values and beliefs, they may become the focus of behavioral and cognitive intervention aimed at "doing less."

Doing Less: Decreasing Spiritually Inconsistent Behavior

Another general enhancement approach is to remove obstacles (including competing responses) that impede spiritual development. Other chapters in this book offer some examples, including overcontrolling behavior (chap. 9) and unresolved resentment and bitterness (chap. 10), which themselves border on ways of being as well as doing. In a more general sense, spirituality requires space to grow, and part of the task is clearing away other behaviors that compete with "doing more" and "being more."

A good starting point in clearing space by "doing less" is to learn what competes with time and motivation for spiritual development. A daily activity journal, for example, can help to identify how time is currently spent, a first step toward altering time use. This may be accomplished by initiating self-monitoring or "journaling" of those elements, experiences, or reactions in the person's daily living that seem to block spirituality. More focused self-monitoring can be helpful in a functional analysis of behaviors that unintentionally displace "doing more" and "being more" time (watching TV, playing computer games, or "surfing" the Web, etc.). Self-monitoring may also identify responses that seem to suppress the pursuit of spirituality (e.g., unwanted thoughts, heavy drinking or illicit drug use, feelings of resentment).

The power of associative (classical or respondent) learning can apply here. For many people, specific stimuli (e.g., particular music, visual meditative symbols, or the smell of incense) have been associated with spiritual experience and expression in the past and tend to evoke or enhance the experiences of peace, comfort, joy, and awe. These stimuli, and the well-being responses associated with them, may be helpful in the counterconditioning (e.g., systematic desensitization) of other stimuli that interfere with spiritual experience. Meditation training in many ways resembles a process for extinction or counterconditioning of intrusive thoughts and feelings that inhibit spiritual growth. Counterconditioning methods may also be helpful in undoing negative associations linked to unpleasant or traumatic experiences with religion.

Bitterness and Learned Forgiveness

Personal bitterness, resentment, or unforgiveness is often cited as being particularly destructive to physical, mental, and spiritual health (Ornish, 1998). Its opposite and competing force is, in a word, love (Ornish, 1998; Powell et al., 1984). The giving and receiving of love seem to be common denominators in many forms of spirituality and religion.

In our own practice, we have found (as is mirrored in the growing literature on forgiveness, health, and disease) that when clients come in with pockets of bitterness, we have often been unable to effectively alter health, stress, or personal relationship patterns until we systematically address these old wounds and the places of lingering resentment. An embittered person, even in one small area of his or her life or past, is handicapped in his or her efforts to become spiritually fulfilled and free. Guided by a classical desensitization model, we seek to extinguish the conditioned aversive emotion associated with a particular person or set of circumstances. The negative emotion can be evoked by intentional repeated presentations of the evoking stimuli; beyond a straight extinction approach, it can also be useful to evoke additional competing (counterconditioning) states of experienced wellness and to teach behavioral and cognitive behavioral skills (e.g., anger management) for active coping with disruptive situations (e.g., Novaco, 1995; Williams & Williams, 1994).

Reducing Overindulgence

As another "doing less" example, overindulgence in a variety of addictive behaviors (e.g., eating, drinking, risk taking, gambling, and even smoking) tends to undermine in many the motivation for spiritual development (as well as for many other activities). One of the characteristic symptoms of dependence is a giving up of other pursuits, as increasing amounts of time and energy are devoted to the addiction—an "unholy attachment" described by May (1991). A variety of addictive behaviors (e.g., alcohol and other drug dependence, compulsive working) have been conceptualized as being, at their core, spiritual deficits (Alcoholics Anonymous, 1976; May, 1991). The way out, in this view, involves displacing the addictive behavior while enhancing (replacing it with) spirituality. An excellent example (Powell et al., 1984) can be found in the use of cognitive–behavioral interventions to suppress high-risk, coronary-prone (i.e., hostile, unloving, self-absorbed) behavior patterns and replacing them with more spiritually focused practices (e.g., giving and receiving love, patience development, anger management and forgiveness, and reorientations of time and priorities to spiritual and nonmaterial pursuits and others). Our work with recovering alcoholic smokers (Martin, et al., 1997; Patten, et al., 1998) provides another example of the use and importance of spiritual–behavioral integrations in the effective treatment of addictive behavior.

An interesting example is the long-standing spiritual practice of fasting and self-denial. In many spiritual traditions, an important function of fasting is to reduce attachment to (and automatic indulgence in) high-probability responses that are perceived to divert time and effort from spiritual experience and expression. It is not difficult to conceptualize this as an intentional extinction process. Many religious holy times (e.g., Ramadan, Yom Kippur, Lent) have traditionally included fasting for various lengths of time.

It can be difficult to get started with fasting. For those who wish to follow this practice of self-denial as a periodic or regular observance, some gradual shaping is wise (Foster, 1988). For example, if the eventual target fast were an annual 7-day, water-only fast of prayer and solitude, a first approximation might be a 1-day, fruit-juice-only fast. With success in this, one may build to a single-day fast from all nourishment, gradually adding days during which normal activities are diminished and the desired spiritual practices are increased. With regard to fasting, trying to do too much too quickly is a recipe for failure and discouragement.

Other spiritual issues may revolve around displacing high-probability behaviors. Materialism, often described as an impediment to spiritual development, by definition involves potent primary and secondary reinforcers. Spiritual writings and religious history are replete with examples of even highly spiritually developed individuals struggling with choices between the profound pull of immediate reinforcers (distractions, temptations) and the transcendent spiritual path that may not be as immediately rewarding. Some resolve this dilemma by relinquishing control (see chaps. 6 and 9 in this book). Cognitive–behavioral principles can also be applied to establish persistent or rule-governed behavior patterns that override immediate gratification, a common challenge in treating addictive behaviors (Martin, et al., 1997; Patten, et al., 1998). A wide range of useful cognitive–behavioral strategies (e.g., goal setting, fading, Premack principle, contingency management, motivational interviewing, public commitment, and social support) can be applied in pursuit of a simpler lifestyle that leaves space for spirituality to grow. As with most "do less" approaches, it is wise while decreasing one response to "do more" of the previously lower probability behavior that is meant to replace it.

CONCLUSION

In conclusion, we point to three general insights from this topic and discussion. First, there is much shapable behavior in spirituality. Most spiritual belief systems specify core practice components intended to draw the adherent into higher levels of spiritual identity, strength, and expression. Second, psychology, particularly cognitive–behavioral therapy, has much to offer in helping individuals strengthen their spirituality and religious adherence. Third, spiritual behavior enhancement may be approached from three basic directions that involve increasing spiritual practice (doing more), strengthening spiritual identity (being more), and decreasing spiritual barriers (doing less). In each category, we have presented examples of cognitive–behavioral strategies and examples to illustrate how behavioral science can be applied in helping to enhance desired spiritual and religious practices.

Behavioral interventions were founded on learning theory (Chance, 1994; Holland & Skinner, 1961; L. K. Miller, 1980) and have been successfully applied to general problems (Sulzer-Azaroff & Reese, 1982), as well as health behavior (Elder, Geller, Hovell, & Mayer, 1994). In a pragmatic approach, practices such as prayer, meditation, worship, scriptural study, and even love and humility may be operationally defined as voluntary (operant) behaviors that are subject to the principles of learning. We have illustrated how cognitive–behavioral approaches can be adapted to help motivate, shape, alter, and maintain spiritual practices and lifestyle.

We recognize that "spirituality" and "behavioral technology" can seem strange companions in the same sentence. Yet, as illustrated throughout this book, at least the behavior in spirituality merits serious attention in science and practice. A number of empirically validated behavioral interventions have incorporated spiritual components, with salutary effects on health across a variety of individuals, settings, and religious affiliations. These studies have been reviewed elsewhere in detail (Larson, 1994; Larson, et al., 1998; Martin & Carlson, 1988; Booth & Martin, 1998, 1999; Ornish, 1998) and in other chapters in this book. Research consistently reflects a relationship of spiritual and religious involvement with better health and quality of life. Nevertheless, spirituality has remained at the outskirts of clinical practice, research, and education (Bergin, 1991). We believe that spirituality and behavioral psychology can benefit from a sharing of perspectives. Behavioral approaches can be applied in various ways to promote spiritual as well as mental and physical health. The relatively unexplored terrain of spirituality, in turn, may reveal new insights and approaches from which to forge a more complete behavioral science.

REFERENCES

Alcoholics Anonymous. (1976). *Alcoholics Anonymous*. New York: Alcoholics Anonymous World Services.

Bandura, A. (1986). *Social foundations of thought and action: A social-cognitive theory*. Englewood Cliffs, NJ: Prentice-Hall.

Beck, A. T., Rush, A. J., Shaw, B. F., & Emery, G. (1979). *Cognitive therapy of depression*. New York: Guilford Press.

Bergin, A. E. (1991). Values and religious issues in psychotherapy and mental health. *American Psychologist, 46*, 394–403.

Booth, J., & Martin, J. E. (1998). Spiritual and religious factors in substance use, dependence, and recovery. In H. Koenig (Ed.), *Handbook of religion and mental health* (pp. 175–200). New York: Academic Press.

Booth, J., & Martin, J. E. (1999). *Church-based cardiovascular risk behavior interventions in high-risk African-Americans: Current status and future directions*. Manuscript submitted for publication.

Brownell, K. D., Marlatt, G. A., Lichtenstein, E., & Wilson, G. T. (1986). Understanding and preventing relapse. *American Psychologist, 41*, 765–782.

Chance, P. (1994). *Learning and behavior* (3rd ed.). Pacific Grove, CA: Brooks/Cole.

Elder, J., Geller, S., Hovell, M., & Mayer, J. (1994). *Motivating health behavior*. Albany, NY: Delmar.

Foster, R. J. (1988). *Celebration of discipline: The path to spiritual growth*. New York: HarperCollins.

Holland, J. G., & Skinner, B. F. (1961). *The analysis of behavior*. New York: McGraw-Hill.

Larson, D. B. (1994). *The faith factor: An annotated bibliography of systemic reviews and clinical research on spiritual objects* (Vol. 1). Rockville, MD: National Institute of Healthcare Research.

Larson, D. B., & Larson, S. S. (1994). *The forgotten factor in physical and mental health: What does the research show?* Rockville, MD: National Institute for Healthcare Research.

Larson, D. B., Swyers, J. P., & McCullough, M. E. (1998). *Scientific research on spirituality and health: A consensus report*. Rockville, MD: National Institute of Healthcare Research.

Levin, J. S., & Vanderpool, H. Y. (1991). Religious factors in physical health and the prevention of illness. *Prevention in Human Services, 9*, 41–64.

Martin, J. E., Ameika, C., & Lydston, D. (1999, March). *Effects of a spiritually based diet program in high-risk African Americans*. Paper presented at the meeting of the Society of Behavioral Medicine, San Diego, CA.

Martin, J. E., Calfas, K. J., Patten, C. A., Plarek, M., Hofstetter, R., Noto, J., & Beach, D. (1997). Prospective evaluation of three smoking interventions in 205 recovering alcoholics. *Journal of Consulting and Clinical Psychology, 65*, 190–194.

Martin, J. E., & Carlson, C. R. (1988). Spiritual dimensions of health psychology. In W. Miller & J. E. Martin (Eds.), *Behavior therapy and religion: Integrating spiritual and behavioral approaches to change* (pp. 57–110). Newbury Park, CA: Sage.

Martin, J. E., & Dubbert, P. M. (1984). Behavioral management strategies for improving health and fitness. *Journal of Cardiac Rehabilitation, 4*, 200–208.

May, G. (1991). *Addiction and grace*. San Francisco: HarperCollins.

Miller, L. K. (1975). *Principles of everyday behavior analysis*. Monterey, CA: Brooks Coles.

Miller, L. K. (1980). *Principles of everyday behavior analysis*. Pacific Grove, CA: Brooks/Cole.

Miller, W. R., & C'de Baca, J. (1994). Quantum change: Toward a psychology of transformation. In T. Heatherton & J. Weinberger (Eds.), *Can personality change?* (pp. 253–280). Washington, DC: American Psychological Association.

Miller, W., & Martin, J. E. (Eds.). (1988). *Behavior therapy and religion: Integrating spiritual and behavioral approaches to change*. Newbury Park, CA: Sage.

Miller, W. R., & Rollnick, S. (1991). *Motivational interviewing*. New York: Guilford Press.

Moss, R. A., Prue, D. M., Lomax, B. D., & Martin, J. E. (1982). Implications of self-monitoring for smoking treatment. *Addictive Behaviors, 7*, 381–385.

Novaco, R. W. (1995). Clinical problems of anger and its assessment and regulation through a stress coping skills approach. In W. O'Donohue & L. Krasner

(Eds.), *Handbook of psychological skills training: Clinical techniques and applications* (pp. 320–338). Boston: Allyn & Bacon.

Nowinski, J., Baker, S., & Carroll, K. (1992). *Twelve step facilitation therapy manual: A clinical research guide for therapists treating individuals with alcohol abuse and dependence* (DHHS Publication No. ADM 92-1893). Rockville, MD: National Institute on Alcohol Abuse and Alcoholism.

Ornish, D. (1998). *Love and survival: The scientific basis for the healing power of intimacy.* New York: HarperCollins.

Patten, C. A., Martin, J. E., Myers, M. G., Calfas, K. J., & Williams, C. D. (1998). Effectiveness of cognitive-behavioral therapy for smokers with histories of alcohol dependence and depression. *Journal of Studies on Alcohol, 59,* 327–335.

Persons, J. B. (1989). *Cognitive therapy in practice.* New York: Norton.

Powell, L., Friedman, M., Thoresen, C. E., Gill, J. J., & Ulmer, D. K. (1984). Can the Type A behavior pattern be altered after myocardial infarction? A second year report from the Recurrent Coronary Prevention Project. *Psychosomatic Medicine, 46,* 293–313.

Project MATCH Research Group. (1997). Matching alcoholism treatments to client heterogeneity: Project MATCH posttreatment drinking outcomes. *Journal of Studies on Alcohol, 58,* 7–29.

Propst, L. R., Ostrom, R., Watkins, P., Dean, T., & Mashburn, D. (1992). Comparative efficacy of religious and nonreligious cognitive-behavioral therapy for the treatment of clinical depression in religious individuals. *Journal of Consulting and Clinical Psychology, 60,* 94–103.

Richards, P. S., & Bergin, A. E. (Eds.). (1997). *A spiritual strategy for counseling and psychotherapy.* Washington, DC: American Psychological Association.

Salkovskis, P. M. (Ed.). (1996). *Frontiers of cognitive therapy.* New York: Guilford Press.

Shamblin, G. (1997). *The weigh down diet.* New York: Doubleday.

Sulzer-Azaroff, B., & Reese, E. (1982). *Applying behvaioral analysis.* New York: Holt, Rinehart & Winston.

Virkler, M. (1986). *Dialogue with God.* South Plainfield, NJ: Bridge Publishing.

Voorhees, C. C., Stillman, F. A., Swank, R. T., Heagerty, P. J., Levine, D. M., & Becker, D. M. (1996). Heart, body, and soul: Impact of church-based smoking cessation interventions on readiness to quit. *Preventive Medicine, 25,* 277–285.

Williams, R. B., & Williams, V. (1994). *Anger kills: Seventeen strategies for controlling the hostility that can harm your health.* New York: HarperCollins.

III

SOME SPIRITUAL ISSUES
IN TREATMENT

9

SPIRITUAL SURRENDER: A PARADOXICAL PATH TO CONTROL

BRENDA S. COLE AND KENNETH I. PARGAMENT

It is in the gray area between the possible and the futile that the battle of coping with stress has to be fought. (Breznitz, 1980, p. 265)

In clinical practice therapists typically work with clients to increase personal control. They help clients to "take charge" of the situation and their emotions. There are, however, limits to personal control in any situation. As strange as it may seem, at times the only way to enhance personal control may be to give up control: the paradoxical path of *surrender*. Take, for example, Donna's story.

Donna was adopted when she was only an infant. Separated from her biological sister and brother, Donna grew up regretting the missed opportunity to be a part of a "family." So later in life when her biological sister's five children entered foster care and faced adoption, it was especially important to her that they remain together. It became evident, however, that the siblings would be separated unless she and her husband adopted all five of the children. As difficult as this change would be for their already large family of five children, she and her husband began adoption proceedings. Donna put tremendous effort into the adoption process: (a) providing a loving home for three of the children as an initial foster care parent; (b) working out visitations with her sister, the biological mother, who was hostile to her adoption plans; and (c) working through the bureaucratic paperwork and legal system. As their temporary foster mother, Donna experienced the joy of seeing the children happy and together in her own home, but her feelings turned to anguish and despair when her efforts to ensure the success of the adoption were threatened by the biological mother and court system. She distinctly recalled a moment of overwhelming helplessness in the midst of this struggle. Try as she might, she knew that the control over her children's future was out of her hands. At that moment she had a realization, "If anyone is going to play King Solomon, it should be God and not me." With this insight she prayed to God, "With your help I'll do all that I can for as long as they're mine." She identified this change as an experience of surrender, an experience through which she shifted her focus from controlling the adoption to fulfilling God's purpose for her in the children's lives. Out of this experience emerged a sense of peace. She was able to continue, more patiently and more calmly, letting go of trying to make the adoption happen through being a "perfect" mother in the eyes of the court, and focusing instead on what she could do to provide loving care for these children.

The paradox of spiritual surrender is evident in Donna's story. Only through the subjective experience of giving up control was she able to enhance her control over her emotions and actions. Once she let go of her search for control, she experienced feelings of relief, the ability to think more clearly, and the ability to work more productively toward her goal of adoption. Paradoxically, however, these benefits were unintended. Donna surrendered the outcome of the adoption into God's hands not to gain relief but to give life to her spiritual values. She surrendered her desire for control for the sake of the sacred. Happily in this case, she became the "official mother" of all five of the children.

In this chapter we explore the relationship between spiritual surrender and control in more detail. The discussion is divided into four sections. In the first section, we discuss the importance of control or mastery in the coping process and the different types of control-oriented coping. We then consider how beliefs about the individual's relationship with God or a higher power can enhance personal control. We also note, however, that the pursuit of personal control to the exclusion of other goals and values can become dysfunctional. There are, after all, limits to what individuals are able to master on their own in virtually every situation. We suggest that spirituality offers an alternative and unique response to human limitations, one in which the ends of coping are transformed from the secular to the sacred. Control is surrendered for the sake of spiritual ends. Yet, in the process, control may be paradoxically increased. In the second section, we consider the qualities that mark this experience of spiritual surrender and the paradoxical ways in which control is simultaneously enhanced through the process of letting go. In the third section, we evaluate the helpfulness of surrender as a coping method. We explore relevant studies and case reports that suggest spiritual surrender may be beneficial. In the fourth section, we present some ways therapists might facilitate the process of surrender in clinical settings.

THE IMPORTANCE OF CONTROL IN THE COPING PROCESS

Coping involves what Pargament (1997) has described as a "search for significance in times of stress" (p. 90). When faced with a traumatic event, people strive toward what they perceive to be of significance in their lives. The object of significance may vary across people and situations, but control is commonly one overriding concern (e.g., Thompson, Collins, Newcomb, & Hunt, 1996). When stressful situations severely threaten the ability to control the substance and course of life, people strive to reestablish a sense of mastery and self-determination.

Researchers have suggested that there are two types of control that are especially important in the coping process. Lazarus and Folkman (1984) have distinguished between problem-focused and emotion-focused coping efforts. Problem-focused coping involves activities directed externally at controlling aspects of the environment. Emotion-focused coping, on the other hand, is directed at controlling emotional reactions and the ability to adjust to distressing situations. Problem-focused coping and emotion-focused coping correspond, in part, to what others have called "primary control" and "secondary control," respectively (Rothbaum, Weisz, & Snyder, 1982). Primary control involves "attempts to change the world so that it fits the self's needs" (Rothbaum et al., 1982, p. 8), and secondary control involves attempts to change the self to "flow with the current" of life. Although there are some differences between these two models (problem-focused and emotion-focused vs. primary and secondary control), both models note that control can be directed outwardly, inwardly, or both. For the sake of simplicity, we use the constructs of primary and secondary control to capture this distinction.

Researchers have paid considerable attention to the role of primary and secondary control in times of stress (e.g., Band & Weisz, 1988; Lazarus & Folkman, 1984; Rothbaum et al., 1982; Thompson et al., 1996; Thompson, Nanni, & Levine, 1994; Weisz, McCabe, & Dennig, 1994; Weisz, Rothbaum, & Blackburn, 1984; for a critique, see Skinner, 1996). Until recently, however, researchers have given little attention to the ways in which beliefs about the transcendent are involved in the coping process, specifically how these beliefs affect the search for control.

Pargament and colleagues (Pargament et al., 1988; Pargament, Smith, Koenig, & Perez, 1998) have studied how beliefs about the individual's relationship with God are involved in the coping process. They have identified four control-related coping styles: self-directing, collaborative, deferring, and pleading. Each style represents a different approach to the search for primary and secondary control. When using the *self-directing approach*, the individual perceives the self as being the center of control. Although the person may believe in God, the individual sees the self as having free choice, agency, and responsibility to direct the course of life events and to adapt to difficult life situations. In this approach, primary and secondary control are sought through the individual's own efforts. The *collaborative approach* rests on a view of God as a partner in the coping process. The person works with God to find meaning in difficult situations, to generate and implement solutions to problems, and to sustain the self emotionally. Thus, from this perspective, primary and secondary control are achieved through the relationship between the individual and God. The *deferring approach* differs from the above two in that personal responsibility is relinquished. In the search for primary or secondary control, the individual turns over the responsibility for dealing with the entire situation to God. Finally, in the *pleading approach*, the individual seeks control indirectly. Through petitioning and pleading, the person asks God to intervene in the situation to bring about a more favorable outcome, one more in line with personal wishes. This coping approach seems to be directed more at primary than secondary control. Assimilation to the state of the world is rejected in favor of changing the world through God.

How can you tell which coping style best describes clients? Pargament and colleagues (1988, 1997) have developed measures to assess these four styles (see Table 9.1 for illustrative items).

Research on these coping styles suggests that they differ in terms of their helpfulness (Bransfield, Ivy, Rutledge, & Wallston, 1991; Casebolt, 1990; Hathaway & Pargament, 1990; Kaiser, 1991; McIntosh & Spilka, 1990; Schaefer & Gorsuch, 1991; Sears & Greene, 1994; Winger & Hunsberger, 1988). Generally, the collaborative approach has been associated with better outcomes than the deferring (Pargament et al., 1988), self-directing (Pargament et al., 1990), and pleading approaches (Pargament, 1997), especially in low-control situations (Bickel et al., 1998). For example, Bickel et al. found that under high-stress situations (i.e., situations that are less predictable and controllable), the self-directing approach was associated with increases in depression, whereas the collaborative approach was associated with decreases in depression.

What are the practical implications of these findings? Comments by clients that they turn to God for help or guidance in the midst of their most difficult moments may raise concerns among many clinicians about overdependence, passivity, or avoidance (Pargament & Park, 1995). These results, however, suggest that there is no need for alarm. In fact, there is every reason to consider encouraging a client's sense of partnership or collaboration with transcendent dimensions of life in coping.

TABLE 9.1
Illustrative Items From Control-Oriented Coping and Spiritual Surrender Scales

Deferring
1. Didn't do much, just expected God to solve my problems for me.
2. Knew that I couldn't handle the situation, so I just expected God to take control.
3. Didn't try to do much; just assumed God would handle it.

Pleading
1. Pleaded with God to make things turn out okay.
2. Bargained with God to make things better.
3. Prayed for a miracle.

Self-directing
1. Tried to deal with my feelings without God's help.
2. Tried to make sense of the situation without relying on God.
3. Made decisions about what to do without God's help.

Collaborative
1. Tried to put my plans into action together with God.
2. Worked together with God as partners.
3. Tried to make sense of the situation with God.

Spiritual surrender
1. Did my best and then turned the situation over to God.
2. Did what I could and put the rest in God's hands.
3. Took control over what I could and gave the rest up to God.

Note. People respond to the items in terms of the way they cope with either a specific major life stressor or with major life stressors in general. For a copy of the full RCOPE, contact the second author. From Pargament, K. I., Smith, B. W., Koenig, H. G., & Perez, L. (1998, August). *The Many Methods of Religious Coping: Development and Initial Validation of the RCOPE.* Paper presented at the meeting of the American Psychological Association, San Francisco, CA. Adapted with permission of the authors.

THE LIMITS OF CONTROL IN COPING

These four styles of coping reflect the variety of ways one's perceived relationship with the sacred can be involved in the search for primary control, secondary control, or both within the coping process. There is, however, more to coping than control. After all, the amount of personal control that is possible in any situation is always constrained by other forces. Focusing exclusively on the search for added control, then, may become problematic. Consider, for instance, the following case:

> [Mike] does not believe in any power higher than himself, is relatively focused on personal achievement and material possessions (e.g., money accumulation), and he does not pray or meditate (though he exercises regularly and takes generally good care of himself physically); he feels that he must always be in control of himself and nearly every situation, and tends to struggle frequently with his own perfectionism; he believes only in himself and in the competitive marketplace—that he must strive against others to "rise to the top" and achieve all of which he is capable. (Martin & Carlson, 1988, p. 64)

Most clinicians are familiar with someone like Mike and recognize the potential negative consequences of a preoccupation with personal control. These include negative emotions (e.g., anxiety, anger, sadness); stress-related disorders such as headaches, hypertension, and coronary-prone behavior; and the addictive overconsumption of food, tobacco, and alcohol. Because people are finite, because personal resources are bounded, and because the possibilities in any situation are necessarily limited, a preoccupation with personal control will often lead to frustration and failure.

The religions of the world offer an alternative to efforts to conserve the sense of control. They provide mechanisms to transform significance (i.e., what is taken to be worthy of pursuit) in times of stress (Pargament, 1997). Spiritual surrender represents one such method of transformation particularly relevant to control. Through spiritual surrender, control is abandoned for the sake of the sacred, be it a transcendent purpose, ideal, relationship, or commitment. In the process, however, both primary and secondary control may be inadvertently enhanced. We turn now to a more detailed discussion of the nature of spiritual surrender.

QUALITIES OF SPIRITUAL SURRENDER

It is important to be clear about the meaning of the words *spiritual surrender* and the qualities of this experience within the coping process. Before we begin, however, we must stress that spiritual surrender is not simply a coping mechanism. Religious traditions do not solely teach surrender as part of the survival kit for when things get tough. Surrender is a profound spiritual practice within many different religious traditions that transcends times of crises. Consider these examples:

> *Muslim:* Whosoever surrenders himself to Allah, doing good meanwhile, has taken hold of the surest hand-grip, and towards Allah is the outcome of affairs. (The Qur'an 31:21)

> *Hindu:* O scion of Bharata's clan! Seek refuge in Him, making a total surrender of your being—body, mind and soul. By His grace you shall attain to supreme peace and the everlasting abode. (Srimad-Bhagavad-Gita 18:62)

> *New Age:* When peace comes at last to those who wrestle with temptation and fight against the giving into sin; when the light comes at last into the mind given to contemplation; or when the goal is finally achieved by anyone, it always comes with just one happy realization; "I need do nothing." (A Course in Miracles, 1985, p. 363)

Thus, any consideration of the role of surrender within difficult times should reflect an appreciation for the value of surrender as a general aspect of spiritual life.

If we think back to Donna's determined effort to adopt her five children, we can identify some salient aspects of surrender. First, surrender involves a recognition of a higher value or greater good in the seemingly negative situation. In Donna's story, we heard how she became aware of something more important than her own desire to adopt the children. The greater good was broader than her personal concerns and was known only by God. What was most important, she realized, was to trust God and care lovingly for the children in spite of the fact that things might not work out as she thought best. This awareness of a higher value is essential to the process of surrender. It is an awareness that is also evident in 12-step recovery programs for alcoholism (see chap. 6 in this book).

Second, and in many ways related to the recognition of a higher value, surrender involves an experience of self-transcendence. The individual begins to see the self in relationship to a higher purpose or transcendent reality rather than as the center of the world. What motivates this shift, however, is not a search for control, either primary or secondary. Instead, the individual begins to look for a connection with a transcendent reality, a goal that requires relinquishing all forms of control. In a sense, the person stops "playing God" and starts "seeking God." This shift from control to transcendence reflects what Pargament (1997) has referred to as a "transformation of significance." The focal point of the search for significance, a search that organizes and directs one's thoughts and behavior, changes from control to the sacred.

Spiritual surrender is much more than a cognitive shift. It is an experiential shift as well, one that involves changes in motivation, affect, values, perception, thought, and behavior. The individual experiences an enlarged sense of existence, the self as immersed in the divine. In Judeo-Christian religious terms, the person begins to "live, move, and have one's being in God." From a Zen perspective, the individual realizes Buddha nature. In the process, the person's own desires are released or set aside for the sake of a greater good or existence, often framed in terms of spiritual beliefs or commitments. Donna experienced this transformation as she put aside her desire to be the mother of her sister's children and instead focused on God and loving the children for as long as they were with her.

Third, the subjective experience following surrender is characterized by an enhanced state of being. People often describe this state as one of total acceptance resulting in feelings of completeness, serenity, gratitude, and compassion. Donna described greater awareness of her situation, a sense of calm, and the ability to focus more effectively on the things that were under her control.

Even though Donna's experience of surrender reflects a Judeo-Christian religious tradition, other religious traditions also view surrender as an important aspect of life. Dogen Zenji, a Zen master and considered by some to be the major founder of the Zen Buddhist tradition in Japan, said let go of and forget your body and mind. Throw your life into the abode of the Buddha, living by being moved and led by the Buddha. When you do this without relying on your own physical and mental power, you become released from life and death and become a Buddha. (cited in Beck, 1989, pp. 149–150)

Speaking on the meaning of this passage, Beck (1989), an American Zen teacher, commented that

since Buddha is none other than this absolute moment of life (which is not the past or the present or the future), [Dogen Zenji] is saying that this very moment is the abode of the Buddha, enlightenment, paradise. It is nothing but the life of this very moment. . . . Wisdom is to see that there is nothing to search for. If you live with a difficult person, that's nirvana. Perfect. If you're miserable, that's it. And I'm not saying to be passive, not to take action; then you would be trying to hold nirvana as a fixed state. It's never fixed, but always changing. There is no implication of "doing nothing." But deeds done that are born of this understanding are free of anger and judgment. No expectation, just pure and compassionate action. (pp. 150–151)

Here, too, we can identify the three common themes of surrender, albeit with different metaphors and images. (a) *Recognition of a higher value*: In his own words Dogen Zenji called others to reach for a higher value than what is normally perceived to be worthy of pursuit. Beck referred to this as "enlightenment" or "paradise." (b) *Self-transcendence*: Dogen Zenji affirmed the importance of transcendence in the metaphor "throw your life into the abode of the Buddha." He encouraged students to transcend their normal way of thinking and experiencing life when he says "forget your body and mind." (c) *Enhanced state of being*: Dogen Zenji suggested that through the process of surrendering one's life, the individual realizes the highest state possible, becoming a "Buddha." This state, according to Beck, is marked by a deeper satisfaction in life, "free of anger and judgment" and filled with compassion. Thus, the experience of surrender is not limited to Judeo-Christian traditions. Surrender plays an important role in other religious traditions as well.

What is the relationship between control and surrender? The act of surrender is, by its very nature, an act of relinquishing control as an object of significance. Significance is shifted away from control to one's relationship to sacred realities and the living out of spiritual commitments in light of those relationships. There is an important point that follows here: Surrender cannot be intentionally used as a means of gaining either primary or secondary control; however, a greater sense of control may ensue from the act of surrender to the sacred. In terms of secondary control, the act of surrender may help the individual adapt to reality. The focus on the sacred puts worldly concerns into a broader perspective and may generate feelings of acceptance. Similarly, spiritual surrender may assist rather than undermine the exercise of primary control. Surrender, Beck (1989) clearly warned the Buddhist disciple, is not a path of avoidance or irresponsibility. She suggested that acceptance that leads to "doing nothing" is as much an error as not accepting life as it is. Similarly, Donna's surrender did not mean ending her efforts to adopt the children. Thus, for people working from both Judeo-Christian and Buddhist traditions, surrender should not be equated with passivity or avoidance. The clarity of mind that often follows spiritual surrender may enhance both the ability to take constructive action and the ability to adapt to life situations.

Note that we are talking specifically about spiritual surrender here. Clearly, it makes a difference to whom the individual surrenders. The surrender to other forces, such as a dictator or abusive spouse, is likely to lead to much different outcomes in terms of primary and secondary control as well as well-being.

HOW HELPFUL IS SPIRITUAL SURRENDER?

Several lines of empirical study suggest that spiritual surrender may be helpful to people not only psychologically but also spiritually. First, there are particular contexts in which surrender is likely to be helpful in the coping process. Surrender is likely to be of particular value when people are faced with situations that have few controllable aspects (e.g., death, chronic illness, accidents). In situations like these, the options for personal control, especially primary control, are severely limited. Moreover, attempts to exert primary control may be not only nonproductive but also counterproductive; misplaced attempts to exert primary control in the pursuit of problem-focused goals may interfere with the pursuit of other, more attainable goals. In this vein, research suggests that people tend to engage in emotion-focused, compared with problem-focused, coping in low-control situations (Folkman & Lazarus, cited in Folkman, 1984; Vitaliano, De-Wolfe, Maiuro, Russo, & Katon, 1990) and find the former more helpful under these conditions (e.g., Strentz & Auerbach, 1988). Attempts to exert secondary control also appear to be more helpful than attempts to exert primary control under life-threatening conditions (Weisz et al., 1994, p. 324). As noted earlier, spiritual surrender offers another alternative to the search for primary control. Thus, it, too, is likely to be especially helpful in conditions affording low objective control.

Second, two studies on the helpfulness of prayer offer indirect support for the importance of surrender in coping with distress. The studies examined the effects of different types of prayer on anxiety. The first study focused on the effects of reflective and intercessory prayer in a sample of members of a Baptist congregation (Elkins, Anchor, & Sandler, 1979). Intercessory prayer was described as praying for "a spiritual intervention in one's personal life or in the lives of others" (Elkins et al., 1979, p. 81). Reflective prayer was described as "communicating private feelings to a supreme being" (Elkins et al., 1971, p. 81). Both types of prayer were oriented toward either primary control, attempting to influence the outcome of events (intercessory prayer), or secondary control, expressing feelings to the sacred as a means of adjusting better to the situation (reflective prayer). Neither type of prayer, however, significantly reduced anxiety or tension when compared with a control group.

Although this study alone does not speak to the effects of surrender, these results are more interpretable when integrated with those found by Carlson, Bacaseta, and Simanton (1988). Carlson et al. also focused on the effects of prayer and devotional meditation on anxiety and tension. Participants were college students from a Christian liberal arts college. In contrast to the Elkins et al. (1971) study, this study examined contemplative prayer, or prayer in which the individual focused on "development of Christian virtues" (Carlson et al., 1988, p. 363). This type of prayer was not oriented toward primary or secondary control; instead, it embodied self-transcendence, the surrender of self-concerns. The objective of this prayer, Carlson et al. (1988) stated, was "to relate to God in a quiet, non-verbal and open manner" (p. 363). Interestingly, participants who used this type of prayer experienced reductions in anxiety and anger more so than did members of a control group or a group using progressive muscle relaxation. Unfortunately, because the participants in this study were also instructed to contemplate scriptures reflecting "God's care and concern," it is unclear whether the results were due solely to the experience of surrender (Carlson et al., 1988, p. 363). Spiritual support, which could have increased secondary control, may also have played a beneficial role. Nevertheless, when these two studies are considered together, they suggest that spiritual surrender may be helpful in reducing distress in some situations and may be more helpful than other spiritual and religious practices or progressive muscle relaxation. Moreover, Carlson et al. (1988) offered a ready means for incorporating spiritual surrender into the therapy process. Contemplative prayer may be an appropriate intervention for spiritually interested clients whose goals include letting go.

Third, studies of the effects of transcendent experiences provide some support for the helpfulness of surrender. Hood, Hall, Watson, and Biderman (1979) found that scores on a mysticism scale were associated with a range of positive psychological variables, such as broad interests, creativity, innovation, tolerance of others, and social adeptness. In their study, mysticism was defined by eight subscales that assessed a sense of oneself as "[absorbed] into something greater than the mere empirical ego"; an experience of all things having an "inner subjectivity" beyond material form (e.g., experiencing all things having consciousness); a modification of time and space (e.g., experiencing timelessness); receiving knowledge that is "nonrational, intuitive, insightful," an experience that cannot be communicated through "conventional language"; positive affective quality; and experiences marked by a sacred or holy quality. In other studies, mysticism has been associated with strong ego strength, self-actualization experiences, and ego permissiveness. The latter is said to encourage "regression in service of the ego," or the use of unconscious material for the purposes of ego development or adaptive functioning (for a review, see Hood, Spilka, Hunsberger, & Gorsuch, 1996). In addition, Yates, Chalmer, St. James, Follansbee, and McKegney (1981) found that cancer patients who had recently experienced feelings of closeness to God or nature experienced decreased levels of pain. Self-transcendence measured in less traditionally spiritual terms (i.e., "expanded self-boundaries that help to discover or make meaning," Coward, 1996, p. 117) has also been associated with indexes of well-being: emotional well-being, sense of coherence, hope, self-esteem, and cognitive well-being (Coward, 1996; Reed, 1991).

The results of these studies suggest that the transcendent experiences, so typical of spiritual surrender, have positive associations with psychological and physical well-being and may be particularly helpful in times of crisis. Thus, clinicians may do well to explore transcendence with clients for whom surrender seems to be an appropriate intervention. Ask clients, "Have you ever had transcendent experiences in which you felt connected to something beyond yourself?" "What was that like for you?" "What helped you feel connected?" "When was the last time you felt this connection?" "What would it be like for you to spend a little time each day relating to [God, Allah, a higher power, etc]?"

Fourth, a few researchers have begun to measure spiritual surrender directly and to evaluate its effects. The results of this research have also been promising. Wong-McDonald and Gorsuch (1997) found that spiritual surrender was negatively related to self-directing coping and positively associated with both collaborative and deferring coping approaches. However, when the effects of the other coping approaches were controlled, spiritual surrender predicted increases in intrinsic religiousness, importance of spirituality, belief in control by God, and religious as well as existential well-being. These results suggest that spiritual surrender plays a unique and helpful role in the coping process. The scale used to measure surrender in this study reflected a conservative Christian orientation. Because the participants in this study were conservative Christians, the orientation of this scale was not problematic; however, questions remain about whether a construct of surrender more compatible with diverse religious traditions and administered to a more diverse population would yield similar results. Results of another investigation suggest the answer to both questions may be yes.

Pargament et al. (1998) conducted a validation study of the RCOPE, a comprehensive, theoretically based measure of spiritual coping that assesses, among other methods, several approaches to control (i.e., collaborative, deferring, pleading, self-directing) and spiritual surrender. Spiritual surrender was measured by items such as "Did my best and then turned the situation over to God" and "Did what I could and put the rest in God's hands" (see Table 9.1). Consistent with previous research and theory about the control-oriented constructs, the items of these dimensions loaded on distinct scales in a factor analysis. Moreover, these scales related to adjustment in different ways in a population of hospitalized patients coping with serious medical illnesses (Koenig, Pargament, & Nielsen, in press). Spiritual surrender, in particular, predicted several measures of positive adjustment (e.g., lower depression, better quality of life, stress-related growth, cooperativeness in the interview, and positive religious outcomes) more strongly than did the deferring, pleading, and self-directing scales. Spiritual surrender, like the collaborative approach, was associated with positive adjustment. However, spiritual surrender was more likely to be used than a collaborative approach in more distressing situations as measured by the patient's number of medical diagnoses.

Overall, these findings suggest that spiritual surrender plays a distinctive role in people's lives. Moreover, like the collaborative approach, it is associated with more positive adjustment than the deferring, pleading, and self-directing approaches. Consider, then, assessing a client's spiritually oriented coping style and its implications for psychological and spiritual well-being. To conduct an assessment, consider the RCOPE (see Table 9.1). Help your client weigh the advantages of adopting either a more collaborative approach to control or embracing spiritual surrender.[1] Finally, if it seems desirable, based on discussions with your client, explore ways to increase spiritual surrender or collaborative coping. The items on these respective scales offer a starting point for this discussion.

Although the research findings presented above are encouraging, they are still preliminary. Until additional research is conducted, perhaps the most compelling evidence of the effectiveness of spiritual surrender will have to come from the stories of people who have experienced relief through surrender in times of great personal loss or tragedy. Donna's adoption of her five children is one such story. The benefits of spiritual surrender are also evident in the story told by Janet, a cancer survivor.

Janet grew up with an alcoholic father and a chaotic home situation. She recalled her childhood as a time when, more than anything, she wanted to be loved. Although her mother later remarried, things did not improve for Janet. She was sexually abused by her stepfather. In addition

---

[1]Editor's note: For a secular discussion of these clinical issues, see Steven C. Hayes, Neil S. Jacobson, Victoria M. Follette, and Michael J. Dougher (Eds.), *Acceptance and change: Content and context in psychotherapy* (1994). Reno, NV: Context Press.

to these stressors, every woman in Janet's family, including her mother, died from cancer before Janet was an adult. In spite of these life challenges, Janet was anything but bitter, unloving, or dysfunctional. An accomplished businesswoman, loving mother, and woman who had been deeply committed to helping children for most of her life, Janet was a model of how to face adversity with dignity, compassion, and a marvelous sense of humor, all in spite of the fact that she, too, was diagnosed with cancer at the age of 35.

When asked about her response to her diagnosis, Janet described initially feeling devastated. Throughout her life she had learned to cope by being "in control." Now she was faced with the ultimate loss of control, control over her own body. She recalled the frightening recognition, "I could die." Moreover, throughout the treatment process, she remembered feeling at the mercy of others. Medical decisions were made for her by doctors, and she felt helpless to direct her own treatment. When asked how she coped with this loss, Janet described how there gradually came a point when she realized that she had to surrender control over the final outcome of her cancer treatment. In a moment of surrender, she drew on her Catholic tradition and prayed "Thy will be done." As she began to accept the limits of her control, she decided that she would not give up. She would "go out kicking and screaming" but draw on faith that everything was happening for a higher purpose. Janet focused on her belief that "everything that comes into our lives is a training ground for something that happens on a higher level." From that perspective, she began to explore what it was that her cancer had to teach her. In our terms, Janet experienced a transformation of significance. She shifted her primary concerns from controlling and curing her cancer to the sacred, toward living her life in a way that reflected God's purpose. However, her surrender did not prevent her from doing all that she could to influence her health.

Janet did not claim that spiritual surrender erased the pain of dealing with cancer, but she did describe greater peace, more self-acceptance, and a clearer focus on the important things in life. She declared, "I am not what I do anymore. I am who I love." Much of her attention these days is invested in her family. So, for Janet, surrender also involved a transformation of how she saw and valued herself. In addition, her ability to surrender control helped her make important decisions that have enabled her to live more fully. She quit her job working for an abusive employer and eventually opened a store selling items for women with cancer. In reference to this latter change, Janet stated, "Cancer put me in training to learn how to help other cancer patients." Thus, through the experience of spiritual surrender, Janet was able to see her situation and her life differently. Today she can say, "I guess I'm glad I had cancer. It got me off my butt and made me change my life." Stories like those of Janet and Donna offer powerful testimony to the helpful role of spiritual surrender in the coping process.

SPIRITUAL SURRENDER IN THE CLINICAL SETTING

Given that surrender can play a helpful role in the coping process, how can you help a client for whom surrender seems appropriate? Before attempting such assistance there are some important points to keep in mind. First, some preparatory work is needed to understand the client's orientation to spirituality and whether the client is likely to find the concept of surrender meaningful. Part of this work requires learning about the words and images that the client finds meaningful in reference to the sacred. Second, be careful to avoid framing surrender in terms of utility. Although the goal may be to decrease distress and increase adaptive functioning, that goal runs counter to the ontological nature of spiritual surrender. One cannot surrender control to intentionally gain control. To paraphrase Frankl (1948/1984), control cannot be "pursued" through surrender, but, paradoxically, it may "ensue" from the search for the sacred. Third, acknowledge that spiritual surrender is an appropriate response to human limitations and the exigencies of life. That people are not in fact in total control of their own fates is likely to be realized in the most extreme moments: the death of a loved one, violent assault, sexual abuse, or being stricken with a life-threatening disease. Here and in many other life situations, the ultimate healing response may be one of surrender.

It is also important to be alert to problematic behaviors that are masquerading as spiritual surrender. Deferral, pleading, relinquished control that is more akin to "learned helplessness"—each of these responses to crisis may, at first glance, appear to be spiritual surrender. However, unlike spiritual surrender, these responses are likely to undermine active problem solving. Help the client differentiate spiritual surrender from these other approaches and explore the implications of each for effective coping. Some degree of active problem solving is possible and desirable in most situations. Clients should be helped to find the common ground where spirituality and active problem solving meet.

With these points in mind, there are several ways that you can introduce spiritual surrender into the therapy process. First, help the client consider the appropriateness of spiritual surrender by a well-framed comment or question. Inserting the client's word for the transcendent where people have used the word God below, ask questions like, "Is there something here that you need to surrender to God?" or "You seem to be struggling to let go of this tragedy. What would it be like for you to surrender this to God?" Questions such as these affirm that surrender is an appropriate response for many people, and you initiate a discussion of whether it is appropriate for a particular client in a particular situation. Second, many religious traditions have their own specific practices or sacred readings oriented toward the theme of spiritual surrender. Explore with the client aspects of his or her own tradition that may be helpful. Consider facilitating this process by working in collaboration with the client's clergy. Third, look into structured activities that facilitate a surrender response. For example, consider the two activities below. The first is directed at helping clients identify uncontrollable aspects of a situation. The second facilitates an experience of surrender.

To help clients differentiate the controllable from the uncontrollable aspects of a situation, you might offer them a piece of paper titled "circles of control." Draw two circles on the page: one labeled "things under my control" and the other labeled "things not under my control." The clients should think of concerns they have and write each concern in the correct circle. This exercise is modeled after one described by Baugh (1988). It is, as he pointed out, a tool for expressing the Serenity Prayer in one's life. We use an exercise like this in our spiritually focused therapy groups for cancer patients titled "re-creating your life." During the session on control, the therapist has the participants fill in the circles and then share these with the group. The therapist then urges group members to challenge each other's decisions if it appears that someone placed a concern in the wrong circle. The therapist also identifies and challenges two possible errors: either aborting primary control when control is possible or attempting to direct the course of uncontrollable aspects of their lives. As part of this process, the therapist helps participants explore the consequences of trying to control the uncontrollable in terms of anxiety and loss of energy to invest in things under their control.

Within this same session, the therapist discusses potential ways to cope with things beyond personal control. The group discusses spiritual surrender as a potentially helpful response. To help participants better identify things they need to surrender and to facilitate the experience of surrender, the therapist leads the participants through a guided imagery. Because the participants to date have all had a theistic perspective of the sacred, the imagery has involved surrendering aspects of their lives to God. The components of the imagery include relaxation instructions, visualizing God's presence, asking God what needs to be surrendered, visualizing placing the surrendered concern in God's hands, and then visualizing oneself bathed in a white light.

Martin and Carlson (1988) provided two case examples of other means of integrating surrender within clinical practice. In one instance, one of the authors was co-conducting a smoking cessation program that was floundering. Many of the participants were noncompliant and disruptive. The clinicians decided to take a different tack. Drawing on the 12-step program of Alcoholics Anonymous, Martin and Carlson (1988) "encouraged giving up control to God, praying for deliverance from the habit, and praying for success for each other, while also following the behavioral steps of the program" (p. 98). They reported that this new approach was widely accepted by group members and that it appeared to be instrumental in maintaining a zero dropout rate and successful smoking cessation by a majority of the participants.

In a second case example, Martin and Carlson (1988) worked with a young woman who was overweight and having difficulty beginning an exercise program. Having tried behavioral procedures without success, they decided to integrate a spiritual perspective that included a strong surrender component. They instructed her to

> (a) admit that, on her own at least, she didn't currently have the "power" or motivation to get up and exercise; (b) pray at night for God to help her arise in time and have the desire to go exercise; (c) completely turn the outcome over to God after praying and putting the matter in God's hands; and then (d) follow the previously tried behavioral techniques that had not helped (i.e., contracting with loved one, posting exercise graph, laying exercise clothes out night before . . .). (Martin & Carlson, 1988, p. 99)

The authors reported that this intervention was successful in modifying her exercise behavior. Additionally, it clearly exemplifies the interplay between surrender and active coping. She was not only instructed to relinquish control over the outcome to God but also to take control over those things that she could do to reach her goal.

The structured activities and case examples above demonstrate ways to integrate surrender within clinical situations. The key ingredient among them is the therapist's affirmation of surrender as a viable option and willingness to explore the appropriateness of spiritual surrender within the client's life.

CONCLUSION

Clinicians generally are masters of the "art of control." Explicitly or implicitly, therapists from diverse theoretical orientations often convey to their clients the value of controlling their internal and external environments and help their clients exert more control in their lives. This is often a desirable goal. However, the search for control can become a problem in itself when it excludes other balancing values and goals. If therapists help the client already overly preoccupied with control, to focus further on control, they may make a bad situation worse. An alternative approach is needed that recognizes the limits of personal powers, the humanly impossible as well as the humanly possible. Spiritual surrender offers one such alternative healing pathway. Through spiritual surrender, the search for control is transformed into a search for the sacred, but in the process primary and secondary control can be paradoxically enhanced. Practices such as "letting go and letting God" (from a Judeo-Christian perspective) or mindfulness meditation (from the Zen Buddhist tradition; see chap. 4 in this book) free the individual to focus on spiritual commitments, experiences, or ideals and invest energy only in those aspects of life that are amenable to change. Perhaps one of the reasons for the success of programs like the 12-step recovery program for alcoholic individuals is just this blend of spiritual surrender and active problem solving (see chap. 6 in this book). In addition, spiritual surrender may be one of the critical ingredients of other transformational processes, such as conversion (Ullman, 1989; Zinnbauer & Pargament, 1998) and forgiveness (McCullough, Worthington, & Rachal, 1997; see chap. 10 in this book). Certainly, the research and life stories reviewed here suggest that spiritual surrender is a viable path to positive mental health outcomes and greater spiritual well-being.

We hope that this chapter encourages clinicians to further explore the helpful role of surrender in the coping process. Just as important, we hope this chapter stimulates further studies of spiritual surrender as an important response to human limitations and human suffering. There is much to learn about this paradoxical path.

REFERENCES

Band, E., & Weisz, J. (1988). How to feel better when it feels bad: Children's perspectives on coping with everyday stress. *Developmental Psychology, 24,* 247–253.

Baugh, J. (1988). Gaining control by giving up control: Strategies for coping with powerlessness. In W. L. Miller & J. E. Martin (Eds.), *Behavior therapy and religion: Integrating spiritual and behavioral approaches to change* (pp. 125–138). Newbury Park, CA: Sage.

Beck, C. (1989). *Everyday Zen: Love and work.* San Francisco: Harper.

Bickel, C. O., Ciarrocchi, J., Sheers, N. J., Estadt, B. K., Powell, D. A., & Pargament, K. (1998). Perceived stress, religious coping styles, and depressive affect. *Journal of Psychology and Christianity, 17,* 33–42.

Bransfield, D., Ivy, S., Rutledge, D. & Wallston, K. (1991, August). *A religiously-oriented program to promote breast cancer screening.* Paper presented at the 99th Annual Convention of the American Psychological Association, New York.

Breznitz, S. (1983). The noble challenge of stress. In S. Breznitz (Ed.), *Stress in Israel* (pp. 265–274). New York: Van Nostrand Reinhold.

Carlson, C., Bacaseta, P., & Simanton, D. (1988). A controlled evaluation of devotional meditation and progressive relaxation. *Journal of Psychology and Theology, 16,* 362–368.

Casebolt, J. (1990, October). *The role of religion in problem-solving and decision-*

making: *Reliance on God*. Paper presented at the meeting of the Society for the Scientific Study of Religion, Virginia Beach, VA

A course in miracles: Combined volume. (1985). Glen Ellen, CA: Foundation for Inner Peace

Coward, D. (1996). Self-transcendence and correlates in a healthy population. *Nursing Research, 45*, 116–121.

Elkins, E., Anchor, K., & Sandler, H. (1979). Relaxation training and prayer behavior as tension reduction techniques. *Behavioral Engineering, 5*, 81–87.

Folkman, S. (1984). Personal control and stress and coping processes: A theoretical analysis. *Journal of Personality and Social Psychology, 46*, 839–852.

Frankl, V. (1984). *Man's search for meaning*. New York: Washington Square Press. (Original work published 1948)

Hathaway, W., & Pargament, K. (1990). Intrinsic religiousness, religious coping, and psychosocial competence: A covariance structure analysis. *Journal for the Scientific Study of Religion, 29*, 423–441.

Hood, R., Jr., Hall, J., Watson, P. J., & Biderman, M. (1979). Personality correlates of the report of mystical experience. *Psychological Reports, 44*, 804–806.

Hood, R., Jr., Spilka, B., Hunsberger, B., & Gorsuch, R. (1996). *The psychology of religion: An empirical approach* (2nd ed.). New York: Guilford Press.

Kaiser, D. (1991). Religious problem-solving styles and guilt. *Journal for the Scientific Study of Religion, 30*, 94–98.

Koenig, H. G., Pargament, K. I., & Nielsen, J. (in press). Religious coping in medically ill hospitalized older adults. *Journal of Nervous and Mental Diseases*.

Lazarus, R., & Folkman, S. (1984). *Stress, appraisal, and coping*. New York: Springer.

Martin, J. E., & Carlson, C. R. (1988). Spiritual dimensions of health psychology. In W. R. Miller & J. E. Martin (Eds.), *Behavior therapy and religion: Integrating spiritual and behavioral approaches to change* (pp. 57–110). Newbury Park, CA: Sage.

McCullough, M. E., Worthington, E. L., Jr., & Rachal, K. C. (1997). Interpersonal forgiving in close relationships. *Journal of Personality and Social Psychology, 73*, 321–336.

McIntosh, D., & Spilka, B. (1990). Religion and physical health: The role of personal faith and control. In M. Lynn & D. Moberg (Eds.), *Research in the social scientific study of religion* (Vol. 2, pp. 167–194). Greenwich, CT: JAI Press.

Pargament, K. (1997). *The psychology of religion and coping: Theory, research, practice*. New York: Guilford Press.

Pargament, K., Ensing, D., Falgout, K., Olsen, H., Reilly, G., Van Haitsma, K., & Warren, R. (1990). God help me: 1. Religious coping efforts as predictors of the outcomes to significant negative life events. *American Journal of Community Psychology, 18*, 793–825.

Pargament, K., Kennell, J., Hathaway, W., Grevengoed, N., Newman, J., & Jones,

W. (1988). Religion and the problem-solving process: Three styles of coping. *Journal for the Scientific Study of Religion, 27, 90–101.*

Pargament, K. I., Smith, B. W., Koenig, H. G., & Perez, L. (1998). Patterns of positive and negative religious coping with major life stressors. *Journal for the Scientific Study of Religion, 37,* 711–725.

Pargament, K., & Park, C. (1995). Merely a defense? The variety of religious means and ends. *Journal of Social Issues, 51,* 13–32.

The Qu'ran: Translated, with a critical re-arrangement of the Surahs (R. Bell, Trans.). (1939). Edinburgh, Scotland: Clark.

Reed, P. (1991). Self-transcendence and mental health in oldest-old adults. *Nursing Research, 40,* 5–11.

Rothbaum, R., Weisz, J., & Snyder, S. (1982). Changing the world and changing the self: A two process model of perceived control. *Journal of Personality and Social Psychology, 42,* 5–37.

Schaefer, C., & Gorsuch, R. (1991). Psychological adjustment and religiousness: The multivariate belief-motivation theory of religiousness. *Journal for the Scientific Study of Religion, 30,* 448–461.

Sears, S., & Greene, A. (1994). Religious coping and the threat of heart transplantation. *Journal of Religion and Health, 33,* 221–229.

Skinner, E. (1996). A guide to constructs of control. *Journal of Personality and Social Psychology, 71,* 549–570.

Srimad-Bhagava-Gita. (Swami Tapasyananda, Trans.). (1988). Mylapore, Madras, India: Sri Ramakrishna Math. (Original work published c. 150 B.C.).

Strentz, T., & Auerbach, S. (1988). Adjustment to the stress of simulated captivity: Effects of emotion-focused versus problem-focused preparation on hostages differing in locus of control. *Journal of Personality and Social Psychology, 55,* 652–660.

Thompson, S., Collins, M., Newcomb, M., & Hunt, W. (1996). On fighting versus accepting stressful circumstances: Primary and secondary control among HIV-positive men in prison. *Journal of Personality and Social Psychology, 70,* 1307–1317.

Thompson, S., Nanni, C., & Levine, A. (1994). Primary versus secondary and central consequence-related control in HIV-positive men. *Journal of Personality and Social Psychology, 67,* 540–547.

Ullman, C. (1989). *The transformed self: The psychology of religious conversion.* New York: Plenum.

Vitaliano, P., DeWolfe, D., Maiuro, R., Russo, J., & Katon, W. (1990). Appraised changeability of a stressor as a modifier of the relationship between coping and depression: A test of the hypothesis of fit. *Journal of Personality and Social Psychology, 59,* 582–592.

Weisz, J., McCabe, M., & Dennig, M. (1994). Primary and secondary control among children undergoing medical procedures: Adjustment as a function of coping style. *Journal of Consulting and Clinical Psychology, 62,* 324–332.

Weisz, J., Rothbaum, F., & Blackburn, T. (1984). Standing out and standing in. *American Psychologist, 39*, 955–969.

Winger, D., & Hunsberger, B. (1988). Clergy counseling practices, Christian orthodoxy and problem solving styles. *Journal of Psychology and Theology, 16*, 41–48.

Wong-McDonald, A., & Gorsuch, R. (1997, November). *Surrender to God: An additional coping style?* Paper presented at the meeting of the Society for the Scientific Study of Religion, San Diego, CA.

Yates, J., Chalmer, B., St. James, P., Follansbee, M., & McKegney, R. (1981). Religion in patients with advanced cancer. *Medical and Pediatric Oncology, 9*, 121–128.

Zinnbauer, B. J., & Pargament, K. I. (1998). Spiritual conversion: A study of religious change among college students. *Journal for the Scientific Study of Religion, 37*, 161–180.

10

ACCEPTANCE AND FORGIVENESS

CYNTHIA SANDERSON AND MARSHA M. LINEHAN

On purely scientific grounds, these recipes for living might be regarded as better tested than the best of psychology and psychiatry's speculations on how lives should be lived. (Donald Campbell, 1975, p. 1103)

Donald Campbell (1975), best known for his hard-nosed writings on experimental design and research methodology, lamented contemporary psychology's hasty dismissal of religious and spiritual traditions, or "recipes for living." He used the occasion of his presidential address to call for a scientific approach to these formulas for a well-lived life. In this chapter we examine two elements in those formulas: acceptance and forgiveness. We explore them as spiritual practices, psychological constructs, and strategies in psychotherapy. We draw on both Western and Eastern traditions, highlighting their similarities and differences. We offer practical examples for their use in psychotherapy as well as suggest the limits of their efficacy and the dangers of misuse that accompany each. Our goal is to provoke readers to consider the place acceptance and forgiveness have in their lives and in the psychological treatment offered to others.

ACCEPTANCE

An Overview of Spiritual Practice

The Middle English root for the word *accept* is *kap-*, meaning to take, seize, or catch. This root meaning more closely embodies the spirit of this discussion and is more accurate for our purposes than the modern word *receiving*. Receiving, an aspect of acceptance, may fail to convey how the practice of active acceptance requires careful observation, openness to experience, and tolerance of all that life presents. Acceptance is the developed capacity to fully embrace whatever is in the present moment. It requires a spacious mind, an open heart, and strength to bear one's experience. A strict definition is required to avoid misunderstanding. Acceptance, although it might include the following, does not necessarily mean resignation, agreement, servitude, or passivity.

The discipline of willing acceptance is not for the faint-hearted. Review the life of any major contemplative, any sturdy practitioner of acceptance, and one discovers an individual with deep reserves of mercy, patience, and compassion that he or she has come by the hard way. Gandhi urged his followers to accept blows from the armies of the British colonials without resorting to retaliation. This nonviolent tactic changed India's politics and history, and was instrumental in lessening international support for British occupation. Martin Luther King, His Holiness the Dalai Lama, and Thich Nhat Hanh have imitated this peaceful form of protest in their crusades for social justice. In doing so, they have demonstrated tolerance and understanding of their "enemies." Their spiritual ancestors, be they Buddha, Moses, Jesus, or Mohammed, demonstrated a willingness to bend fully to reality as it is through their example. Buddha accepted the inevitability of old age, disease, and death. Job accepted the silence of God, as he sat covered in sores, rebuked by his oldest friends. Jesus embraced "not my will but thy will" and climbed the cross.

None of these individuals can be described as passive. It is more accurate to view them as actively opening to life as it is while seeking change. Their example returns us to the root meanings of acceptance. It is receiving, seizing, and catching God's will, from a Western perspective, or reality simply as it is, an Eastern view. Although one may think of these leaders as embodying strength and endurance, they all struggled with the same questions that present themselves to each generation: Why is there good and evil? Why is there suffering? How did the world come to be? Each spiritual tradition recognizes the universal experience of being human, in its fullness and its pain, and reflects this in its literature. The Tao Te Ching, Dhammapada, Qur'an, Talmud, Torah, and New Testament speak repeatedly to undeniable aspects of sentient existence: (a) the awareness of the presence of good and evil; (b) the inevitability of suffering, disease, old age, and death; and (c) the struggle to make meaning out of chaos. "The Tao doesn't take sides; it gives birth to both good and evil" (Lao Tzu, "n.d."/1988, p. 5); we are all subject to suffering, disease, old age, and death" (Samyutta Nikaya, "n.d."/1995, p. 270), "and I applied my mind to know wisdom and to know madness and folly. I perceived that this also is but a striving after wind" (Ecclesiastes 1:17, "n.d.," 1994, p.

842). Religious writings may pound the reader with these hard truths or gently allude to them. But they return, again and again, to inescapable and painful facts. The spiritual practice of acceptance, of willingness, of obedience is hard work, requiring the student to "turn the mind" again and again to reality.

But why bother accepting reality? Why confront helplessness, terror, or losses? Why not distract ourselves as much as possible from the inevitable destruction that awaits us and all we love? Spiritual and religious teachers say that a full embrace of reality, in all its glory and horror, is the only way out of even greater suffering. This is not an idea that enjoys popularity in secular culture. Rather, popular culture encourages people to distract themselves from ultimate reality with work, achievement, financial success, Internet "surfing," or sports. These are positive addictions and distractions. People who distract themselves with vodka, a line of cocaine, credit card debt, or promiscuous sex may be diagnosed with a psychiatric disorder. It is easy to miss the boat all people share: To paraphrase Arme Sexton (1975), many people are frantically rowing toward something or someone that will get them out of their pain. Spiritual traditions teach people to let go of this pointless venture. Only the individual who can embrace reality as it is will find peace of mind, equanimity, or a state of grace.

Of course, we do not mean that Christians or Zen Buddhists or Hindus or Muslims have the same experience when practicing obedience to a supreme being or opening themselves to the emptiness of form. There are dramatic and irreconcilable differences both within and between the world's spiritual traditions. These differences, in turn, affect the content and type of acceptance that is practiced. Brief comparisons of Christian contemplative prayer and Zen meditation easily make the point. The Catholic contemplative, kneeling at meditative prayer, opens his or her heart and mind not only "to the knowledge and even to the experience of the transcendent and inexpressible God" but also to the recognition of "our illusions, [including those that] feed the roots of sin" (Merton, 1961, p. 67). Sin, signifying human imperfection and failure, is distinctly Western. Christians believe that Jesus is the incarnation of God; Buddhists do not have the concept of a personal savior. Buddhists may take a vow to save all sentient beings from the endless cycle of rebirth; Christians hope for "the resurrection of the body and life everlasting" (Book of Common Prayer, 1952, p. 71). By contrast, the Zen monk engages in mindfulness meditation, bringing his full attention to any object—feelings, thoughts, sensations, urges, memories—observing their ebb and flow within. His aim is the development of nonattachment, the attitude of neither clinging to things as he wants them to be or pushing away the things he does not want.

It is not our intent to engage in a lengthy comparison of spiritual belief systems. We acknowledge these differences to protect ourselves from overdrawing the similarities among contemplative or meditative disciplines. Psychotherapists attempting to integrate spiritual and psychological techniques must be careful to avoid the pitfalls of overgeneralization and a muddy conceptualization of spiritual life.

Whether we are speaking of a Christian accepting the will of God, a Buddhist accepting the cycle of birth and death, or a Muslim accepting the judgment of Allah, we must consider the discipline required to embrace reality—however it is defined—as it is. Eastern meditative and Western contemplative traditions offer the student structured practice, individual instruction, supervision by a mentor, and the support of a like-minded community. And both emphasize practice, practice, practice. Practice: It cannot be overemphasized. Any honest portrayal of any kind of monastic life is replete with stories of monks and nuns barely tolerating each other or themselves (Bianco, 1992). It can be easier to accept the grand scheme of things than the fact that one's brother monk makes annoying noise when eating, sings off key, or talks in a high-pitched tone. Those engaged in a spiritual path require the support and consultation of the community, and its senior members, to tolerate the emotions, thoughts, and urges that arise in meditation and contemplation (Epstein, 1996; Goldstein & Kornfield, 1987; Gunaratana, 1993). Otherwise, escape and avoidance occur. The monk hardens his heart against his brother. The nun drops out when she becomes afraid of her fear of loneliness. The support of the community is critical, balanced with the effort and commitment of the seeker. Acceptance is an endeavor requiring individual courage and a society of support.

Acceptance: Strategies for Psychotherapy

> It costs so much to be a full human being that there are very few who have the enlightenment or the courage to pay the price. . . . One has to abandon altogether the search for security, and reach out to the risk of living with both arms. One has to embrace the world like a lover. One has to accept pain as a condition of existence. One has to court doubt and darkness as the cost of knowing. One needs a will stubborn in conflict, but apt always to total acceptance of every consequence of living and dying. (West, 1991, p. 254)

Acceptance has deep roots in the history of psychology and psychotherapy. Psychoanalysis, existential psychotherapy, cognitive–behavioral therapy (CBT), and humanistic treatment all require the client to confront, approach, or endure the pain that is part of life. Indeed, a fair number of psychiatric problems are thought to result from the avoidance of pain or denial of reality. Anxiety, despair, panic, dissociation, substance abuse, alcoholism, and parasuicide may be the result of a collision with terrifying experiences in life, such as rape or cancer. They also may arise as a result of genetic or biological vulnerabilities or in the context of ordinary life events: leaving home for college, losing a parent, being passed over for a job, or marital strife. Then there is the existential anxiety that accompanies the awareness of the fragile nature of life and questions regarding its meaning (Becker, 1973). Once the sole province of religion, it has become part of the psychotherapist's job to lead his or her clients into, and through, pain with the goal of helping the client experience life more fully and with greater mastery (Kabat-Zinn, 1990; Kohlenberg & Tsai, 1991; Linehan, 1993a; Hayes, Jacobson, Follette, & Dougher, 1994).

Linehan (1993a, 1997) elucidated how strategies for acceptance of reality are helpful to the client, the therapist, and the treatment team. Likewise, Hayes, et al. (1994) formulated *acceptance and commitment therapy*, in part as a means to treat clients' avoidance of emotional experiencing. Recently Hayes, et al. (1994) also edited a book devoted exclusively to the use of acceptance and change in psychotherapy. Furthermore, in the latest edition of a classic text on behavior therapy, Goldfried and Davidson (1996) included a commentary on the importance of incorporating acceptance into behavioral treatments. Empirically supported psychotherapies for anxiety disorders implicitly incorporate acceptance in the form of exposure and emotional processing (Craske & Barlow, 1993; Foa & Kozak, 1986). That is, they require the client to approach his or her fears, or associated cues, while tolerating moderate-to-severe distress.

All major psychotherapy approaches openly acknowledge that pain is an unavoidable aspect of existence. Psychotherapists must help clients tolerate the aspects of reality that will not yield to change: abuse suffered in childhood, opportunities lost to illness, natural transitions in life, and death. Rather than surveying how each of the above authors would use acceptance, we focus our discussion on acceptance strategies in one treatment approach: dialectical behavior therapy (DBT).

Although DBT now is being applied to individuals with eating disorders, psychotic disorders, and substance abuse, it was originally designed to address the problems of women with chronic suicidality and self-injury—in short, the problems of women experiencing intense shame, guilt, depression, anxiety, and anger. Linehan (1997) has observed that the application of standard CBT to this population, although helpful, ran the risk of driving clients out of treatment. Standard behavioral emphasis on change bypassed the needed acknowledgment of clients' profound emotional suffering. Hurt, angry, and ashamed, clients felt misunderstood and reacted by verbally attacking or dropping out. However, as her work with these clients developed, Linehan noted that focusing solely on their pain and desperation could be equally frustrating for them. Acceptance, without the balance of change, communicated inadvertent passivity or hopelessness on the part of the therapist. The therapist did not "get" the extreme suffering of the client and the client's desperate struggle to escape it. This had the same effect that a firefighter would have if, climbing the ladder to the window of a burning building, he or she empathized with the person about to burn to death instead of snatching the person to safety.

In DBT, acceptance strategies help therapist, client, and treatment teams tolerate themselves and one another as they struggle together for change. The balance between acceptance and change is the fundamental dialectic in DBT. If therapists could simply push their clients nonstop into a life of less pain and greater satisfaction, they would do so; however, therapists who relentlessly emphasize only change may discover too late that the client has had enough and is dropping out, literally or figuratively. Change, including improvement, can be frightening to clients. Therapists must know their clients intimately and have the capacity to simply be with clients, as clients struggle with fear of change or hopelessness or terror of the unknown. The basic acceptance strategies are validation, consultation to the environment, and reciprocal communication. Validation is the act of verifying, corroborating, or confirming another's experience.

Why validate in psychotherapy? The reasons are several-fold. Validation balances the emphasis on change, preventing clients from feeling pushed too far too fast. Second, validation teaches clients self-acceptance and balanced self-assessment; as a result, they experience increased confidence in their judgment. Third, validation can strengthen behaviors through the principles of positive reinforcement. Finally, with validation of normative responses, the therapist communicates to the clients when and how their behavior is reasonable, appropriate, and sensible. Taken together, these functions strengthen the alliance between therapist and client.

In DBT, the therapist uses six levels of validation with clients. The term *levels* is somewhat misleading because one level does not necessarily precede or preclude another. The six levels of validation include the following acceptance behaviors: (a) staying awake and alert to the client; (b) communicating accurate empathy (Rogers, 1980); (c) articulating for the client thoughts, feelings, or other behaviors that he or she cannot yet articulate; (d) affirming that a client's current behavior makes sense in terms of past learning or current vulnerabilities (i.e., major depression, specific phobia, traumatic stress, etc.); and (e) affirming a client's current behavior by verifying that it is reasonable, or justifiable, in terms of biological functioning, current antecedents, or as a step toward a long-term goal. The sixth level of validation, radical genuineness, refers to treating the client with respect in an interpersonal atmosphere of equal status. It is the opposite of responding to the client as if he or she were a child, "second class," or fragile. It requires the therapist to be his or her authentic self with the client, within standard ethical boundaries, meeting the client as a person, not an illness (Rogers & Truax, 1967). Radical genuineness counters the tendency of the mental health system and its members to induce individuals seeking treatment into the role of wholly incompetent, frail, and subordinate people.

Acceptance strategies are used by the therapist in individual treatment, whereas skills for reality acceptance can be taught to clients in a group or individual format. Core mindfulness and distress tolerance skills comprise the two modules that emphasize acceptance of self and acceptance of reality. Based largely in Zen, these principles teach clients that emotional suffering is often created because people cling to things as they wish they would be, or think they should be, instead of accepting things as they are. People's attachment to their wishful thinking, longings, and ideas of fairness can trap them in cycles of pointless longing and despair. The practice of nonattachment is frequently misunderstood as some effort to extinguish love, interpersonal attachment, warmth, and personal meaning. Our concept of attachment, drawn from Zen, is not a synonym for love, warmth, closeness, or intimacy. Rather, it refers to the mind's habitual clinging to feelings, thoughts, and behaviors that are ineffective or not reality based. Emotional suffering is created through this form of attachment and is distinct from the pain of accepting that what one wants cannot be. In addition to orienting clients to these principles, DBT leads them in the guided practice of behaviors that enhance acceptance. These include mindfulness practices (see chap. 4 in this book) as well as exercises designed to cultivate a willingness to "be" with whatever reality presents.

Therapists cannot teach acceptance skills unless they practice them. Furthermore, unless they practice them on difficult problems in their own lives, they cannot advise clients how to use them on their difficult problems. To paraphrase Kohlenberg and Tsai (1991), therapists cannot recognize or reinforce behaviors lacking in their own repertoires. DBT programs require therapists to learn the skills they teach to clients. Moreover, therapists implicitly embrace acceptance tactics in the way they structure their team meetings. Therapists agree in advance that they will acknowledge their own foibles, limitations, shortsightedness, incomplete understanding, and tendency to fall out of the treatment. In the context of six formal agreements (see Linehan, 1993a, pp. 117–119), therapists conducting DBT agree to have diverging viewpoints, to struggle for empathic understanding of clients and each other, and to keep within their own personal limits. Designed to motivate therapists to keep doing treatment while enhancing therapists' competence, the team also provides therapists with rich opportunities to accept the perspective of other team members with whom they passionately disagree. The team structure creates an atmosphere of scientific humility and nondefensiveness balanced against passionately held and argued positions.

Case Example

Miriam[1] comes to psychotherapy deeply unhappy in her marriage. In her first three sessions, she relates her frustration with a recently completed marital therapy in which she felt that she was "crazy" not to be satisfied with her spouse. Her husband, David, a well-known local minister beloved in his church and community, is reportedly handsome, friendly, and hard-working. It was obvious to Miriam that the couple's therapist was as charmed by him as are his parishioners. David has never given her a moment's doubt about his fidelity and is a devoted father to their four sons. Her acquaintances regularly remark that Miriam is lucky to have "nabbed" David. Miriam, less educated than David, regularly defers to his "superior" knowledge and capitulates in household decisions. She cannot understand why she does not feel "madly in love" anymore. Furthermore, she expresses guilt about her preference to return to work instead of staying home with her two younger boys. In her therapy sessions, Miriam is overly apologetic for any perceived failing (i.e., arriving a few minutes late, closing the office door loudly, accidentally knocking a magazine off a table) and her non-verbal behavior communicates shame and low self-regard.

In treating this client, the therapist strongly biased toward change will need the team's help in assessing how hard to push Miriam to become more assertive and how much to accept Miriam's subordinate behaviors. Team members will help the therapist accept the pace of change that is comfortable for Miriam. Of course, this discussion presumes that Miriam wants to improve her assertion skills. The therapist should take care to discover Miriam's values and goals rather than imposing her own. One thing the therapist might have to accept is that Miriam does not aspire to the level of assertiveness that the therapist would choose for her. The consultation team can help the therapist "come clean" about any subtle attempts to override Miriam's values with her own. Because one of the consultation team agreements acknowledges all therapists' fallibility, the therapist does not have to pretend to be unbiased. She relies on the group to correct her.

Miriam's propensity to invalidate herself will be an important target in psychotherapy. She insults herself with self-descriptors like "crazy," "bad," or "inferior." She avoids making plans to return to school because she thinks she is selfish; she avoids challenging David's household budgets because she thinks she is stupid; and she thinks she should adore him as his parishioners do. A primary therapeutic task will be to help Miriam identify and accept her feelings and opinions about her husband. Additionally, the therapist will have to help Miriam discover whether there are feelings she is avoiding by behaving subserviently to others. Perhaps she

---

[1] Names, demographics, and clinical material have been changed to protect client confidentiality.

avoids the guilt or the fear she will experience if she opts for change. The therapist will probably have to help Miriam tolerate the guilt she feels about wanting something of her own, something unrelated to her husband and sons. Or, the therapist may have to help Miriam tolerate the sadness she experiences when she feels estranged from and misunderstood by her husband.

It may be that Miriam will consider divorcing David as a way out of her dissatisfaction. In the absence of abuse and neglect, the therapist will suggest that instead Miriam gather "data" about her marriage before making that decision. She will do this in the context of agreeing with Miriam that divorce is a viable option. In the meantime, Miriam will closely observe her feelings and thoughts about her husband using core mindfulness skills. She can hone her tolerance of his interest in sports while working to make him more receptive to her interest in gardening. The therapist will continue to use the team to access her own balance of acceptance and change. Consistently, with her colleagues' help, she can ask questions such as "Am I subtly influencing Miriam to stay in an unhappy marriage because I am opposed to divorce?" "Am I suggesting that she take more responsibility for the marriage than is reasonable?" "Should I keep insisting they resume couples' therapy or give in to her resistance to that suggestion?"

Throughout the treatment, the therapist will work on her acceptance of Miriam as she is, balanced against Miriam's desire for change. Furthermore, the therapist will target Miriam's lack of acceptance skills and teach her methods for tolerating her husband "as he is." The therapist will balance this against the possibility that her client might decide to leave her husband if her dissatisfaction becomes intolerable to her. Finally, the therapist will use the team's support to struggle with her reactions and responses to Miriam. In a well-functioning team, the therapist's blindspots will be respectfully addressed, but no team member will assume that he or she has the absolute truth about what Miriam should do or the absolute interventions for her problems.

FORGIVENESS

An Overview of Spiritual Practice

Forgiveness is a very old word. Unlike its sisters *pardon, absolve,* and *excuse, forgiveness* refers specifically to a change in emotion. In contrast to the words *accepting* and *embracing, Ghabh-,* the Indo-European root of *forgiveness,* means to give up or give away anger and the actions associated with it, *retribution* and *revenge.* The roots of the word, as old and deep as language itself, reflect its centrality to human relations and humans' life in community. Without the ability to let go of anger, life would be hell. Take a moment to imagine the state of one's life if one could neither forgive nor expect forgiveness for all the hurts, wrongs, or disappointments given and received. One would be caught in perpetual punishment, personal despair, social chaos, and war. The spiritual practice of forgiveness, with its deep roots in all world religions, points a way out of destructive retribution and offers practical guidelines for effective reconnection with oneself and others.

The world's spiritual traditions abound with examples of forgiveness and its close companions: compassion and tolerance. The demand for a sincere change of heart is integral to all religions and is present in the teachings for all spiritual paths: "Subvert anger by forgiveness" (Samusattan 136); "One who forgives an affront fosters friendship, but one who dwells on disputes will alienate a friend" (Proverbs 17:9); "Forgive us our trespasses, as we forgive those who trespass against us" (Matthew 6:12); and "Where there is forgiveness, there is God Himself" (Sikhism, Adi Granth, Shalok, & Kabir). Tales of great spiritual teachers highlight their capacity for forgiveness, even when meeting personal and extreme injury. We marvel at the forgiving words of Gandhi toward his assassin, of Jesus toward his executioners, of Martin Luther King toward his jailers. We are stirred by their capacity to let go of anger and hate in the face of humiliation or death. As with acceptance, we note that their examples of forbearance, and, in some instances outright forgiveness, do not reflect capitulation to a world filled with suffering, injustice, murder, and genocide. Rather, forgoing the impulse for revenge reflects the strength to absorb injury without being poisoned by it.

In this exploration of forgiveness, we highlight similarities and differences between major religious beliefs and their bearing on related spiritual practice. Denying the stark contrasts between and within Eastern and Western traditions does nothing to help the psychotherapist develop refined clinical acumen. This brief overview in no way substitutes for the hours of study and pragmatic experience required to stand in another's shoes, particularly when his or her religious and spiritual traditions differ from one's own. Nor can it replace, or even begin to survey, the extensive literature on philosophical, religious, and spiritual responses to the problem of evil. For that discussion, readers are referred to the works of individuals who, having survived imprisonment, torture, degradation, and unimaginable loss, have discussed the problem of crimes against humanity: Primo Levi, Nelson Mandela, Elie Wiesel, and Henry Wu. Those writers provide a starting point for the ontological and theological questions raised by unspeakable human behavior, past, present, and undoubtedly future. We hope that the individual intent on finding the intersection of psychology and spiritual practice will not flinch at the questions those authors raise.

Spiritual practices and religious traditions present many differences on principles for forgiveness. In the following discussion, we touch on two:

(a) the difference between Judaism and other religious traditions, Western and Eastern, on who can forgive, and (b) the salience of belief in a supreme being, whether one is asking for or granting forgiveness. In Judaism, a man or woman does not ask God to forgive a transgression against another person, nor does he or she grant forgiveness on behalf of others, except at the request of others. Only the injured person can grant forgiveness. The Holocaust provides six million examples of this principle. Jews, Nazi soldiers, German civilians, and members of the world community cannot be forgiven for any part played in the Holocaust because no repair is possible: The murdered cannot be raised from the dead nor the memories erased from the minds of the survivors. Indeed, attempts at revisionist history are redoubled efforts to assault victims. In a well-known example of the problem of forgiveness, Simon Wiesenthal, an inmate in a death camp, was asked by an SS guard to grant absolution at the time of the guard's death. Wiesenthal refused, in keeping with Jewish tradition, but he remained haunted by his response. In *The Sunflower: On the Possibilities and Limits of Forgiveness*, Wiesenthal (1998) surveyed 53 men and women—religious scholars, philosophers, writers, and political figures—on the question of whether he should have forgiven the soldier. Several Christian and Buddhist writers responded with, "I believe one should forgive the person or persons who have committed atrocities against oneself and mankind" (Wiesenthal, 1998, p. 129) and "the question of whether there is a limit to forgiveness has been emphatically answered by Christ in the negative" (Wiesenthal, 1998, p. 129). The Jewish writers, in stark contrast, are consistent in their argument that it was not in Wiesenthal's power to forgive. The clinician attempting to help a client struggle with seeking or granting forgiveness must understand the spiritual context of the offended and the offender. He or she cannot presume to know the guidelines for forgiveness in the client's life or the differences that exist within spiritual and religious communities.

Furthermore, belief in a supreme being influences the practice of forgiveness. Judaism, Christianity, and Islam posit a hierarchical construction of the spiritual realm, with God as divine judge and ultimate arbiter of human behavior, right and wrong. God is on high, humans below, and forgiveness flows from the immortal to his creatures of clay. Eastern belief systems such as Buddhism or Taoism do not recognize a supreme being. They are less hierarchical in their view of the universe and people's place in it; there is no God after whom one models forgiveness. Furthermore, the wrongdoing and the injuries people inflict on one another stem more from ignorance than evil. In Eastern philosophy, forgiveness is born of compassionate understanding: The Buddhist views all phenomena as interconnected, with no event rising in isolation from all other events. Therefore, a man or woman who harms another does so as a result of innumerable prior actions, in the context of a web of influences, and as a result of ignorance about the human condition. Forgiveness is referred to in Buddhism, but compassion is emphasized. Forgiveness emerges naturally with a comprehensive understanding of the universal cause of human suffering. As we will see in our discussion of clinical interventions, compassion plays a key role in the development of forgiveness.

Before discussing forgiveness and psychotherapy, however, we want to reemphasize the day-to-day, sometimes grindingly slow, nature of any spiritual practice. Forgiveness, like acceptance, is not a state of grace that one achieves. It is a skill; it is a capacity; it is a practice. Each person may be born with the potential to forgive, but even great spiritual teachers must hone their ability to forgive, particularly when they face great duress. The Vietnamese Buddhist monk, Thich Nhat Hanh, is a living example of spiritual practice in action. Yet, he reminds his readers of his intense struggles with feelings of anger when he toured the United States during the Vietnam war (Nhat Hanh, 1976). Pleading for peace before Midwest audiences, he sometimes was subjected to outbursts of hatred. Exhausted by worries for his home and bewildered by the anger, he felt the urge to retaliate; instead, he excused himself from the podium to recover through the practice of mindful breathing. Clearly, Nhat Hanh was not filled with automatic compassion, but he was able to draw on a long history of mindfulness practice, catch his feelings of anger, and act opposite to them.

With this example in mind, it is interesting that all religious traditions offer similar practical instructions for forgiveness. The offender, regardless of his or her belief system, must accomplish five steps: (a) personal responsibility must be acknowledged; (b) sincere regret must be expressed; (c) suitable reparation must be made if possible; (d) a promise must be made to stop the offending behavior; and (e) forgiveness must be requested. An apology that lacks personal, sincere, or suitable qualities, or one that is followed by repeated offenses, is usually deemed inadequate and unacceptable. Although there is variation on these rules (e.g., one must forgive when asked three times, one should forgive before sundown, etc.), the fundamental guidelines are consistent across traditions. More interesting, they are mirrored in research and writing on contemporary psychotherapy practice.

Forgiveness: A Guide to Interventions

Forgiveness, or the inability to forgive, is linked to people's concepts of mental well-being and mental disorder. Individuals who have trouble forgiving slights or who hold grudges over minor hurts are viewed as being psychologically troubled. So are people who, according to cultural norms, do not care whether, or recognize when, they have injured someone: They lack the motivation to request forgiveness. Psychotherapists also encounter clients who cannot forgive themselves for personal limits and failing or who let go understandable but ineffective anger toward a family member, friend, or acquaintance. By contrast, it is not uncommon to wonder about people who seem to forgive too much or too easily, letting go of anger in response to emotional hurts that appear unbearable. Furthermore, cultural norms vary in the degree to which one *should* feel secondary guilt or shame in reaction to anger or humiliation when asking for forgiveness. Social codes about anger and forgiveness are embedded in the psychiatric diagnostic nomenclature: One who "persistently bears grudges, i.e., is unforgiving of insults, injuries, or slights," has "inappropriate, intense anger" followed by bouts of severe guilt, "lacks remorse, as indicated by being indifferent to or rationalizing having hurt . . . another" is viewed as suffering from distinct psychiatric symptoms (American Psychiatric Association, 1994, p. 276–277).

Within the past decade, interest in forgiveness has grown among social scientists. Social psychologists, sociobiologists, and political scientists have been the first to examine forgiving behavior (Axelrod, 1984; Barkow, Cosmides, & Tooby, 1992). Clinical and counseling psychologists have followed suit (Enright & the Human Development Study Group, 1996; McCullough & Worthington, 1994). They have provided a number of definitions that largely depend on the context: The context may be intrapersonal or interpersonal or at the level of the social group. In sociobiology, forgiveness is the resumption of a cooperation and collaborative relationship with an individual who has previously cheated, betrayed common interests, or "defected" (Axelrod, 1984). Interpersonal forgiveness is defined as "a willingness to abandon one's right to resentment, negative judgement, and indifferent behavior toward one who unjustly injured us" (Enright, Freedman, & Risque, 1988, pp. 46–49). Finally, clinical and counseling psychologists extend the definition to include intrapersonal behavior: Forgiveness may involve a personal change in thoughts and feelings that result in reduced anger and enhanced emotional processing, regardless of whether a relationship is continued or severed (Coyle & Enright, 1997). Finally, intrapersonal forgiveness also includes letting go of anger at oneself over limitations, imperfections, and errors. What is clear in all of these descriptions is that forgiveness is not simply a change in the internal experience of feeling: Rather, forgiveness can result from a willing effort to change one's thoughts about, and actions toward, someone who has been hurtful.

Early research demonstrates that the practice of forgiveness has benefits and is adaptive at the level of the individual, the dyad, and the social group. Forgiveness appears to be correlated with a decrease in depression, anxiety, and Type A hostility in men and women who formally practice a forgiveness protocol (Coyle & Enright, 1997). Additionally, when anger is a secondary emotional response to a primary emotion such as fear, it inhibits adaptive emotional processing and can circumvent recovery from an emotional trauma (Foa, Riggs, Massen, & Yarczower, 1995). If forgiveness involves letting go of anger, forgiving might help individuals engaged in exposure therapy access primary emotions such as fear. In terms of dyads, forgiveness functions to repair bonds that have been broken by injury. In fact, it appears essential to the maintenance of close friendships, romantic relationships, and marriages. Moreover, research results are clear that the maintenance of close supportive relationships has benefits for both mental and physical health. Finally, the good news is that forgiveness is a winning strategy in geographically stable social groups. Repetitive computer simulations of the competition between purely selfish strategies (always taking more than one gives) versus cooperative–collaborative strategies (fair exchange) have proved the superiority of forgiveness based social exhange. (For a full treatment of forgiveness as a social exchange strategy, see Axelrod, 1984, and Wright, 1994.)

Practical Steps for Forgiveness

Guidelines for forgiveness, instructions for forgiveness, and the components of forgiveness are under development. Enright et al. (1996) and McCullough and Worthington (1994) have developed forgiveness protocols. With regard to forgiveness in an ongoing relationship, the degree of apology one receives has a great deal to do with increasing the likelihood that forgiveness will occur. The term *degree of apology* refers to how well the sincerity of remorse and acknowledgment of responsibility is elaborated. In other words, a perfunctory "I'm sorry" is ineffective when compared with a validating statement such as, "I made a critical remark to you in front of your friends; I'm so sorry that I did that and caused you embarrassment. I won't do it again, I promise." Implicit in apology is the concept of reparation or repentance. *Repentance* in its spiritual sense means a distinct change in behavior, not an apology divorced from behavioral repair. Sociobiologists, social psychologists, and certain religious traditions agree here: Be wary of forgiving an offending behavior that does not change. Prager (1997) has noted the tendency of current social discourse to exclude reparations from the process of forgiveness. Misused, forgiveness without the expectation of repair is poor contingency management and ineffective social modeling.

Apologies and repairs are not the only components of forgiveness. Forgiveness is strongly correlated with cognitive and emotional aspects of empathy as well as with conciliatory acts on the part of the person who has been injured. Enright et al. (1996) and McCullough, Worthington, & Rachal (1997) agreed that forgiveness is helped by taking the perspective of the one who has done the harm and recognizing the emotional pain that he or she is experiencing as a result of the breakdown in the relationship. Enright et al. (1996) defined forgiveness to clients, provided didactic information on how holding onto anger may be hurting them, and presented forgiveness as one option among several. If a client chooses to practice forgiveness, he or she is asked to commit to refraining from revenge behaviors. The clients then collaborate in cognitive exercises that reframe their view of the person who has hurt them. Empathy and compassion arise partly from cognitive reframing, and forgiveness is facilitated by the development of feeling with and for the offending person. When forgiveness occurs in the context of an ongoing relationship, conciliatory behaviors help forgiveness develop and unfold. The research of Mc-Cullough et al. (1997) supports the conceptual distinction of empathy from forgiveness and the role of empathy as a precursor to forgiveness. Additionally, deciding to reconnect with the offending person, in the absence of abuse or neglect, helps empathy and forgiveness occur.

To summarize, we present succinct guidelines for forgiveness based on the research literature. Here are the rules for asking for forgiveness: Give a sincere and validating apology; if possible, repair the hurt; commit to not engage in the injurious behavior again; follow through on the commitment by changing the behavior; and engage in conciliatory acts. A note of caution is required: Overapologizing, self-castigation, and behaviors that convey disrespect for the self are not part of our behavioral definition for effective apologies (Linehan, 1993b). Here are the guidelines for letting go of anger and giving forgiveness: Consider the pros and cons of forgiving the person versus not forgiving the person, including the effects of anger on one's psychological and physical health; use cognitive reframing to understand the offending person's behavior; if the offending person is sincerely sorry, practice validation of his or her distress; finally, act opposite to angry feelings by engaging in conciliatory behavior. If reconciliation is not desired, letting go of anger can still be practiced for the welfare of the client and in keeping with his or her spiritual or religious values.

Clinical Example

Returning to Miriam and David, suppose that David reveals to Miriam that he had an affair with a parishioner. Miriam reacts with understandable hurt, fear, shame, and anger: She is hurt by the betrayal of trust; she is afraid that David may leave her; she is ashamed that others may know her husband has cheated on her; and she is angry in response to the painful feelings that result from David's infidelity. In helping Miriam bear her feelings and come to a decision about what action she will take, we would help her examine a number of questions: Is David offering a sincere apology? If not, how is that affecting her? If so, is she willing to forgive? We would help her explore the pros and cons of forgiving, her doubts about restoring trust, her concerns that he might have another affair, and the question of whether irreparable damage has been done to the relationship.

As therapists, we would not have **predetermined** answers to any of these questions. Rather, our job would be to guide Miriam through her own process without imposing our values. Still, we would offer her information on normative behavior and the consequences of forgiving versus not forgiving. Certainly, if Miriam's angry feelings appear to interfere with processing other emotions, we would point out to her that anger may be preventing her from understanding and accepting sadness, fear, and grief. Furthermore, if Miriam lives according to a set of spiritual values that require her to forgive David, even if they are values with which we disagree, our job is to help her self-validate, not convert her to our perspective. Should Miriam decide to forgive and work on relinquishing her anger with David, we would suggest that she engage in opposite action when she is angry and that she learn to let anger go (see Linehan, 1993b, pp. 160–161). We would remind her that forgiveness is process, not stasis, and that if she decides to forgive, she probably will have to "turn her mind" again and again to letting go of the anger.

A Last Word

In this chapter we have presented a brief overview of how acceptance and forgiveness, practices based on religious tenets and honed in spiritual practice, have been integrated into psychotherapy. Our reviews of religious texts and spiritual disciplines are not meant to substitute for the reader's experience. Indeed, we think that psychotherapists cannot teach or reinforce behaviors for which they lack intrinsic understanding. We therefore urge readers to closely consider their own expertise in accepting and forgiving and to be cautious in assuming that these concepts have the same meaning to their clients.

We did not provide a detailed discussion of whether some injuries are so terrible as to be unacceptable or unforgivable. The reason? The degree to which individuals develop their capacities for acceptance and forgiveness depends entirely on personal goals. Some individuals lead lives wholly committed to spiritual practice; they serve as models of understanding, compassion, acceptance, and forgiveness. For them, the development of capacities such as a full embrace of reality as it is, or forgiveness for even the most egregious injuries, is the purpose of existence. Most individuals we see in psychotherapy will not have the same goals. They may have no spiritual goals or may be courageously struggling just to stay alive, much less forgive someone who has abused or neglected them. What is critical for good clinical practice is that clinicians "stay awake" to their clients and assess, rather than assume, what goals their clients may have. We also must continually reexamine what we know about the constraints on the human spirit while endeavoring to bring a scientific perspective to the "recipes for living" that we inherit.

REFERENCES

American Psychiatric Association. (1994). *Diagnostic and statistical manual of mental disorders* (4th ed.). Washington, DC: Author.

Axelrod, R. (1984). *The evolution of cooperation.* New York: Basic Books.

Barkow, J. H., Cosmides, L., & Tooby, J. (1992). *The adapted mind: Evolutionary psychology and the generation of culture.* New York: Oxford University Press.

Becker, E. (1973). *The denial of death.* New York: Simon and Schuster.

Bianco, F. (1992). *Voices of silence: Lives of the Trappists today.* New York: Anchor Books.

The book of common prayer. (1952). New York: Oxford University Press.

Campbell, D. (1975). On the conflicts between biological and social evolution and between psychology and moral tradition. *American Psychologist 30,* 1103–1126.

Coyle, C. T., & Enright, R. D. (1997). Forgiveness intervention with postabortion men. *Journal of Consulting and Clinical Psychology, 65,* 1042–1046.

Craske, M. G., & Barlow, D. (1993). Panic disorder and agoraphobia. In D. Barlow (Ed.), *Clinical handbook of psychological disorders: A step-by-step treatment manual* (2nd ed., pp. 1–47). New York: Guilford Press.

Ecclesiastes. (1994). In B. M. Metzger & R. E. Murphy (Eds.), *The new Oxford annotated bible* (pp. 842–851). New York: Oxford University Press. (Original work published n.d.)

Enright, R. D., Freedman, S., & Risque, J. (1988). The psychology of interpersonal forgiveness. In R. D. Enright & J. North (Eds.), *Exploring forgiveness* (pp. 46–47). Madison: University of Wisconsin Press.

Enright, R. D., & The Human Development Study Group. (1996). Counseling within the forgiveness triad: On forgiving, receiving forgiveness, and self-forgiveness. *Counseling and Values, 40,* 107–146.

Epstein, M. (1996). *Thoughts without a thinker: Psychotherapy from a Buddhist perspective.* New York: HarperCollins.

Fleischman, P. R. (1990). *The healing spirit: Explorations in psychotherapy and spirituality.* New York: Paragon Press.

Foa, E. B., & Kozak, M. S. (1986). Emotional processing of fear: Exposure to corrective information. *Psychological Bulletin, 46,* 20–35.

Foa, E. B., Riggs, D. S., Massie, E. D., & Yarczower, M. (1995). The impact of fear activation and anger on the efficacy of exposure treatment for PTSD. *Behavior Therapist, 26,* 487–499.

Goldfried, M. R., & Davidson, G. C. (1996). *Clinical behavior therapy.* New York: Wiley.

Goldstein, J., & Kornfield, J. (1987). *Seeking the heart of wisdom: The path of insight meditation.* San Francisco: Shambala Press.

Gunaratana, H. (1993). *Mindfulness in plain English.* Boston: Wisdom Publications.

Hayes, S. C., Jacobson, N. S., Follette, V. M., & Dougher, M. J. (Eds.) (1994).

Acceptance and change: Content and context in psychotherapy. Reno, NV: Context Press.

Kabat-Zinn, J. (1990). *Full catastrophe living*. New York: Doubleday.

Kohlenberg, R. J., & Tsai, M. (1991) *Functional analytic psychotherapy*. New York: Plenum.

Lao Tzu. (1988). *Tao te ching*. (S. Mitchell, Trans.). New York: Harper & Row. (Original work published n.d.)

Linehan, M. M. (1993a). *Cognitive behavioral treatment of borderline personality disorder*. New York: Guilford Press.

Linehan, M. M. (1993b). *Skills training manual for treating borderline personality disorder*. New York: Guilford Press.

Linehan, M. M. (1997). Validation and psychotherapy. In A. Bohart & L. Greenberg (Eds.), *Empathy reconsidered: New directions in psychotherapy* (pp. 353–392). Washington, DC: American Psychological Association.

Merton, T. (1961). *New seeds of contemplation*. New York: New Directions.

McCullough, M. E., & Worthington, E. L. Jr. (1994). Encouraging clients to forgive people who have hurt them: Review, critique, and research prospectus. *Journal of Psychology and Theology, 22*, 3–20.

McCullough, M. E., Worthington, E. L., & Rachal, K. C. (1997). Interpersonal forgiving in close relationships. *Journal of Personality and Social Psychology, 73*, 321–336.

Nhat Hanh, T. (1976). *The miracle of mindfulness*. Boston: Beacon Press.

Prager, D. (1997). *Forgiveness and the dumbing down of christianity: The Prager perspective*. Unpublished manuscript.

Rogers, C. R. (1980). *A way of being*. Boston: Houghton Mifflin.

Rogers, C. R., & Truax, C. B. (1967). The therapeutic conditions antecedent to change: A theoretical view. In C. R. Rogers (Ed.), *The therapeutic relationship and its impact: A study of psychotherapy with schizophrenics* (pp. 97–108). Madison: University of Wisconsin Press.

Samyutta Nikaya. (1995). In A. Wilson (Ed.), *World scripture: A comparative anthology of sacred texts* (p. 270). New York: Paragon House. (Original work published n.d.)

Sexton, A. (1975). *The awful rowing towards God*. Boston: Houghton Mifflin.

West, M. L. (1991). *Shoes of the fisherman*. New York: St. Martin's Press.

Wiesenthal, S. (1998). *The sunflower: On the possibilities and limits of forgiveness*. New York: Random House.

Wright, R. (1994). *The moral animal*. New York: Vintage Books.

11

EVOKING HOPE

CAROLINA E. YAHNE AND WILLIAM R. MILLER

There is no such thing as false hope.
—Mary Pipher

Abandon all hope, you who enter here.
—Dante

What may be history's first controlled outcome trial of a psychotherapy was conducted in 1784 by Benjamin Franklin. Then residing in Paris, he had been appointed by the King of France to investigate the practices of one Anton Mesmer, who claimed to heal physical and mental maladies by manipulating animal magnetism, an invisible fluid allegedly perfused in nature. "His patients increased rapidly," Franklin reported. "His cures were numerous and of the most astonishing nature" (Franklin, 1785, p. xii). These reports led Franklin's delegation to design a clever series of single-subject experiments to test Mesmer's method. Although Mesmer himself declined to participate, other practitioners of mesmerism were engaged. Because people (as well as animate and inaminate objects) could allegedly be magnetized by Mesmer's disciples without touch contact, patients were blindfolded for the first version of what is now called a "balanced placebo" experiment. The dramatic effects observed during face-to-face visual contact also occurred when blindfolded individuals were led to believe that they were being magnetized, even though there was no mesmerist in the room. On the other hand, no effects at all were observed with a mesmerist exerting "magnetism" a foot and a half away from a blindfolded person as long as the person was unaware of his or her presence. Similar results were found when individuals were exposed to a series of trees or basins of water, only one of which had been secretly "magnetized" by mesmerism. Dramatic results followed but were not specifically associated with the magnetized object. Franklin (1785) reflected that

this new agent might be no other than the imagination itself, whose power is as extensive as it is little known. . . . The imagination of sick persons has unquestionably a very frequent and considerable share in the cure of their diseases. . . . In [the physical world] as well as religion, [we] are saved by faith . . . under the genial influence of hope. Hope is an essential constituent of human life. (pp. 100, 102)

It is a common finding that different psychotherapies, even those intentionally designed to diverge from each other markedly in philosophy and practice, often yield highly similar outcomes. This holds across a wide variety of problem areas (cf. Orlinsky & Howard, 1986). There are various interpretations of this finding, but one is that theoretically different therapies may nevertheless have common essential features. Broadly shared attributes of healing have been termed *nonspecific elements* to distinguish them from specific or active ingredients hypothesized to be responsible for the success of a particular treatment approach. The contents of a medication capsule, such as an antibiotic, may exert a specific beneficial effect, but there is also a well-known, more general (nonspecific) benefit of taking a medication that one believes to have healing properties. These nonspecific healing properties are often described as the *placebo effect*. So potent and pervasive is this effect that in demonstrating the efficacy of a new medication, drug manufacturers are required to show that it imparts a specific benefit above and beyond the placebo effect.

Despite its long history, the placebo effect is often maligned, as though it were a trick played on the simple-minded. Yet, placebo effects are widespread and impressively persistent (Shapiro, 1971). A substantial proportion of the pain relief imparted by opiates also occurs when the sufferer takes a compound believed to alleviate pain. The impact of disulfiram, a medication once widely used in treating alcoholism, is illustrative. Disulfiram is taken by the drinker in an attempt to stop drinking. It is designed to create feelings and symptoms of physical illness if alcohol is consumed, and this it does with reasonable success when dosage is adequate. Yet, the beneficial effects that clients show when this medication is taken can include such a large placebo effect that it makes relatively little difference whether the capsule—or even surgical implant—contains disulfiram or an inert powder as long as the clients believe it is the real thing. Like the people in Franklin's experiments, both groups show substantial improvement (W. R. Miller, Andrews, Wilbourne, & Bennett, 1998).

In a study from our own research group (Harris & Miller, 1990), problem drinkers presenting for treatment were randomly assigned (with their knowledge) to one of several conditions. Some started therapy immediately with an outpatient counselor. Others were told that they had an excellent chance of succeeding on their own and were given specific guidelines to follow in changing their problematic drinking. We told these individuals to get started and that we would check back with them in 10 weeks to see how they were doing. Still others were told that we could not see them right away but that they were on a waiting list and we would treat them in 10 weeks. Both the therapist-directed and the self-directed clients showed significant improvement by markedly reducing their alcohol use during the 10-week period. Those on the waiting list, however, showed no improvement at all. They did exactly what we told them to do: They waited for us to help them.

Consider yet another study (Leake & King, 1977) in which people entering three alcoholism treatment programs were tested by a psychologist for various prognostic signs. When the testing was completed, the psychologist shared the results with therapists in the programs, letting them know which individuals in particular showed excellent potential for recovery—those who were truly ready to "bloom." The accuracy of the psychologist's tests was remarkable. During the course of treatment, the high-potential clients showed more motivation for change and involvement in treatment, as perceived by their therapists. A year after discharge, the "high-potential" clients were more likely to be sober and employed. The psychologist's secret, however, was that the "high-potential" clients had actually been chosen at random. They differed from other clients in the same treatment program only in that they had been identified to staff as having excellent possibilities for recovery.

What is going on in this odd collection of studies? Even for clients not receiving what was believed to be the "actual" treatment, the benefits were real enough and lasted just as long as those receiving "the real thing." Those touching "magnetized" trees or taking "medications" expected to get better, and did. Clients who were told that they could get better did so, whereas those who were told they had to wait for us to make them better languished. Clients identified to their therapists as having excellent recovery potential were more likely to recover. What all of these groups had in common was hope.

WHAT IS HOPE?

Hope has long been recognized as a vital element in healing and has been known by many other names, including optimism, the placebo effect, self-efficacy, and positive expectancies. What is this quality of hope, and how is it involved in treatment and change?

Hope as Will

Hope has often been described as having two components (e.g., Snyder, 1994). The first of these is the more spiritual, the element of hope that people speak of when they say that they have been inspired. It has been called *willpower* or *will*, as in the will to live, to survive, to recover, or to learn. As spirit, it can be likened to wind or fire, which is without substance and yet varies in measurable intensity. Without this element of desire or willfulness, there is no hope, and hopelessness in this sense is a synonym for depression, demoralization, and meaninglessness (Kierkegaard, 1849/1941). Too often, hope is equated with the promise of a cure or remission. Hope can also be understood as meaningfulness and dignity even in the face of disease or death, as maintaining one's individuality in adversity (Nuland, 1995).

Nurses are intimately familiar with this broader sense of hope and have written eloquently about it. Hope constitutes an essential experience of the human condition. It functions as a way of feeling, a way of thinking, a way of behaving, and a way of relating to oneself and one's world. Hope has the ability to be fluid in its expectations, and if the desired object or outcome does not occur, hope can still be present (Farran, Herth, & Popovich, 1995, p. 6).

Hope as Way

The second oft-recognized component of hope is what Snyder (1994) called *wayfulness*. Hope is seldom groundless but is attached to something or someone. People hope *in*, people place their hope. A part of understanding spirituality is to know what one hopes in, where one places trust and confidence.

Much has been written of hope placed in oneself, in one's own abilities and resources. This form of hope is spoken of as self-efficacy and self-confidence. One can also place confidence in others. "You are my only hope," a desperate client may tell a therapist, saying that the tide is out on self-hope. The eldest child, the expected cavalry, or the star of the sports team may be invested with hope. The classic American poem "Casey at the Bat" captures such a moment. Slender hope is frequently the element of suspense in film and theater.

There is a third placement of hope that must not escape attention because it is often the net that catches one when all else fails. Such hope is that vested not in oneself or in another human being but in a higher power, in something more ultimate (Tillich, 1958). By this we mean, as in the international 12-step tradition of Alcoholics Anonymous (1976), a power outside of and greater than oneself, that is, a transcendent and in this sense spiritual power. One cannot begin to comprehend the 12-step movement without grasping this, for the program's first three steps involve accepting the limits of self-hope, recognizing a higher source of hope, and opening to that source (see chap. 6 in this book). Hope in a higher power exemplifies how hope encompasses much more than locus of control, an appraisal of personal abilities or those of others. It includes the broader personal sense of way, of direction and meaning. Transcendent spirituality can be the source and basis of hope (Gorsuch, 1993).

It could be debated which of these two, will and way, is the more important in hope. One can speak of "hoping against hope" when no possible way is seen, an act of sheer will or faith. Here, will-hope endures against (in the absence of) way-hope; in aphorism, "where there's a will, there's a way." Such hope is an enduring and ultimate trust beyond evidence of a way. Nevertheless, the way element of hope remains implicit even here, in an overriding sense of faith or meaning.

Hope as Wish

Hope can also be highly specific, a wish for a particular outcome. Here, one speaks of having "a hope." In this context, a hope is a specific desire accompanied by some expectation of fulfillment: "I hope to get out of this abusive relationship alive." "I hope my daughter will recover from her cocaine addiction." "I hope I can help this family bear their loss." "I hope my presence will help my father die with dignity." Again, even at this specific level, the elements of will and way can be discerned.

Hope as Horizon

A fourth important sense of hope is the ability to see beyond the present circumstances. From the windows of our office building at the University of New Mexico, Mount Taylor rises on the horizon 80 miles to the west. Looking to that peak, long held sacred by Native Americans, somehow evokes the longer vision beyond our daily tasks. Hope is a vision that transcends the present, like that mountain beyond the Rio Grande. This longer view may perceive a plan (way), even if it involves no immediate action. It may also be simply the perspective that whatever the present experience is, it too will pass (see chap. 4 in this book). Hope as horizon implies an openness to experience, to imagined or unimagined possibilites, and to transcendence (Myers, 1980).

Hope as Action

Finally, hope is manifest in action. Acting in spite of current circumstances, "against all hope," is perhaps the deepest expression of hope. Through a lifetime of writings, Holocaust survivor Elie Wiesel has struggled with how to deal with the enormity of evil of which humans are capable. Integrity is found not in denying, ignoring, or shrinking from evil but by living and acting against and in spite of it (Brown, 1983). Another survivor, psychotherapist Viktor Frankl (1963), vividly recalled those in the concentration camps who, despite their own severe privations, spent their days encouraging and bringing hope to others. Such hope moves from the realm of thought and feeling into expressed action. It is seen in living as if a new reality has already occurred (W. R. Miller, 1985).

Hope as action can be particularly powerful in communal form, as evidenced in the life of Gandhi. Writing of communal hope, Daly (1973) envisioned God as summoning women and men to act out of their deepest hope and to become who they can be. For example, a group of women with breast cancer decided to expand beyond their medical and support functions to address community issues of prevention as well as detection and treatment. Reasoning that environmental pollution was contributing to the community's current breast cancer epidemic, they challenged narrow individual-focused reactive (rather than proactive) strategies. By taking action and working collectively to challenge the status quo, they also increased their own hope as will, way, wish, and horizon. Whether taken in individual or collective form, hopeful action has a way of renewing hope and inspiring change.

RESEARCH ON HOPE

Measures of Hope

How one goes about measuring hope would obviously depend on which of the above definitions is being used. Attempts to operationalize hope as a critical psychiatric or psychological concept (Averill, Catlin, and Chon, 1990; Stotland, 1969) have served as inspiration for various quantitative measures. Thorough reviews have been published, reflecting a wide array of measurement approaches (Farran et al., 1995; Nunn, Lewin, Walton, & Carr, 1996). Hope has been conceived of both as a trait (e.g., being hopeful most of the time) and as a state (feeling hopeful at the moment), as has its opposite, hopelessness. The various forms of hope described above have also been measured as state and trait constructs with other names such as optimism, empowerment, internal locus of control, self-efficacy, coherence, mindfulness, and purpose in life.

Here we briefly describe several methods that have been used in measuring hope. One interesting approach has been content analysis of natural language. In an early study, Gottschalk (1974) analyzed 5 min of each participant's description of an interesting and dramatic personal life experience. Spontaneous references to the kinds and degrees of hopefulness were coded. Significant negative correlations with depression scales and significant positive correlations with belongingness scales were found. It predicted favorable outcome among patients in a mental health crisis clinic, survival time in patients with terminal cancer, and patients likely to follow treatment recommendations. Similar psycholinguistic systems have been used to code causal attributions (Schulman, Castellon, & Seligman, 1989) and commitment language (Amrhein, 1992).

A more common approach, of course, is the pragmatically simpler paper-and-pencil questionnaire. There is a plethora of such scales of hope and hopelessness, mostly short (8–30 items) and using Likert scaling (Beck, Weissman, Lester, & Trexler, 1974; Erickson, Post, & Paige, 1975; Fibel & Hale, 1978; Herth, 1992; Hinds & Gattuso, 1991; J. F. Miller & Power, 1988; Obayuwana et al., 1982; Scheier & Carver, 1985; Snyder et al., 1991; Staats, 1989; Stoner, 1982). For example, "In the future I plan to accomplish many things" is answered with strongly agree, agree, disagree, or strongly disagree (Nowotny, 1989). Psychometric analyses, when provided, have usually suggested reasonable internal consistency and reliability. Some authors have provided normative data helpful to clinicians in interpreting individual scores (e.g., Gottschalk, 1974; Snyder et al., 1991). Rarely, hope has been measured as a multidimensional construct (e.g., Nunn et al., 1996).

Within a clinical interview, one can use a simple Likert scale to measure clients' hopefulness (cf. Rollnick, Butler, & Stott, 1997). One might ask, for example, "On a 0–10 scale, where 0 is feeling completely hopeless and 10 is feeling very hopeful, where are you right now?" (The same format can be used to ask where a person generally is, emphasizing trait rather than state aspects.) This can be followed by inquiry and reflection to explore sources of hope. If the person gives a score higher than zero, for example, one can ask, "Why are you at (current score) instead of zero? In other words, what is it that gives you some hope?" Another option is to inquire, "What would it take for your hope to increase from (current score) to (higher score)?" Exploring spiritual and other sources of hope can be important in understanding a client's dilemma and resources (Gorsuch, 1993).

Correlates of Hope

Measures of hope have been found to correlate with a broad range of positive outcomes. Summarizing this literature, Snyder (1994) concluded that "high hope persons have a greater number of goals, have more difficult goals, have greater happiness and less distress, have superior coping skills, recover better from physical injury, and report less burnout at work" (p. 24). Burnout on the job, for example, and subsequent staff turnover were reduced in a nursing home when psychologists, as part of a mindfulness experiment, encouraged caregivers to question their assumptions about what patients could not do independently (Langer, 1989). When the staff realized that patients were able to do many things for themselves that the staff had been doing for them, the workload was lightened and caregivers felt less overwhelmed. They felt more hopeful about patients' abilities, about the manageability of their own responsibilities, and about the work setting in general. Reframing and reevaluating beliefs allowed workers to perceive a less limited, more hopeful view, paralleling the alcoholism treatment study described above. With such renewed hope, workers were more likely to stay on the job.

Can hope be explained away as being only the shadow of other factors? Research indicates that hope continues to make a significant independent contribution to outcomes even after other factors such as intelligence and previous achievement are taken into account (Snyder, 1994). A source of confusion here, too, is that hope is a common thread running through many other constructs (e.g., empowerment, placebo, locus of control, self-efficacy, and acceptance of responsibility).

HOPE IN TREATMENT

How Is Hope Relevant to Treatment?

If hope exerts an independent influence on outcomes, it deserves attention during treatment if only for prognostic reasons. Inspiring hope has been described as the practitioner's first duty to the client and a major contribution to treatment (Pipher, 1996). Effective treatment combats hopelessness by strengthening the therapeutic relationship, inspiring expectations of help and recovery, awakening emotional responsiveness, providing new learning experiences, enhancing a sense of mastery or self-efficacy, and affording opportunities for rehearsal and practice (Frank & Frank, 1993).

Gorsuch (1993) opined that regardless of the pathway one has followed into alcohol abuse, hope is one element necessary for a person to find a way out. Without hope the individual quickly gives up trying to change. Within 12-step programs (see chap. 6 in this book), hope comes from relying on a higher power rather than on one's own control (cf. chap. 11). Prayer or other appeals for divine help often occur long before a person seeks formal treatment (Willoughby, 1996). Understanding and cooperating with a client's sources of hope can be an important process in treatment.

In one sense, inspiring hope involves a way of being with clients (Rogers, 1951; Rollnick & Miller, 1995). A long list of practitioner characteristics has been linked to the evocation of hope and change: warmth, friendliness, interest, supportiveness, empathy, credibility, and a positive attitude toward one's clients (Orlinsky & Howard, 1986; Turner, Deyo, Loeser, Von Korff, & Fordyce, 1994).

Yet, like hope itself, evoking hope has to do with action as well as being. We describe three practical ways of fostering clients' hope: educating, eliciting, and lending.

Educating

Hopelessness sometimes has to do with a lack of information and perspective. "What does it mean?" clients wonder about their current dilemma. Hopelessness emanates from explanations that attribute one's suffering to causes that are "personal, permanent, and pervasive" (Seligman, 1990, p. 43). Giving accurate information and reframing may enhance hope by educating clients that their situation is not uniquely personal, unchangeable, or generalized to all aspects of life.

Another fundamental bit of education to consider is that no matter what the situation, one has the freedom to choose how to perceive and understand it. This is where it is important to have a broader understanding of hope than the probability of a cure or other particular outcome. Frankl's (1963) classic and passionate statement of this truth affirms that even in the midst of hopeless (way) circumstances, the person chooses meaning and how she or he will respond (hope as will). A more recent, inspiring account can be found in Ritterman's (1991) work with families of political prisoners subjected to torture in Chile. Her story of one prisoner in particular, Daniel Rodriguez, exemplifies the tenacity of spirit that can maintain hope and unity in the face of evil. Her own contagious sense of hope, maintained despite witnessed atrocities, is itself an inspiration for therapists.

Treatment and mutual-help groups can provide a particularly powerful context within which to evoke hope. Sharing day-to-day experiences in a supportive group setting can reduce shame and isolation, and foster practical problem solving (Herman, 1992). Clients report that one of the most helpful aspects of group psychotherapy is instilling hope (Whalan & Mushet, 1986; Yalom, 1975). In a structured support group (Yahne & Long, 1988), women found hope in seeing other members solve problems and grow. Such persuasive modeling of hope can be a distinct advantage of group experience over individual psychotherapy.

Reminiscence groups for women in nursing homes illustrate how elderly institutionalized women can give something meaningful to others, reinforcing their own sense of hope (C. A. Brody, 1990; C. M. Brody & Semel, 1993). The female participants in one study were asked to take turns in the group reminiscing about key experiences of a lifetime. Some landmark themes included their first day at school, graduations, going to work or getting married, a pet they cherished, the birth of a child, the loss of loved ones, or some other theme of their mutual choosing. In so doing, they wove their own tapestry of hope and meaning about their lives while witnessing the weaving process of other group members (W. R. Miller,

Yahne, & Rhodes, 1990). Groups and families can serve to reinforce a sense of community, give meaning to individual experience, and nurture hope.

Eliciting

In English, *to educate* has the connotation of passing something (in this case, hope) from provider to recipient. The Latin root of *educate* means to draw out. Thus, an alternate image for evoking hope is that of the midwife, coaxing and pulling it from the person who already has it within. Feminist therapy, for example, focuses on finding and using the person's own strengths while also recognizing the many sociopolitical factors that influence one's well-being (Hawley & Sanford, 1992). These ideas suggest two considerations for the practitioner: understanding the internal and external world within which the person lives and calling forth the person's own bases of hope.

Happily, the clinical methods by which one pursues these two goals are similar. Empathic, reflective listening is a time-honored way of establishing a therapeutic relationship and developing an accurate understanding of the client's world (Rogers, 1951; Truax & Carkhuff, 1967). W. R. Miller and Rollnick (1991) have developed a directive adaptation of this client-centered approach to elicit and consolidate clients' own self-motivational statements of commitment and hope. In a series of clinical trials, this motivational interviewing approach has been found to evoke significant change in persistent problems, even with relatively brief counseling (Rollnick & Miller, 1995).

Such an approach assumes, of course, that people do have within them the seeds of hope and change, a view that we share. Psychological and psychiatric writings are rich with anecdotal examples. Sacks (1985), a consummate storyteller, helped clients find meaning in their experiences by identifying patterns of their personal values to provide inner structure. A psychiatrist recounted his conversation with a 6-year-old girl—a Black child initiating school desegregation in New Orleans against great odds, including mobs, violence, daily threats to her life, and ostracism—who said she hoped she would get through one day and then another. She also observed that if she managed to do so with success, it would be "because there is more to me than I ever realized" (Dugan & Coles, 1989, p. xiv–xv). Evoking hope has to do with helping clients discover that there is more to them than they currently realize.

Lending

One of our clients brought to her final session a colorful framed, hand-stitched quilt sampler on the back of which she had written, "Thank you for believing in me until I could believe in myself." It was as though she had borrowed her therapist's hope until she regained her own.

It is a powerful gift to see someone not merely as they are but as they can be. The transforming effect of such vision lies at the heart of Cervantes's (1605/1905) classic tale of Don Quixote, rendered more recently as *The Man of La Mancha*. An experiment described earlier (Leake & King, 1977) demonstrated the self-fulfilling prophecy of believing in clients' possibilities. Hope for the client's progress is an element that Karen Horney found particularly lacking in Freud's psychoanalysis (Manrique, 1984).

One child development specialist discovered a creative way to foster hope in children undergoing medical treatment. She became a "fortune teller" who, after careful homework with the parents, focused on the children's strengths and interests, and envisioned their future related to those. For example, she learned that one second grader loved riding his bike, so her "palm reading" for him was that when he graduated from high school, he would bicycle across the country with his team. The fortunes she told were imaginary, and therein was their strength. They were also based on a reality: Children need to hear about their own competence and about their ability to grow and master challenges. Especially in times of stress and discouragement, such fostering of hope is invaluable (Dudley, 1986).

Therapists are sometimes concerned not to raise false hopes. Certainly lying to one's clients is unethical. The underlying concern here is usually linked to a limited conception of hope: the probability of cure. However, as discussed earlier, there are important and much broader conceptions of hope. Consider a woman at age 75 just diagnosed with early Alzheimer's disease. Averages suggest that she has perhaps a year or two of reasonable mental faculties. What would be false and true hope in her situation? False hope would be to deny the diagnosis (assuming that it has been arrived at competently) or to promise a cure (there is none at this writing). Such promises are false because they ask her to trust in that which is not true or trustworthy. Some empirical room for optimism can be found in the highly variable course of the disease and in measures that may retard its progression. What is most important to see, however, is that these are limited ways of understanding what hope is. They focus on hope as way. A broader conception of hope and health is needed here, one that accepts the truth and lives through it. Here, for example, are paths that a clinician might follow with this client in discovering and nurturing her hope.

Hope as Will

In what does this woman place her ultimate hope and trust? This requires exploring her sense of meaning in life in general and in her life in particular through past, present, and future. With regard to the past, it can involve helping her to look backward with pride and gratitude (Pipher, 1996). There may also be unfinished business to address for closure or completion of the past. For the present, one can help her in choosing her attitude and actions in difficult circumstances. To face adversity with dignity and compassion is not only of personal benefit but often is also meaningful to others. What is her hope-as-will in this circumstance?

Hope as Horizon

For the future, beyond whatever hope is in the material world (who will care for her, how her individuality and wishes will be honored after she can no longer choose), one's deepest strength is often found in that which transcends material existence. What does she believe about spirit, afterlife, and her connection with that which is larger than her self? What is there of meaning that will survive the material life of her mind and body? What is her hope horizon?

Hope as Wish

Whatever her own future may hold, she may also hope *that* or hope *for* certain things. What are these hopes? Some might be particular wishes that could yet be fulfilled for her. (She always hoped to see the Grand Canyon.) Some may be particular wishes for family or others that could be enabled through requests or bequests. Acting on these specific hopes-as-wishes can be a source of meaning. What does she wish?

Hope as Action

The enactment of wishes is only one possible form of hope-as-action. A larger question is, "How do I want to act, to be in the time remaining for me?" Some have found personal meaning and hope through reaching out to others (e.g., to other victims or those at risk). Some have willfully chosen to act with caring and cheerfulness through their own illness. Caregivers say of such people with amazement, "She gave hope *to us!*" How will she choose to act and be?

Helpers as Hopers

The practice of counseling and psychotherapy, like that of pastoring, is a remarkable privilege: to be intimately present with other human souls at some of their darkest and brightest moments (Gilmore, 1973). With that privilege also comes a profound responsibility. It is neither a responsibility to "fix it" for the client (for ultimately one cannot) nor the heady image of being the upper rock climber who holds a lifeline. Rather, it is a responsibility of presence and of awareness (Shafranske & Malony, 1996). On our clearest days, we bring to these encounters a vision of God-in-the-other, a deep and numinous respect for that center that is whole and holy in the person sitting next to us (Buber, 1958). The therapist is sometimes the only person in the room conscious of it and has the important task of imparting that vision again to the client. Part of the privilege of the therapist is to witness firsthand the remarkable change that is possible in a human life. It sometimes comes in sudden and stunning transformations (W. R. Miller & C'deBaca, 1994). More often, it occurs in small steps, in cumulative change with times of surging ahead and of falling back (James, 1902/1985). Beyond whatever technical expertise we can bring to psychotherapy, clients need our vision of a sacred centered will in them and our knowledgeable assurance that change is not only a possibility but is the normal music of life. Said differently, therapists evoke hope by calling forth the will that is within and shedding light on the way onward.

This means that it is the therapist's vitality to experience and manifest hope, which cannot be done without some difficult and ongoing work of one's own. This is echoed in the traditional requirement, now often bypassed, that no one should become a psychotherapist without first walking the road of a client. We cannot give that which we have not received. Neither is this a one-time procedure, a laying on of hope that is then forever retained. Rather, it is an ongoing journey of discovering and embracing one's own sources of hope.

CONCLUSION

The evocation of hope can be one of the most important and central elements of healing. Too often equated with the particular promise of a cure, hope is better understood in its broader meanings that involve will, way, wish, action, and horizon. Whether there are empirical grounds for an optimistic prognosis, this richer and deeper context of hope is a vital perspective for the therapist.

In Spanish, the verb for hope, *esperar*, also means to wait. Helping clients to find and realize their sources of hope can be a process of waiting together for a clearer vision to emerge from clouds, as of a distant mountain. It is important to remember that the task is not one of installing hope as much as evoking it, calling it forth from the client's own rich resources. You may lend hope to a client who has little, but it is only a loan until his or her own can be reborn. In this sense, hope is not given as much as found. What we give our clients is, at most, a lens or mirror through which their own vision is clarified. That in itself can be a remarkable gift.

REFERENCES

Alcoholics Anonymous. (1976). *Alcoholics Anonymous: The story of how many thousands of men and women have recovered from alcoholism* (3rd ed.). New York: Alcoholics Anonymous World Services.

Amrhein, P. C. (1992). The comprehension of quasi-performative verbs in verbal commitments. New evidence for componential theories of lexical meaning. *Journal of Memory and Language, 31,* 756–784.

Averill, J. R., Catlin, G., & Chon, K. K. (1990). *Rules of hope.* New York: Springer-Verlag.

Beck, A. T., Weissman, A., Lester, D., & Trexler, L. (1974). The measurement of pessimism: The Hopelessness Scale. *Journal of Consulting and Clinical Psychology, 42,* 861–865.

Brody, C. A. (1990). Women in a nursing home: Living with hope and meaning. *Psychology of Women Quarterly, 14,* 579–592.

Brody, C. M., & Semel, V. G. (1993). *Strategies for therapy with the elderly: Living with hope and meaning.* New York: Springer.

Brown, R. M. (1983). *Elie Wiesel, messenger to all humanity.* Notre Dame, IN: University of Notre Dame Press.

Buber, M. (1958). *I and thou* (R. G. Smith, Trans., 2nd ed.). New York: Scribner.

Cervantes Saavedra, M. (1905). *Don Quixote* (J. M. Cohen, Trans.). New York: Hispanic Society of America. (Original work published 1605)

Daly, M. (1973). *Beyond God the father: Toward a philosophy of women's liberation.* Boston: Beacon Press.

Dudley, M. N. (1986). *Nurturing hope in times of stress.* Albuquerque, NM: Childlife Program, Presbyterian Hospital.

Dugan, T. F., & Coles, R. (Eds.). (1989). *The child in our times: Studies in the development of resiliency.* New York: Brunner/Mazel.

Erickson, R. C., Post, R. D., & Paige, A. B. (1975). Hope as a psychiatric variable. *Journal of Clinical Psychology, 31,* 324–330.

Farran, C. J., Herth, K. A., & Popovich, J. M. (1995). *Hope and hopelessness: Critical clinical constructs.* London: Sage.

Fibel, B., & Hale, W. D. (1978). The Generalized Expectancy for Success Scale: A new measure. *Journal of Consulting and Clinical Psychology, 46,* 924–931.

Frank, J. D., & Frank, J. B. (1993). *Persuasion and healing: A comparative study of psychotherapy* (3rd ed.). Baltimore: Johns Hopkins University Press.

Frankl, V. (1963). *Man's search for meaning.* Boston: Beacon Press.

Franklin, B. (1785). *Report of Dr. Benjamin Franklin, and other commissioners, charged by the King of France, with the examination of the animal magnetism, as now practised in Paris.* London: J. Johnson.

Gilmore, S. K. (1973). *The counselor-in-training.* Englewood Cliffs, NJ: Prentice Hall.

Gorsuch, R. L. (1993). Assessing spiritual variables in alcoholics anonymous research. In B. S. McCrady & W. R. Miller (Eds.), *Research on Alcoholics Anonymous: Opportunities and alternatives* (pp. 301–318). New Brunswick, NJ: Rutgers Center of Alcohol Studies.

Gottschalk, L. A. (1974). A hope scale applicable to verbal samples. *Archives of General Psychiatry, 30,* 779–785.

Harris, K. B., & Miller, W. R. (1990). Behavioral self-control training for problem drinkers: Components of efficacy. *Psychology of Addictive Behaviors, 4*, 82–90.

Hawley, N. P., & Sanford, W. (1992). Psychotherapy. In The Boston Women's Health Book Collective (Eds.), *The new our bodies, ourselves: A book by and for women* (pp. 100–104). New York: Touchstone.

Herman, J. L. (1992). *Trauma and recovery: The aftermath of violence—From domestic abuse to political terror*. New York: Basic Books.

Herth, K. A. (1992). An abbreviated instrument to measure hope: Development and psychometric evaluation. *Journal of Advanced Nursing, 17*, 1251–1259.

Hinds, P., & Gattuso, J. (1991). Measuring hopefulness in adolescents. *Journal of Pediatric Oncology Nursing, 8*, 92–94.

James, W. (1985). *The varieties of religious experience: A study in human nature*. Cambridge, MA: Harvard University Press. (Original work published 1902)

Kierkegaard, S. (1941). *The sickness unto death* (W. Lowrie, Trans.). Princeton, NJ: Princeton University Press. (Original work published 1849)

Langer, E. J. (1989). *Mindfulness*. Reading, MA: Addison-Wesley.

Leake, G. J., & King, A. S. (1977). Effect of counselor expectations on alcoholic recovery. *Alcohol Health and Research World, 1*, 16–22.

Manrique, J. F. D. (1984). Hope as a means of therapy in the work of Karen Horney. *American Journal of Psychoanalysis, 44*, 301–310.

Miller, J. F., & Power, M. J. (1988). Development of an instrument to measure hope. *Nursing Research, 37*, 6–10.

Miller, W. R. (1985). *Living as if: How positive faith can change your life*. Philadelphia: Westminster Press.

Miller, W. R., Andrews, N. R., Wilbourne, P., & Bennett, M. E. (1998). A wealth of alternatives: Effective treatments for alcohol problems. In W. R. Miller & N. Heather (Eds.), *Treating addictive behaviors: Processes of change* (2nd ed., pp. 203–216). New York: Plenum.

Miller, W. R., & C'deBaca, J. (1994). Quantum change: Toward a psychology of transformation. In T. Heatherton & J. Weinberger (Eds.), *Can personality change?* (pp. 253–280). Washington, DC: American Psychological Association.

Miller, W. R., & Rollnick, S. (1991). *Motivational interviewing: Preparing people to change addictive behavior*. New York: Guilford Press.

Miller, W. R., Yahne, C. E., & Rhodes, J. M. (1990). *Adjustment: The psychology of change*. Englewood Cliffs, NJ: Prentice Hall.

Myers, D. G. (1980). *The inflated self: human illusions and the biblical call to hope*. New York: Seabury Press.

Nowotny, M. L. (1989). Assessment of hope in patients with cancer: Development of an instrument. *Oncology Nursing Forum, 16*, 57–61.

Nuland, S. B. (1995). *How we die: Reflections on life's final chapter*. New York: Vintage.

Nunn, K. P., Lewin, T. J., Walton, J. M., & Carr, V. J. (1996). The construction and characteristics of an instrument to measure personal hopefulness. *Psychological Medicine, 26*, 531–515.

Obayuwana, A. O., Collins, J. L., Carter, A. L., Rao, M. S., Mathura, C. C., & Wilson, S. B. (1982). Hope Index Scale: An instrument for the objective assessment of hope. *Journal of the National Medical Association, 74*, 761–765.

Orlinsky, D. E., & Howard, K. I. (1986). Process and outcome in psychotherapy. In S. L. Garfield & A. E. Bergin (Eds.), *Handbook of psychotherapy and behavior change* (3rd ed., pp. 311–381). New York: Wiley.

Pipher, M. (1996). *The shelter of each other: Rebuilding our families*. New York: Ballantine Books.

Ritterman, M. K. (1991). *Hope under siege: Terror and family support in Chile*. Norwood, NJ: Ablex.

Rogers, C. R. (1951). *Client-centered therapy, its current practice, implications and theory*. Boston: Houghton Mifflin.

Rollnick, S., Butler, C. C., & Stott, N. (1997). Helping smokers make decisions: The enhancement of brief interventions from general medical practice. *Patient Education and Counselling, 31*, 191–203.

Rollnick, S., & Miller, W. R. (1995). What is motivational interviewing? *Behavioural and Cognitive Psychotherapy, 23*, 325–334.

Sacks, O. (1985). *The man who mistook his wife for a hat, and other clinical tales*. New York: Harper & Row.

Scheier, M. F., & Carver, C. S. (1985). Optimism, coping and health: Assessment and implications of generalized outcome expectancies. *Health Psychology, 4*, 219–247.

Schulman, P., Castellon, C., & Seligman, M. E. P. (1989). Assessing explanatory style: The content analysis of verbatim explanations and the Attributional Style Questionnaire. *Behavior Research and Therapy, 27*, 505–512.

Seligman, M. E. P. (1990). *Learned optimism: How to change your mind and your life*. New York: Pocket Books.

Shafranske, E. P., & Malony, H. N. (1996). Religion and the clinical practice of psychology: A case for inclusion. In E. P. Shafranske (Ed.), *Religion and the clinical practice of psychology* (pp. 561–586). Washington, DC: American Psychological Association.

Shapiro, A. K. (1971). Placebo effects in medicine, psychotherapy, and psychoanalysis. In A. E. Bergin & S. L. Garfield (Eds.), *Handbook of psychotherapy and behavior change: An empirical analysis* (pp. 439–473). New York: Wiley.

Snyder, C. R. (1994). *The psychology of hope*. New York: Free Press.

Snyder, C. R., Harris, C., Anderson, J. R., Holleran, S. A., Irving, L. M., Sigmon, S. T., Yoshinobu, L. R., Gibb, J., Langelle, C., & Harney, P. (1991). The will and the ways: Development and validation of an individual-differences measure of hope. *Journal of Personality and Social Psychology, 60*, 570–585.

Staats, S. (1989). Hope: A comparison of two self-report measures for adults. *Journal of Personality Assessment, 53*, 366–375.

Stoner, M. (1982). Hope and cancer patients. *Dissertation Abstracts International, 13,* 1983B. (University Microfilms No. 83–12,213)

Stotland, E. (1969). *The psychology of hope.* San Francisco: Jossey-Bass.

Tillich, P. (1958). *The dynamics of faith.* New York: HarperCollins.

Truax, C. B., & Carkhuff, R. R. (1967). *Toward effective counseling and psychotherapy: Training and practice.* Chicago: Aldine.

Turner, J. A., Deyo, R. A., Loeser, J. D., Von Korff, M., & Fordyce, W. E. (1994). The importance of placebo effects in pain treatment and research. *Journal of the American Medical Association, 271,* 1609–1614.

Whalan, G. S., & Mushet, G. L. (1986). Consumers' views of the helpful aspects of an inpatient psychotherapy group: A preliminary communication. *British Journal of Medical Psychology, 59,* 337–339.

Willoughby, K. V. (1996). *Progression of alcohol-related behaviors in a Navajo sample.* Unpublished master's thesis, University of New Mexico, Albuquerque.

Yahne, C. E., & Long, V. O. (1988). The use of support groups to raise self-esteem for women clients. *Journal of American College Health, 37,* 79–84.

Yalom, I. D. (1975). *Theory and practice of group psychotherapy.* New York: Basic Books.

12

SERENITY

GERARD J. CONNORS, RADKA T. TOSCOVA,
AND J. SCOTT TONIGAN

Although the concept of serenity appears intermittently in the psychological literature, it is a notion that has received much wider consideration in the popular press. It is difficult to view a rack of magazines without seeing references to serenity or related topics such as calmness, peace of mind, repose, or tranquility. This is often done in two contexts: to facilitate coping with stress or other life challenges and to facilitate enlightenment or spiritual growth.

Although serenity is a concept with psychological overtones, it is also a central construct that warrants coverage in a book on spirituality. One can be serene without a sense of spirituality, but spiritual practices are widely recommended to enhance serenity. In the three sections of this chapter, we explore definitions of serenity, how can it be measured, and what can be done to engender it.

DEFINING SERENITY

A Global Amorphous Concept?

Most individuals have no difficulty in using the words *serene* or *serenity* in their conversations or writings. Although there is sometimes a

235

loss for words on how to define "serene" or "serenity," when people do apply the terms there is a consistent colloquial usage that equates serenity with a variety of generally positive experiences, emotions, and states of being. Thus, in psychological terms, one can equate it with experiencing positive mood states.

One starting point for defining serenity is the *Oxford English Dictionary* (1989). When used to describe personal comportment, dating back to the late 1500s, the term denoted an inward calm and cheerful tranquility. Its main other use during this period was in describing weather, such as calm, clear, and tranquil skies. Additional insights on the nature of serenity are offered by a review of the term's synonyms. A brief listing includes calmness, composure, cool, patience, peace, peace of mind, placidity, quiescence, quietness, quietude, stillness, tranquil mind, and tranquility. On the flip side, antonyms include agitation, disquietude, restlessness, and upset.

Serenity in Psychology

Within the psychological literature as well, the term *serenity* has been used to specify peace of mind or inner peace, often in the face of external or difficult circumstances. As examples, serenity has been equated with peace amid the storms of life (Katz, 1980), quieting the mind (McKenna, 1977), and experiencing an inner peace despite external or difficult circumstances (Gerber, 1986; Roberts & Cunningham, 1990). Bailey (1990), writing in the context of recovery from addictive behaviors, defined serenity as "feelings of tranquility, gratitude, contentment, affection for others, and a deep inner peace" (p. 1).

Within the context of psychotherapy, Masserman (1989) identified three "ultimate and urgent human aspirations" (p. 258). The first two aspirations were physical (referring to capabilities associated with controlling one's material milieu) and social (referring to interpersonal alliances necessary for group securities). The third aspiration was labeled *existential* and pertained to "the beliefs and faiths essential to metapsychological serenity" (Masserman, 1989, p. 258).

Maslow identified serenity as a component of what he termed the "plateau experience" (see Cleary & Shapiro, 1995). As described by Hoffman (1988) in his biography of Maslow, the plateau experience is a "serene and calm, rather than intensely emotional, response to what we experience as miraculous or awesome. The high plateau always has a noetic and cognitive element, unlike the peak experience, which can be merely emotional" (p. 340). According to Cleary and Shapiro (1995), "Maslow emphasized the need to bring calmness into one's psychological state—that we need the serene as well as the poignantly emotional, and he called attention to the plateau experience as an example of serenity" (pp. 10–11).

Serenity in 12-Step Programs

Another context in which serenity plays a central role is in 12-step recovery programs (described in greater detail in chap. 6 in this book). Such groups, regardless of problem focus (e.g., alcohol, drugs, gambling, codependency), in almost all cases embrace serenity as a core component, outcome, or both of the recovery process. Bailey (1990), for example, identified serenity as "the cure for all addictions" (p. 1). In this context, Kurtz and Ketcham (1992) described the term *being at home* as the "place where we find peace and harmony that comes from learning to live with the knowledge of our own imperfections and from learning to accept the imperfections of others" (p. 232). To find this state of harmony and balance, Kurtz and Ketcham endorsed the practice of self and other forgiveness.

The most tangible expression of appreciation for the importance of serenity in 12-step programs is the Serenity Prayer, which is shown in Table 12.1. The origins of the Serenity Prayer are uncertain. Its composition is often credited to Reinhold Niebuhr, a 20th-century Christian theologian. However, Niebuhr is quoted as crediting the prayer to Friedrich Oetinger, an 18th-century theologian. Nevertheless, Niebuhr is clearly responsible for its popularization in the United States, and it has been used within Alcoholics Anonymous (AA) since the 1940s. Although the term *serenity* is not formally defined in the AA literature, the text of the prayer includes elements of acceptance, letting go of control over certain elements of life, developing trust in and surrendering to God's will, discerning when to take

TABLE 12.1
The Serenity Prayer

God, grant me the serenity to accept the things I cannot change,
the courage to change the things I can,
And the wisdom to know the difference.

Living one day at a time,
Enjoying one moment at a time,
Accepting hardship as a pathway to peace,
Taking this sinful world as it is,
Not as I would have it.

Trusting that you will make all things right
If I surrender to your will,
So that I may be reasonably happy in this life
And supremely happy with you forever in the next.

Note. In the public domain.

appropriate action, accepting life on life's terms, having a present-day orientation, and experiencing joy.

A Concept Analysis

A detailed exposition on defining serenity has been provided by Roberts and Cunningham (1990). Their starting point was an impression from the literature that the meaning of serenity was at best ambiguous. Furthermore, they perceived two distinct research needs. The first was for the meaning of serenity to be clarified and articulated. Their second research need was to establish a mechanism for measuring serenity. At whatever point these needs are met, clinicians will be in a better position to explore influences on and correlates of serenity and apply them in clinical practice.

Roberts and Cunningham (1990; see also Roberts & Fitzgerald, 1991) began their endeavors on serenity by performing a "concept analysis" of serenity. They first generated a list of all previous uses of the term. They then identified the particulars associated with previous uses of the term, including defining attributes, antecedents, and consequences. The authors recruited five experts on serenity (three had written on the topic, one taught on the topic in the context of tai chi classes, and one had studied serenity through involvement with members of AA) to assist in the process. The experts reviewed and critiqued materials on serenity, and later participated in roundtable discussions that focused on the concept analysis of serenity. The experts responded to proposed definitions of serenity and components of the concept analysis until consensus was achieved by at least four of the five experts.

The concept analysis discussed by Roberts and Cunningham (1990) focused overall on serenity in the context of "a human experience that involves a positive mood state, feeling, thought, state of being, or level of consciousness" (p. 580). Their endeavor led them to the identification of 10 critical attributes that they felt represented the defining characteristics of serenity. These defining characteristics are listed in Table 12.2.

The defining characteristics, described in greater detail by Roberts and Cunningham (1990), are only highlighted here. One important characteristic identified was to detach from or become distinct from emotions and surrounding circumstances. In this regard, some researchers acknowledged detachment as a vehicle for attaining serenity and experiencing calmness, tranquility, and evenness. Gerber (1986), for example, identified detachment as being central to serenity. The term *detachment* does not refer to being unaware of surrounding realities. Instead, there is a recognition and acceptance of such realities, but in a manner that permits keeping them distinct and in perspective.

Another important feature of serenity concerns the ability to find a secure inner space or haven. All of the experts contributing to Roberts

TABLE 12.2
Defining Characteristics of Serenity

1. The ability to detach from desires and/or emotion and feelings.
2. The ability to be in touch with an inner haven of peace and security.
3. A sense of connectedess with the universe.
4. A trust in the wisdom of the universe.
5. The habit of actively pursuing all reasonable avenues for solving problems.
6. An ability to accept situations that cannot be changed.
7. A way to give unconditionally of one's self.
8. Forgiveness of self and others.
9. The ability to let go of the past and the future and to live in the present.
10. A sense of perspective as to the importance of one's self and life events.

Note. From "Serenity: Concept Analysis and Measurement," by K. Roberts and G. Cunningham, 1990, Educational Gerontology, 16, 577–589. Copyright 1990 by Taylor & Francis, Inc. Adapted with permission of the author.

and Cunningham's (1990) concept analysis concurred that "the ability to reach this inner haven even in the midst of turmoil" (p. 581) was central to attaining serenity.

Several more of the defining characteristics proposed by the above-mentioned researchers warrant highlighting. Two of these pertain to one's relationship with the universe, broadly defined. These specifically deal with one's connection with the universe and faith or trust in the orderliness of this universe that exists beyond oneself.

Two other characteristics of serenity, according to Roberts and Cunningham (1990), reflect personal responsibilities. The first is proactively addressing situations that can be changed in a positive manner. Related to this is an acceptance of situations that cannot reasonably be altered despite one's efforts. Both of these notions are central to the Serenity Prayer, which was described earlier.

The consolidation of these defining characteristics by Roberts and Cunningham (1990) led them to propose the following working definition of serenity: "a spiritual experience of inner peace, trust, and connectedness that exists independently of external events" (p. 582). Additional components to the definition could include detachment and letting go of needing to be in control of others, reduced preoccupation with material gain (i.e., distinguishing needs from wants; Hiltner, 1972), appropriate sense of self-importance, and humility (Kurtz & Ketcham, 1992). We have elected to use the working definition provided by Roberts and Cunningham (1990) in this chapter for several reasons. First, this definition was derived from a careful and systematic effort designed to identify and incorporate the elements most central to previous thinking about serenity and what it represents. Although one might raise issues about their definition, Roberts and Cunningham's (1990) work stands out as being the most systematic, comprehensive, and elucidated effort to define serenity. A third attractive feature of this definition, from our perspective, is that the focus is on the presence of positive experiences (e.g., inner peace and connectedness) as opposed to the absence of particular uncomfortable experiences (e.g., anger, tension, or anxiety). Taken together, the definition emphasizes the life enhancement states and qualities to be found through the experience of serenity.

A SERENITY SCALE

Researchers have conducted numerous studies of the assessment of spirituality (see chap. 3 in this book; see also MacDonald, LeClair, Holland, Alter, & Friedman, 1995), driven at least in part by the indication that spirituality is positively related to health. There also have been efforts to assess serenity, and we think the best example to date is reflected in the work of Roberts and her colleagues (Roberts & Aspy, 1993; Roberts & Cunningham, 1990). Those researchers used the concept analysis results on serenity described earlier as the starting point for the development of the Serenity Scale, a measure of serenity.

In an early effort, Roberts and Cunningham (1990) developed an initial set of 62 potential items to tap into the critical dimensions of serenity described earlier (see Table 12.2). The respondents (a group of graduate students and a group of elderly volunteers) were instructed to respond to the items using a 5-point scale ranging from *never had the experience* to *always had the experience*. Analyses revealed that the measure had high overall internal reliability for both samples, mostly satisfactory reliability for the separate scales (e.g., Inner Haven, Detachment, Connectedness, etc.), and the desired modest intercorrelations among the scale scores.

Further work on the measure was conducted by Roberts and Aspy (1993) using a larger and more diverse sample of 542 participants. The majority were clients at an urban, university-based health care clinic; smaller numbers of participants were recruited from settings such as an inner-city ambulatory care center, a middle-class senior citizens' center, an automobile factory assembly line, and a group of health care professionals working at local health care facilities. Fifty-nine percent of the participants were women, 51% were married, and 73% were White. Thirteen percent had less than high school education, 27% had a high school degree, and the remainder had at least some college education. The majority (77%) described themselves as being in good or excellent health. Evaluation of responses to the 65 items on this version of the scale led to a shortening of the original instrument, with the goal of maintaining high internal consistency with the fewest number of items necessary. The result was a 40-item Serenity Scale.

A subsequent factor analysis suggested a nine-factor solution that accounted for just more than 58% of the total variance. Because of the seminal nature of this work, we describe the results of this analysis in some detail, along with representative items of the Serenity Scale that were associated with the factors identified. In this way, it will be possible for readers to develop a sense of the statements used to represent the components of serenity. The factors (and representative Serenity Scale items[1]) were labeled as follows:

1. *Inner Haven* (I experience an inner quiet that does not depend upon events; I experience an inner calm even when I am under pressure; I am aware of an inner peace; I experience peace of mind).
2. *Acceptance* (I take care of today and let yesterday and tomorrow take care of themselves; I live one day at a time; I am forgiving of myself for past mistakes).
3. *Belonging* (I feel isolated [reverse scored]; I have a feeling of not belonging [reverse scored]; I feel lonely [reverse scored]).
4. *Trust* (I trust that life events happen to fit a plan which is larger and more gentle than I can know; Even though I do not understand, I trust in the ultimate goodness of the plan of things; I trust that everything happens as it should).
5. *Perspective* (I take action to change the things that must be changed; I attempt to deal with what is, rather than what was, or what will be; I try to place my problems in the proper perspective in any given situation).
6. *Contentment* (I expect people to repay my help with good behavior [reverse scored]; I wish I had more material goods [reverse scored]; I feel stressed when I cannot have things I want [reverse scored]).
7. *Present Centered* (I wish I could go back and do things differently [reverse scored]; I feel regretful about the past [reverse scored]; I feel angry when I remember certain things that have happened to me [reverse scored]).
8. *Benevolence* (When I remember persons who have caused me pain, I hope that good things will happen to them; I feel forgiving of those who have harmed me).
9. *Cognitive Restructuring/Self-Responsibility* (When I am in a problem situation, I ask whether or not my attitude is part of the problem; I find that changing what I think solves problems).

Two important indications are provided by the results of Roberts and Aspy's (1993) work. The first is that, as expected, serenity is a multidi-

[1]From "Serenity: Caring With Perspective," by K. T. Roberts and L. Fitzgerald, 1991, *Scholarly Inquiry for Nursing Practice, 5,* 127–142. Copyright by Springer Publishing Company, 1991. Adapted with permission.

mensional construct. Second, these results are consistent with the assertion made earlier in this chapter that serenity is predominantly associated with the presence of a variety of apparently positive states and experiences. The scale should be useful in future research with a variety of clinical and nonclinical populations. In clinical settings, for example, the multifactorial Serenity Scale could be used to assess various aspects of serenity among clients who have a wide range of presenting problems, such as stress and adjustment-related difficulties, mood disorders (e.g., anxiety, depression), health problems, or existential problems.

In a recent clinical case, one of us worked with a 45-year-old client. Tom and his wife of 6 years had been separated for 4 months, at her request, before she asked for them to reunite. Tom had accepted this reconciliation excitedly, even though they had both dated other people during the separation. They experienced a passionate 2-month reunion, after which Tom found himself depressed, anxious, mistrustful, and withdrawn from his wife. He was not sleeping well and had lost his appetite and sexual drive. He was obsessing about not being able to trust his wife any more even though she had repeatedly apologized and reiterated her commitment to him. As a long-standing member of AA, Tom was concerned that this event had made him "lose my serenity," which, in turn, he felt, would threaten his sobriety. As described earlier, serenity is regarded as an important state for the successful long-term emotional maintenance of the recovering alcoholic individual. It was clear that Tom had issues related to most of the defining characteristics of serenity. Another client whose treatment included a focus on serenity was Susan, a high school teacher and working mother who described guilt and inadequacy over her inability to meet all of the demands of her family and work. She felt stressed, overwhelmed, and harried, and contemplated giving up a job that she loved and needed financially. We return briefly to these two cases in a discussion of ways for fostering serenity.

APPROACHES FOR ENGENDERING SERENITY

Over the years, a variety of writings on serenity have provided several useful approaches for fostering a sense of serenity. In this section, we revisit several of the critical attributes of serenity described earlier (see Table 12.2) and discuss how psychotherapy can facilitate the development of those particular components of serenity. Within the context of therapy, many of the components of serenity can be described as positive outcomes associated with the successful completion of therapeutic tasks. In a way, the process is one of developing *intrapersonal* skills, including the fostering of inner peace, relaxation, security, trust in self, self-acceptance, self-forgiveness, and the experience of connectedness, balanced by reasonable levels of detachment, letting go of past and future events, and exertion of control. Other aspects of the experience of serenity that may be addressed within therapy are interpersonal skills (e.g., such as empathy, acceptance, tolerance, and forgiveness of others) as well as detachment from needing to control outside events and people. Components of serenity can themselves be observed and experienced as process variables in the context of ongoing therapy. Many "nonspecific" therapist characteristics commonly described as being important to effective treatment can be thought of as manifestations of serenity. For example, therapist empathy, acceptance, and tolerance of client imperfections (Kurtz & Ketcham, 1992) together can provide a "safe haven" for clients that may reduce defensiveness and foster an internalization of the safe haven of serenity.

Detaching

The connection between detachment and serenity has been highlighted by many writers (Gerber, 1986; Kurtz & Ketcham, 1992; Whitfield, 1984). This detachment refers not only to detachment from external events but also to disidentification from disruptive and negative mood states. For many, this detachment reflects a "letting go" phenomenon. Again, this does not mean being in a state of denial, being oblivious to reality issues. In fact, to "let go" first implies being aware of that which must be released (see chap. 10 in this book).

How does one foster such detachment? Gerber (1986) described the use of words in concert with breathing cycles to engender detachment. Others (e.g., Epstein, 1998; Kabat-Zinn, 1994) advocate quietly focusing on and observing unpleasant or disturbing thoughts and feelings while breathing deeply, a process of passive awareness (see chap. 4 in this book). Such processes can reduce the emotional impact of thoughts and feelings and allow them to be released. This resembles the well-researched technique of systematic desensitization (Wolpe, 1969). Others have viewed detachment as the releasing of cravings and never-ending wants (Epstein, 1998; Hiltner, 1972), through the use of cognitive restructuring and values clarification to identify and prioritize core values, distinguishing needs from wants. It was helpful for Susan, the high school teacher and working mother identified earlier, to examine the amount of effort she placed in having her two daughters in 10 different extracurricular activities because she thought they were "enriching" and because she wanted to provide opportunities that she felt deprived of while growing up. She had persisted in this despite the fact that even her daughters felt harassed by the numerous activities and welcomed eliminating some of them.

Another avenue often followed for seeking detachment and serenity is meditation (see chap. 4 in this book). In a review of meditation as a psychotherapeutic strategy, Smith (1975) defined meditation as "mental exercises that generally involve limiting thought and attention. Such exercises vary widely and can involve sitting still and counting breaths, attending to a repeated thought, or focusing on virtually any simple external or internal stimulus" (p. 558). Among the more common forms of meditation are those focusing on awareness, those focusing on emotions, and those based on physical movement (Foster & Shoemaker, 1996; Kabat-Zinn, 1994; Lama Surya Das, 1997; J. P. Miller, 1994). The various types of meditation available (for a review, see Goleman, 1977) are drawn from both Eastern and Western traditions, and there are similarities between these two approaches. Many contemporary writers blend and adapt Eastern spiritual philosophies to Western thinking (Lama Surya Das, 1997). Frequently cited features of the meditative experience include self-transcendence, enlightenment, openness, intensification and changes of consciousness, and meaningfulness (Osis, Bockert, & Carlson, 1973)—all possible correlates of serenity. Others view the benefit and goal of meditation as the quieting of the mind to the influence of destructive, "boring, repetitive, and pointless" cognitions that isolate individuals from real feelings and the ability to connect with others (Epstein, 1998, p. 59). The clients mentioned earlier, Tom and Susan, both benefited from quieting their minds of such thoughts. These and other issues relevant to meditation are described in chapter 4 in this book.

Finding an Inner Haven

Most contributors to the literature on serenity have noted the importance of safe inner haven or sanctuary. Ideally, the individual practices reaching this inner haven on a regular basis and, perhaps more important, can reach it as needed in times of emotional turmoil or stressful life events. When in this inner haven, the person experiences tranquility and freedom from both external and internal disruptions. Some therapists train clients to directly create such a space through the use of guided imagery and visualization. A therapist, for example, may teach breathing techniques to facilitate an initial relaxation and then paint a beautiful and serene picture tailored to the client's needs and experiences using words or relaxing music. Indeed, the demand for such a state is so great that bookstores and music stores stock a variety of resources for the pursuit of serenity. Such books and audiotapes can be particularly useful adjuncts in therapy with individuals experiencing anxiety disorders, depression, withdrawal from drugs, and general environmental stressors. The creation of a visual safe haven was particularly useful to Debbie, a 21-year-old student who had been raped on a college campus 2 years earlier. Despite her ongoing participation in a rape support group, she had continued to have sleep disturbances, anxiety, and concentration problems that prevented her from being able to focus on her studies. In therapy she was able to learn first how to focus on her breathing to induce relaxation. The therapist then was able to elicit from Debbie's past experiences a time in her life when she felt safe, comfortable, and serene. This experience then was described in great detail by the therapist using visual, auditory, and olfactory cues. It was first practiced in the therapy session and then at other places when she felt comfortable. It was to become her safe haven, and eventually she was able to produce the experience when she was extremely stressed and had flashbacks of her attack. This practice was enhanced by the use of an audiotape of calm music with flowing water while visualizing her safe haven. She also used this strategy at night, which improved the quality of her sleep and her general emotional well-being.

Acceptance and Empathy

Acceptance of situations that are beyond one's personal control is an alternative to exerting energies in the pursuit of change efforts that are likely to be futile. Rather than insisting that others change, or seeking to alter what is beyond one's control, a person can focus on what is changeable: one's own attitudes, detachment, and serenity. Accepting that which is beyond personal control is one of the premises of the Serenity Prayer (Kurtz & Ketcham, 1992).

There is a second aspect of acceptance that can also operate in the service of serenity: self-acceptance. Gerber (1986) asserted that people need to have compassion and respect for themselves, embracing their unique competence and worthiness. Such acceptance is one factor leading to serene living.

Acceptance can be greatly enhanced by encouraging empathy toward others. There seems to be a reciprocal relationship between self-acceptance and acceptance of others. In their chapter on empathy, Oliner and Oliner (1995) distinguished between sympathy, a feeling for another based on self-centered feelings, and feeling *with* another person, taking the other's perspective. Oliner and Oliner asserted that encouraging the expression and sharing of feelings in small groups with a facilitator can be particularly helpful in increasing empathy, especially among men. Similarly, increasing empathy has been found to enhance harmony and acceptance in couples therapy (Rampage, 1995). The concept of acceptance is discussed in greater detail in chapter 10 in this book.

As for Tom, the client introduced earlier, accepting his wife's infidelity as well as his own was an important healing component of his therapy. The past could not be changed, but he could change how he felt about the past. A next step would be forgiveness.

Forgiveness and Giving of Self

According to Roberts and Cunningham (1990), the "serene person has made peace with the past and achieved a state of forgiveness of self and others" (p. 582). As reviewed by Hargrave and Sells (1997), *forgiveness* is a term that has been used in three primary contexts: releasing resentments toward someone, restoring or repairing relationships and mending emotional wounds, and releasing an offending party who caused an injury (broadly defined) from potential retaliation. Such forgiveness is hypothesized to counteract bitterness, resentments, and regrets. In fact, Nelsen (1997) asserted that an "unwillingness to forgive is one of the greatest blocks to our inner wisdom" (p. 117).

Encouraging forgiveness is a spiritual intervention frequently used by psychotherapists (Richards & Bergin, 1997). In reviewing the limited evidence regarding its use in psychotherapy, Richards and Bergin (1977) concluded that there is sufficient support "for the belief that forgiveness is an important component of interpersonal and psychological healing" (p. 212) and endorsed its "careful use" in psychotherapy. Forgiveness can be a particularly useful strategy in working with adults who experienced maltreatment, abuse, or neglect while growing up and now are plagued by persistent and unproductive anger and blame. Forty-year-old Rachel, an accountant who had been married and divorced three times and was the mother of two children who lived with their respective fathers, had debilitating headaches, chronic back pain, anxiety, difficulties with her children, and interpersonal relationship problems caused by persistent and chronic anger and rage reactions. Recognizing that her childhood experiences were unacceptable and that she did not deserve the maltreatment she had received, Rachel nevertheless needed to shift her focus from blaming her mother for her current difficulties. In learning to forgive her mother, she also learned to forgive herself for her own parenting deficits and instead focus on strategies to improve her current situation and find some "peace of mind."

In 12-step programs, forgiveness is an important concept because it is seen as the healer of resentment. According to Kurtz and Ketcham (1992), "resentment is the poison of the spiritual life" (p. 213). If not addressed, it exacerbates anger, fear, and sadness and interferes with the person's ability to work through the spiritual steps necessary for maintaining recovery. For this reason, 12-step program members are encouraged to write about their resentments and to share such feelings with another person. Similarly, such feelings can be expressed and explored in the therapy process.

Engaging in a process of forgiveness may also better set the stage for forgiving oneself. Some have postulated that giving of oneself is an innate drive, or at least strongly desired by most people. Accordingly, it would follow that, "serenity results in part from one's ability to express altruism or goodness" (Roberts & Cunningham, 1990, p. 582)—again a reciprocal process. These and other elements of forgiveness are described in chapter 10.

Letting Go and Living in the Present

Experiencing the aspects of serenity described above facilitates letting go and living in the present. Detaching, acceptance, and finding an inner haven all should contribute to the prospects of letting go and focusing on the present moment. The importance of living in the present is highlighted throughout the literature on serenity and is discussed in this book by Cole and Pargament in the broader context of spirituality (chap. 9). Roberts and Cunningham (1990) reported that the "serene person lives fully in the present" (p. 582), and Whitfield (1984) wrote that "living in the here and now is a powerful way to be" (p. 1). Indeed, Whitfield (1984) cited Krishnamurti in suggesting that perhaps the greatest stumbling block on the road to serenity is "being preoccupied with time" (p. 1). Being able to let go and live in the present places the individual at the point of transcending the constraints of time and other burdens. The title of Kabat-Zinn's (1994) meditation guide, *Wherever You Go, There You Are*, itself is a strong reminder about the importance of being in the present, freed from past and future burdens, fears, and worries.

Trust

A trust in others and the sense that no matter what happens one will be fine are based on a belief in the benevolent wisdom of the universe. This type of belief relaxes people's defenses and increases a sense of connection with the universe and with others (Epstein, 1998). In a Christian context, trust is based on a belief in the benevolence who offers forgiveness, with no questions asked, as illustrated in the biblical story of the prodigal son and his father (Hiltner, 1972). Another aspect of trust within a theistic context is that one is guided by God toward some task or predetermined destination. In 12-step programs, this involves turning over one's will to a higher power. The task is to carefully learn to distinguish needs from wants, to give up the struggle for irrelevant and unnecessary wants, and instead to recognize that true needs are provided for by God without a struggle (Borg, 1994; Epstein, 1998; Hiltner, 1972). In therapy, belief in a benevolent universe may be fostered by first developing trust in a benevolent therapist, with a hope of enhancing the client's own tolerance, acceptance, and empathy.

Some Additional Comments

We focused on the domains identified in this chapter because they have the potential for being readily applicable and manageable to address in a wide range of clinical situations. Addressing such domains may also set the stage for clients to experience some of the more abstract components of serenity, such as transcendence, gratitude and grace, surrender to and unity with the universe or some higher power, humility, and a balanced perspective on one's importance (see Hiltner, 1972; Kurtz & Ketcham, 1992; Roberts & Cunningham, 1990). In this way it may serve, as it does in the 12-step programs, as a way of speaking about a final common spiritual pathway to health.

Before leaving this section, it may be useful to identify some possible indications that a given client might be a candidate for assessment or interventions relating to serenity. In some cases, the client may specifically mention such a concern, but this is the exception. More often, the indication is found in a comment or presenting complaint reflecting what Moore (1992) has characterized as the "emotional complaints of our time" (p. xvi). As described by Moore, they include emptiness, meaninglessness, vague depression, disillusionment, loss of values, yearning for personal fulfillment, and hunger for spirituality. All of these complaints have in common the recognition of a void, the absence of serenity.

The client's request is often to make these aversive states go away, as if the absence of pain were the goal of life. The limitations of avoidant coping are widely recognized, and many of the chapters in this book instead emphasize an acceptance of what is. Yet, to a client suffering emptiness of spirit, acceptance of the void offers little completion. The broad concept of serenity, which can be construed in many kinds of secular and religious language, offers something toward which to move. In this view, serenity does not consist in the absence of aversive experiences. Rather, emotional ills bespeak an absence of the positive and vibrant quality of serenity, which one can experience in the midst of aversive circumstances.

People find their own serenity through a diverse range of avenues. Some follow Zen Buddhist paths emphasizing a transcendence of everyday reality to reach enlightenment (e.g., Foster & Shoemaker, 1996; Lama Surya Das, 1997). Some pursue new age spirituality that offers a blending of Western and Eastern religious philosophies (e.g., Borysenko, 1993; R. S. Miller & the Editors of the *New Age Journal*, 1992). Others find a sense of serenity in Judeo-Christian spirituality and communities. For still others, serenity may be pursued through secular methods such as relaxation techniques. Professional respect is warranted for such a diversity of paths toward a common maturity.

SUMMARY

At first blush, the globally positive concept of serenity may seem so amorphous as to be of little more than metaphoric use in psychotherapy or science. Yet, when unpacked, as in the germinal work of Roberts and her colleagues, the construct of serenity contains a number of more specific processes that are widely recognized as therapeutic and health promoting. Far from being the absence of aversive states, serenity involves the practice of vibrant processes that lead toward a final common pathway of spiritual wellness. The processes embedded in this construct include many of those discussed elsewhere in this book: acceptance, forgiveness, letting go, mindfulness, empathy, coping detachment, meditation, and prayer. There seems to be a reciprocal relationship between extending conditions such as acceptance and forgiveness to others and experiencing serenity oneself. Progress has been made toward a multivariate definition and measurement of serenity. The differentiation of processes that make up serenity in turn points toward practices to foster it. Thus, the concept of serenity has both experiential and practical implications for clinicians and may be particularly helpful in understanding broad spiritual aspects of the processes and outcomes of psychotherapy.

REFERENCES

Bailey, J. V. (1990). *The serenity principle*. New York: Harper & Row.

Borg, M. J. (1994). *Meeting Jesus again for the first time: The historical Jesus and the heart of contemporary faith*. San Francisco: Harper.

Borysenko, J. (1993). *Fire in the soul: A new psychology of spiritual optimism*. New York: Warner Books.

Cleary, T. S., & Shapiro, S. I. (1995). The plateau experience and the postmortem life: Abraham H. Maslow's unfinished theory. *Journal of Transpersonal Psychology, 27*, 1–23.

Epstein, M. (1998). *Going to pieces without falling apart: A Buddhist perspective on wholeness—Lessons from meditation and psychotherapy*. New York: Bantam Doubleday Dell.

Foster, N., & Shoemaker, J. (Eds.). (1996). *The roaring stream: A new Zen reader*. Hopewell, NJ: Ecco Press.

Gerber, W. (1986). *Serenity*. New York: University Press of America.

Goleman, D. (1977). *The varieties of the meditative experience*. New York: Dutton.

Hargrave, T. D., & Sells, J. N. (1997). The development of a forgiveness scale. *Journal of Marital and Family Therapy, 23*, 41–62.

Hiltner, S. (1972). *Theological dynamics*. Nashville, TN: Abingdon Press.

Hoffman, E. (1988). *The right to be human: A biography of Abraham Maslow*. Los Angeles: Torcher.

Kabat-Zinn, J. (1994). *Wherever you go, there you are*. New York: Hyperion.

Katz, C. (1980). Reducing stress: Serenity is not freedom from the storm, but peace amid the storm. *Dental Practice, 1*, 59–63.

Kurtz, E., & Ketcham, K. (1992). *The spirituality of imperfection: Storytelling and the journey to wholeness*. New York: Bantam Books.

Lama Surya Das. (1997). *Awakening the Buddha within: Tibetan wisdom for the Western world*. New York: Bantam Doubleday Dell.

MacDonald, D. A., LeClair, L., Holland, C. J., Alter, A., & Friedman, H. L. (1995). A survey of measures of transpersonal constructs. *Journal of Transpersonal Psychology, 27*, 171–235.

Masserman, J. H. (1989). The dynamics of contemporary therapies. *Journal of Contemporary Psychotherapy, 19*, 257–270.

McKenna, M. (1977). *The serenity book*. New York: Rawson.

Miller, J. P. (1994). *The contemplative practitioner: Meditation in education and the professions*. Westport, CT: Bergin & Garvey.

Miller, R. S., & the Editors of the *New Age Journal*. (1992). *As above so below: Paths to spiritual renewal in daily life*. New York: St. Martin's Press.

Moore, T. *Care of the soul*. (1992). New York: HarperCollins.

Nelsen, J. (1997). *Understanding: Eliminating stress and finding serenity in life and relationships* (2nd ed., rev.). Rocklin, CA: Prima.

Oliner P. M., & Oliner S. P. (1995). *Toward a caring society*. Westport, CT: Praeger.

Osis, K., Bockert, E., & Carlson, M. L. (1973). Dimensions of the meditative experience. *Journal of Transpersonal Psychology, 5*, 109–135.

Oxford English dictionary. (1989). Oxford, England: Clarendon Press.

Rampage, C. (1995). Gender aspects of marital therapy. In N. S. Jacobson & A. S. Gurman (Eds.), *Clinical handbook of couples therapy* (pp. 261–273). New York: Guilford Press.

Richards, P. S., & Bergin, A. E. (1997). *A spiritual strategy for counseling and psychotherapy*. Washington, DC: American Psychological Association.

Roberts, K., & Cunningham, G. (1990). Serenity: Concept analysis and measurement. *Educational Gerontology, 16*, 577–589.

Roberts, K. T., & Aspy, C. B. (1993). Development of the Serenity Scale. *Journal of Nursing Measurement, 1*, 145–163.

Roberts, K. T., & Fitzgerald, L. (1991). Serenity: Caring with perspective. *Scholarly Inquiry for Nursing Practice, 5*, 127–142.

Smith, J. C. (1975). Meditation as psychotherapy: A review of the literature. *Psychological Bulletin, 82*, 558–564.

Whitfield, C. L. (1984). Stress management and spirituality during recovery: A transpersonal approach: II. Being. *Alcoholism Treatment Quarterly, 1*, 1–50.

Wolpe, J. (1969). *The practice of behavior therapy*. Elmsford, NY: Pergamon Press.

IV

SPIRITUALITY IN
PROFESSIONAL TRAINING

13

DIVERSITY TRAINING IN SPIRITUAL AND RELIGIOUS ISSUES

WILLIAM R. MILLER

In the preceding chapters the authors have addressed a variety of spiritual issues in psychotherapy. One of my hopes in assembling this book has been to provide perspectives and resources that will be useful not only in practice but also in training future therapists. My own training in a scientist-practitioner psychology program was mostly silent on this subject, leaving me with the impression that it was not a proper topic for discussion among mental health professionals. We owe it to our students and future clients to do better than that. In this final chapter I offer some thoughts on the process of diversity training of future psychotherapists, conscious that they are matters on which reasonable people disagree. I hope that these thoughts will encourage further informed consideration of the training issues involved. Toward this end, I have also proposed a set of practical "take-away messages," found at the end of each section.

As in other health professions, the American Psychological Association and American Medical Association require accredited training programs to prepare students to work knowledgeably and ethically with clients who differ on a number of personal dimensions. One such dimension of diversity has to do with clients' religious and spiritual perspectives, echoing a more general American value on religious freedom and plurality. With regard to psychiatry training, the American Medical Association (1998) specified that

> the curriculum should contain enough instruction about these issues [including religion and spirituality] to enable residents to render competent care to patients from varioius cultural backgrounds. This instruction must be especially comprehensive in those programs with residents whose cultural backgrounds are significantly different from those of their patients. (pp. 265–267)

Yet, clinical training programs typically do little to prepare their students for professional roles with people who vary widely in their spiritual and religious backgrounds, an oversight that has been pointed out for decades (Bergin, 1980; Clement, 1978, Miller & Martin, 1988). The problem has been, in part, a shortage within training programs of role models for such integration. As a group, mental health professionals in general and psychologists in particular tend to report low levels of religious belief and involvement relative to the U.S. population. The historical reasons for this are unclear, but this underrepresentation serves to pass on a deficit in sensitivity from generation to generation of psychotherapists. This is one reason why religious laity and professionals have sometimes been wary of referring to mental health professionals.

To be sure, there are important exceptions to this general trend. Transpersonal psychology has from its inception been centrally interested in spiritual and religious aspects of human nature and has been described as "the melding of the wisdom of the world's spiritual traditions with the learning of modern psychology" (Cortright, 1997, p. 8). There are substantial specialty disciplines in the psychology of religion (Hood, Spilka, Hunsberger, & Gorsuch, 1996) and in pastoral psychology and counseling (Miller & Jackson, 1995). Existential therapy focuses on the broader questions of meaning and existence that have also been key concerns of world religions (Frankl, 1962). Some psychotherapy training does occur within the context of seminaries and other institutions of higher education that have historical ties to religion. Throughout the history of mental health disciplines, many scholars have written thoughtfully on the interface of spirituality and religion with health (e.g., Allport, 1961; James, 1902/1985; Larson, Swyers, & McCullough, 1998; Mowrer, 1961; Pattison, 1978; Peck, 1978), a process continued in this and other recent books (cf. Richards & Bergin, 1997; Shafranske, 1996). Yet, intentional diversity training remains far from normative in mainstream scientist-practitioner or professional-model programs. Clearly it is not for a lack of history, resources, thoughtful scholarship, or broader role models within the disciplines.

IMPORTANCE OF THE TOPIC

There is ample justification for devoting professional training time to preparing students to work competently with spiritual and religious diversity. In the course of their careers, nearly all therapists are likely to be called on to help clients who vary in age, ethnicity, cultural background, gender, sexual preference, and socioeconomic status. It is virtually certain in a pluralistic society that their clients will also vary widely on spiritual and religious dimensions.

The most vital general message to deliver in diversity training is that these differences *matter* in professional practice and deserve careful attention. Silence communicates at least irrelevance, if not a taboo. Open discussion of spirituality, by contrast, gives trainees permission to explore the subject. It is important that respected mentors provide not only permission but also active encouragement to explore spiritual and religious issues openly as a part of professional practice. This includes communicating that there are not only important practical reasons but also scientific reasons for doing so. On the practical side, a majority of clients, at least in the United States, have explicit religious beliefs and practices, and many regard their spiritual faith as being of central importance in their lives. In random general population surveys, as many as 40%–50% of people report having had spiritual–mystical experiences (Greeley & McCready, 1975). On the science side, as discussed in chapter 1, a large body of correlational research documents a generally positive relationship between religious involvement and health outcomes, including mental health. Other studies have shown that with religiously committed clients, the effectiveness of psychotherapy can be increased when their beliefs are not only respected but also actively incorporated in treatment regardless of the therapist's own belief (Propst, 1980; Propst, Ostrom, Watkins, Dean, & Mashburn, 1992).

Message: *Encourage open discussion and exploration of spiritual and religious issues during training and supervision.*

TERMINOLOGY

Many people confuse spirituality with religion. In this book we have all sought to differentiate these constructs, and it is useful to do so in professional training as well. Unlike religion, spirituality is part of every individual, an aspect to be understood in gaining a comprehensive picture of a person. The approach taken in this book is that one's spirituality, like personality, is complex and multidimensional. It encompasses beliefs and motivations, values and meaning, and behavior and subjective experience. Involvement with the social institutions of religion is only one dimension, sometimes a relatively unimportant one, in understanding an individual's spirituality.

It can be a stimulating and thought-provoking exercise to discuss, in the context of training, what spirituality is and what roles it plays in individual psychology, health, and society. This might arise in coursework on personality, interviewing, development, cross-cultural psychology, professional issues, assessment, or psychotherapy. In such discussion, the roles of religion also invariably arise, and provide an opportunity both for education about the scientific literature and for differentiation between spirituality and religion. Spirituality rarely appears in the index of texts currently used in clinical training. Religion, if it appears at all, most often is indexed in relation to particular kinds of psychopathology such as obsessive–compulsive personality. Almost never is there mention of the consistently positive association between religious involvement and mental health. The fourth edition of the *Diagnostic and Statistical Manual of Mental Disorders* (American Psychiatric Association, 1994), however, did include for the first time "religious or spiritual problem" among its V codes (i.e., additional conditions that may be a focus of clinical attention), and its brief description implicitly recognized the differentiation of spirituality from organized religion.

Message: *Help students to think more openly about spirituality as an aspect of individuals and to differentiate it from participation in religious institutions.*

OVERCOMING PREJUDICE

Consistent with the healer's principle of "first, do no harm," training programs have a responsibility to address students' own attitudes toward spirituality and religion. An early step in any diversity training is to explore, increase awareness of, and (to the extent possible) overcome prior prejudices (such as racism or sexism) that may bias professional work. It is professionally unacceptable in most current training and supervision contexts to make or ignore disparaging remarks about a client's race, cultural background, or gender. Sadly, it is not so inconceivable that a client's religious beliefs would be belittled or regarded as a source of pathology (Cortright, 1997). Indeed, there have been influential role models for such denigration. Sigmund Freud regarded religiosity as evidence of developmental immaturity. Albert Ellis (1980), in the *Journal of Consulting and Clinical Psychology*, stated that "the elegant therapeutic solution to emotional problems is to be quite unreligious and have no degree of dogmatic faith that is unfounded or unfoundable in fact. . . . The less religious [people] are, the more emotionally healthy they will tend to be" (p. 637). Similar racist or sexist remarks by a professional would be shunned.

The basic principle is a simple and familiar one: profound acceptance and respect for differences and rejection of prejudices that distort professional judgment and practice. Students may well enter training with strong biases about religion. Some may equate religiousness with pathology, immaturity, authoritarianism, or lack of reflective intelligence. Others may regard a particular religious perspective to be the one and only correct way of perceiving reality. Modeling respect begins with accepting the student's own chosen belief while extending similar respect for other beliefs. These are important but by no means simple training and supervision issues. They are often intertwined with deeply held attitudes and values, emotions, and personal history. To leave such countertransference issues unexplored would be unthinkable in supervision if the content were almost anything else except religion.

Message: *Model and teach professional respect for varying spiritual and religious perspectives. Do not overlook prejudicial statements and attitudes among trainees, any more than one would ignore racist or sexist remarks.*

PROFESSIONAL COMPETENCE

Examining concepts, attitudes, and prejudices and establishing spirituality as a proper topic for clinical dialogue are important steps. Yet, diversity education also commonly includes a cultural competence component providing knowledge and perspectives that are important in understanding differences. For many trainees, familiarity with a range of spiritual and religious perspectives (as with different racial–ethnic perspectives) is quite limited. How can this need be addressed?

First, I do not recommend adding yet another required course to clinical training curricula. Although coursework on world religions, for example, can be informative for clinical research and practice, this amount of attention to a single diversity issue is not justified as a requirement. Neither do I recommend isolated events like a "religious awareness day," although focused presentations and discussions on special topics in this area can be useful, especially when therapists are likely to be working with many clients from a particular religious background (e.g., Richards & Potts, 1995).

Instead, I believe that it makes sense to integrate diversity education into almost every aspect of clinical training. This has the advantage of communicating that sensitivity and attention to diversity issues should be an integral part of professional functioning. The following are just a few examples of places in a typical clinical training curriculum where such issues could be addressed.

Personality

Although spiritual and religious attributes are among the more stable, perhaps even heritable aspects of human nature (Waller, Kojetin, Bouchard, Lykken, & Tellegen, 1990), and many people regard them as being central to their personal identity, these dimensions often receive surprisingly little attention in coursework and training. Spirituality itself is a fascinating, complex phenomenon to approach from the perspective of individual differences. The search for that which is sacred or divine has been a formative influence in virtually every culture throughout history, yet it is a topic often ignored in the study of personality (Cortright, 1997). Spirituality is also an excellent example of a widely shared construct that offers engaging problems for theory and measurement. Students can be challenged to think critically about questions such as "What is spirituality? How is it different from religion?" "What defines something as a spiritual (vs. not spiritual) phenomenon?" "If spirituality is multidimensional, what are its dimensions or factors?" "In what ways would you expect spirituality to be related to various aspects of personality?"

As discussed in the opening chapter of this book, spirituality is in many ways, like personality, a multidimensional latent construct of individual differences. There is a large scientific literature within the psychology of religion, seldom examined in clinical training, regarding definitional and measurement issues related to spirituality and religion.

An example of a contemporary personality issue is the role of spirituality and religion in coping. Chapter 9 and the cited work of Kenneth Pargament and his colleagues illustrate how people draw on spiritual and religious traditions to cope with ordinary as well as difficult situations. Any assessment of a client's strengths should not exclude coping resources in this area.

Message: *Spirituality has always been an important aspect of character and deserves serious consideration in the teaching of personality.*

Assessment and Interviewing

Clinical students are typically trained to be comfortable and competent in conducting a broad range of assessment, including family history, personality, cognitive functions, sexual history, and psychopathology. Yet, we seldom do much even to encourage trainees (let alone teach them how) to understand a client's religious history and current spirituality.

This diversity issue is fertile ground for exploring some fundamental issues in clinical assessment. How would one go about assessing and understanding a client's spirituality? What kinds of information would result from different assessment approaches (e.g., phenomenological, psychometric), and how appropriate is each to the subject?

A simple approach is to include spirituality in the range of areas to be queried in a clinical interview, without entering into formal measures such as those discussed in chapter 3. A few open-ended questions followed by reflective listening will go a long way toward opening up this aspect of a client's life. "Do you consider yourself a spiritual or religious person? In what ways?" "Tell me a little about your religious background." "To what extent is spiritual or religious faith an important part of your life?" The initial inquiry need not be long, but the very asking gives a client permission to include these issues in the course of psychotherapy.

One way to increase comfort and familiarity with spiritual history taking is to practice it directly in the course of training. This can easily be incorporated into routine training, such as practice in clinical interview skills. Having trainees interview each other on this topic not only provides some experience but it also explicitly establishes spirituality as a topic for discussion in therapy, supervision, and training.

Message: *The evaluation of spirituality offers engaging issues and intriguing challenges that can provide excellent material for the teaching of assessment and interviewing.*

Psychopathology

It has been common, in textbooks and teaching, for religiosity to be linked implicitly to psychopathology through anecdotes. Clinical training in this area should include a fair presentation of the empirical literature on the relationship of spiritual and religious variables to mental health and illness. These issues have been discussed elsewhere in this book, and a number of excellent reviews have been published (e.g., Bergin, 1983; Gartner, Larson, & Allen, 1991; Gorsuch, 1995; Larson et al., 1998; Shafranske, 1996; Worthington, Kurusu, McCullough, & Sandage, 1996; cf. Levin, 1994).

Message: *Professional perspectives on spirituality and religion should be guided by the cumulative body of empirical knowledge, not by anecdote and prejudice.*

Professional Issues

Many clinical programs offer coursework and training on ethical and other professional issues. This is an obvious place for diversity training. The following are just three examples of areas in which the subject matter of spirituality can inform and enliven discussions of professional issues.

Limits of Competence

When is a health professional overstepping the limits of her or his professional competence in dealing with spiritual issues in psychotherapy?

Where are the boundaries of competence in dealing with spiritual and religious issues?

Public Statements

It is not uncommon for psychologists to be asked for opinions that touch on matters of spirituality and religion. What standards should be applied in making such public statements? Consider a variety of statements made publicly by health professionals with regard to religion, and apply professional ethical standards in considering their appropriateness. Where are the boundaries between personal opinion and professional opinion?

Professional Relationships

How do ethical standards on showing regard for colleagues and their institutions apply to professional relationships with members of the clergy? When is referral to a spiritual or religious professional appropriate? When and how is collaboration with these colleagues appropriate in the practice of psychotherapy (cf. Richards & Bergin, 1997)? How would clergy *like* to be consulted by health professionals serving those under their care?

Message: *Future therapists should be prepared to handle spiritual and religious issues in an ethical manner and to relate appropriately to professional colleagues with expertise in spirituality and religion.*

Supervision

Finally, the supervision of new therapists' clinical work affords many opportunities to explore training issues related to spirituality. How will the therapist incorporate clients' spirituality and religious beliefs in psychological practice? When and how (if at all) is it appropriate to challenge a client's belief or practice that is rooted in his or her religion? How will the therapist decide whether and what to disclose about his or her own system of values and beliefs? When is such disclosure appropriate, and what are the pitfalls?

Psychotherapy also raises therapists' own spiritual issues as well as their attitudes, beliefs, and emotions with regard to religion. Supervision should encourage awareness of these issues and include open discussion of how they affect therapist–client processes. For therapists who are themselves committed to a particular spiritual belief system (including atheism), boundaries of influence need to be addressed. Neither professional psychotherapy nor training is an appropriate place for religious proselytism. Clinical training placements may be available in community agencies, such as the nationwide Samaritan Centers, where faith issues are broadly addressed and integrated with professional psychotherapeutic services.

Message: *Spiritual and religious issues should be addressed in professional supervision as part of the training of psychotherapists.*

SUMMING UP

In the training of psychotherapists, spirituality deserves neither more nor less attention than other important aspects of human nature. Although the subject matter is much different, it is in some ways similar to issues of substance use—another area for which psychotherapists have often been inadequately prepared (Miller & Brown, 1997). Aware of it or not, clinicians will be dealing with these issues throughout their professional career. To overlook or ignore them is to miss an important aspect of human motivation that influences personality, development, relationships, and mental health. Specialized coursework may be helpful, but a better approach, I think, is to integrate diversity sensitivity into every aspect of clinical training. As with all areas of diversity training, some faculty will be better prepared than others to do this. What matters most is to prepare future psychotherapists to work in a competent, professional, and ethical manner with clients who vary greatly in spirituality.

REFERENCES

Allport, G. (1961). *The individual and his religion.* New York: Macmillan.

American Medical Association. (1998). *Graduate medical education directory, 1997–1998.* Washington, DC: Author.

American Psychiatric Association. (1994). *Diagnostic and statistical manual of mental disorders* (4th ed.). Washington, DC: Author.

Bergin, A. E. (1980). Psychotherapy and religious values. *Journal of Consulting and Clinical Psychology, 48,* 95–105.

Bergin, A. E. (1983). Religiosity and mental health: A critical reevaluation and meta-analysis. *Professional Psychology: Research and Practice, 14,* 170–184.

Clement, P. (1978, June). Getting religion. *The APA Monitor, 9,* p. 2.

Cortright, B. (1997). *Psychotherapy and spirit.* Albany: State University of New York Press.

Ellis, A. (1980). Psychotherapy and atheistic values: A response to A. E. Bergin's "Psychotherapy and religious values." *Journal of Consulting and Clinical Psychology, 48,* 635–639.

Frankl, V. E. (1962). *Man's search for meaning.* Boston: Beacon Press.

Gartner, J., Larson, D. B., & Allen, G. (1991). Religious commitment and mental health: A review of the empirical literature. *Journal of Psychology and Theology, 19,* 6–25.

Gorsuch, R. L. (1995). Religious aspects of substance abuse and recovery. *Journal of Social Issues*, *J*, 65–85.

Greeley, A., & McCready, W. (1975, January 26). Are we a nation of mystics? *The New York Times*, pp. 12–25.

Hood, R. W., Spilka, B., Hunsberger, B., & Gorsuch, R. (1996). *The psychology of religion: An empirical approach* (2nd ed.). New York: Guilford Press.

James, W. (1985). *The varieties of religious experience: A study in human nature*. Cambridge, MA: Harvard University Press. (Original work published 1902)

Larson, D. B., Swyers, J. P., & McCullough, M. E. (1998). *Scientific research on spirituality and health: A consensus report*. Rockville, MD: National Institute for Healthcare Research.

Levin, J. S. (1994). Religion and health: Is there an association, is it valid, and is it causal? *Social Science and Medicine*, *38*, 1475–1482.

Miller, W. R., & Brown, S. A. (1997). Why psychologists should treat alcohol and drug problems. *American Psychologist*, *52*, 1269–1279.

Miller, W. R., & Jackson, K. A. (1995). *Practical psychology for pastors* (2nd ed.). Englewood Cliffs, NJ: Prentice Hall.

Miller, W. R., & Martin, J. E. (Eds.). (1988). *Behavior therapy and religion: Integrating spiritual and behavioral approaches to change*. Newbury Park, CA: Sage.

Mowrer, O. H. (1961). *The crisis in psychiatry and religion*. Princeton, NJ: Van Nostrand.

Pattison, E. M. (1978). Psychiatry and religion circa 1978: Analysis of a decade, Part I. *Pastoral Psychology*, *27*, 8–25.

Peck, M. S. (1978). *The road less traveled: A new psychology of love, traditional values and spiritual growth*. New York: Simon & Schuster.

Propst, L. R. (1980). The comparative efficacy of religious and nonreligious imagery for the treatment of mild depression in religious individuals. *Cognitive Therapy and Research*, *4*, 167–178.

Propst, L. R., Ostrom, R., Watkins, P., Dean, T., & Mashburn, D. (1992). Comparative efficacy of religious and nonreligious cognitive-behavioral therapy for the treatment of clinical depression in religious individuals. *Journal of Consulting and Clinical Psychology*, *60*, 94–103.

Richards, P. S., & Bergin, A. E. (1997). *A spiritual strategy for counseling and psychotherapy*. Washington, DC: American Psychological Association.

Richards, P. S., & Potts, R. W. (1995). Using spiritual interventions in psychotherapy: Practices, successes, failures, and ethical concerns of Mormon psychotherapists. *Professional Psychology: Research and Practice*, *26*, 163–170.

Shafranske, E. P. (Ed.). (1996). *Religion and the clinical practice of psychology*. Washington, DC: American Psychological Association.

Waller, N. G., Kojetin, B. A., Bouchard, T. J., Jr., Lykken, D. T., & Tellegen, A. (1990). Genetic and environmental influences on religious interests, attitudes, and values: A study of twins reared apart and together. *Psychological Science, 1*, 130–142.

Worthington, E. L., Jr., Kurusu, T. A., McCullough, M. E., & Sandage, S. J. (1996). Empirical research on religion and psychotherapeutic processes and outcomes: A 10-year review and research prospectus. *Psychological Bulletin, 119*, 448–487.

INDEX

Numbers in italics refer to listings in the reference sections.

Deyo, R. A., 224, *233*
Dharap, A. S., 99, *103*
Diagnoses, 3, 20, 24, 256
Diagnostic and Statistical Manual of Mental Disorders, 20, 256
Dialectical behavior therapy (DBT)
  acceptance strategies and, 203–204
  case example, 206–207
  validation and, 204–205
Dietary practice, 164
Disease. *See also* Health; Suffering
  differentiated from illness, 4
  prevention, mindfulness and, 71
Disposition, 7, 26
Dissociation, 31, 76, 202
Distress. *See* Suffering
Diversity training
  assessment/clinical interview and, 258–259
  justification for, client diversity and, 255
  lack of, 253–254
  overcoming prejudice, 256–257
  professional competence and, 257–259
  professional issues, ethics and, 253, 259–261
  psychopathology and, 258, 259
  psychotherapy and, 253–254, 256, 257, 259–261
  spirituality measures and, 258, 259
  supervision and, 260–261
  terminology, 255–256
Diverting Attention/Praying and Hoping subscale, 95, 96
Divine, 3, 6, 30, 209, 258. *See also* Deity
  identification of unconscious with, 32
  intervention, 118–120
  personal relationship with, 92
  science, 35
Divorce, 50
Dixon, T., *15*
Doctrine. *See also* Christian thought/doctrine
  Jewish, 31, 37
  religious beliefs and, 61–62
Dodds, E. R., 22, 32, *42*
Doershuk, C. F., 85, *109*
Dogen Zenji, 185, 186
Doherty, W. J., 136, *157*
Dolan, E., 95, *106*
Donahue, M. J., 87, *103*
Don Quixote, 227

Dossey, L., 38, 97, *104*
Dougher, M. J., *215*
Douglas, A., 29, *42*
Drug problems, 11, 12, 50, 80, 149, 237. *See also* Addiction
Dubbert, P. M., 163, 166, *174*
Dubow, E., *108*
Duckro, P. N., 97, *104*
Dudley, M. N., 227, *230*
Dugan, T. F., 226, *230*

Eagleston, J. R., 4, 5, *17*
Eastern traditions, 37, 39. *See also* Asian spirituality; Buddhism; Hinduism; Islam; Western traditions
  meditation practices, 70, 73, 81, 138, 201, 202, 244
Easwaran, E. A., 8, *15*
Eating problems, 67, 79, 171, 194
  behavior therapy and, 203
Ecclesiastes, 200, *215*
Ecstasy, 38
Eddy, Mary Baker, 31
Editors of the *New Age Journal*, 248, *250*
Education, 30, 35. *See also* Training
  hope and, 225–226
Edwards, J., 20, *42*
Ego, 88
  development, 188
  psychology, 37
Eisenhower, D. D., 36
Elder, J., 172, *173*
Eliot, T. S., 34, *42*
Elkins, E., 188, *196*
Ellis, A., 134, 135, *157*, 256, *261*
Ellison, C. G., 85, 86, 88, 89, *104*
Ellison, C. W., 52, 56, 63, *65*
Emery, G., 167, *173*
Emmanuel movement, 31, 33
Emotion, 27, 69, 79. *See also* Emotional problems
  change in, 207
  detachment and, 238, 243
  primary, fear and, 211, 212
  serenity and, 236, 238
  taking charge of, 179
  toleration of, 202
Emotional problems, 36, 256
  alleviation of, 20
  emotional processing and, 211–212

Women, 227, 240
  hostility and, 211
  pastors, acceptance of, 55
  prayer and, 87
  problems of, 203
  reminiscence groups for, 225
Wong-McDonald, A., 57–59, 64, 189,
      198
Woods, T. E., 52, 64
Woody, G. E., 12, 16
Woolfolk, R. L., 135, 146, 160
Worcester, Ellwood, 32, 33
Worship, 3, 57, 172. See also Prayer
Worthington, E. L., Jr., 11, 13, 18, 133,
      138, 160, 195, 196, 211, 212,
      216, 259, 263
Wright, F. D., 69, 81
Wright, R., 212, 216
Wu, Henry, 208
Wulff, D. M., 20, 34, 37, 40, 46, 147,
      160
Wykle, M., 86, 109

Yahne, C. E., 225, 226, 231, 233
Yalom, I. D., 5, 10, 225, 233
Yarczower, M., 212, 215
Yates, J., 189, 198
Yoga, 39
Yoshinoby, L. R., 232
Young, J. L., 93, 105
Young-Ward, K., 85, 109

Zaleski, C., 33, 46
Zeidner, M., 86, 110
Zen Buddhism, 39, 185, 195, 201. See
      also Buddhism
  principles, 205
  serenity and, 248
Zen meditation, 81, 201
Zinnbauer, B. J., 6, 18, 195, 198
Zoroastrianism, 138
Zuttermeister, P. C., 81, 83
Zweben, A., 112, 129

ABOUT THE AUTHOR

William R. Miller, PhD, is Regents Professor of Psychology and Psychiatry at the University of New Mexico, and Director of Research for UNM's Center on Alcoholism, Substance Abuse, and Addictions (CASAA). A Fellow of both the American Psychological Association and the American Psychological Society, he also served as Director of Clinical Training for UNM's APA-approved doctoral program in clinical psychology. He maintains an active interest in pastoral counseling and the integration of spirituality and psychology. Currently, he is supported by a 10-year senior career Research Scientist Award from NIAAA to focus a full-time effort on clinical research. He received his PhD in clinical psychology from the University of Oregon in 1976.